W9-DGX-813

THE AFRICAN
AIDS EPIDEMIC

A History

THE AFRICAN AIDS EPIDEMIC

A History

John Iliffe
Professor of African History
University of Cambridge

Ohio University Press
ATHENS

James Currey
OXFORD

Double Storey / a Juta company
CAPE TOWN

James Currey Ltd
73 Botley Road
Oxford OX2 0BS
www.jamescurrey.co.uk

Ohio University Press
The Ridges, Building 19
Athens, Ohio 45701
www.ohioedu.oupress

Double Storey Books
a Juta company
Mercury Crescent
Wetton, Cape Town,
7780, South Africa
www.juta.co.za

All rights reserved. No part of this book may be reproduced in any form,
or by electronic, or mechanical means, including information storage
and retrieval systems, without permission in writing from the publishers,
except by a reviewer who may quote brief passages in a review.

© James Currey Ltd, 2006
First published 2006
1 2 3 4 5 10 09 08 07 06

ISBN 10: 0-85255-891-0 (James Currey cloth)
ISBN 13: 978-085255-891-1 (James Currey cloth)
ISBN 10: 0-85255-890-2 (James Currey paper)
ISBN 13: 978-085255-890-4 (James Currey paper)
ISBN 0-8214-1668-X (Ohio University Press cloth)
ISBN 0-8214-1689-8 (Ohio University Press paper)
ISBN 1-77013-048-9 (Double Storey Books paper)

British Library Cataloging in Publication Data
Iliffe, John
    The African Aids epidemic : a history
    1. Aids (Disease) - Africa 2. Epidemics - Africa - History -
    20th century 3. Epidemics - Africa - History - 21st Century
    I. Title
    614.5'99392'0096

Library of Congress Cataloging-in-Publication Data
Iliffe, John
    The African Aids epidemic : a history / John Iliffe.
    p. cm.
    Includes bibliographical references and index.
    ISBN 0-8214-1688-X (alk. paper) -- ISBN 0-8214-1689-8 (pbk.: alk. paper)
    1. Aids (Disease)--Africa--History. I. Title.
    RA643.86.A35I43 2006
    614.5'993920096--dc22   2005054660

Typeset in 10/10.5 pt Photina
by Long House, Cumbria
Printed and bound in Britain by
Woolnough, Irthlingborough

Contents

Maps

Preface

I am indebted to the staff of many libraries: University Library, Medical Library, African Studies Centre Library, and St John's College Library, Cambridge; London School of Hygiene and Tropical Medicine; School of Oriental and African Studies, London; British Library for Development Studies, Falmer; British Library, London and Boston Spa; Library of Congress, Washington; South African National Library, Pretoria and Cape Town; University of Cape Town Library; Cullen Library, University of the Witwatersrand; Ministry of Health, Entebbe; Makerere University Library; Albert Cook Memorial Library, Kampala; Medical Library, Kenyatta National Hospital, Nairobi; and Medical Library, Muhimbili Medical Centre, Dar es Salaam.

Among individuals I am especially grateful to Shane Doyle, Pieter Fourie, John Lonsdale, Margie Struthers, David Throup, and Megan Vaughan. James Currey Publishers deserve my thanks for the urgency with which they have undertaken publication.

Writing the book has left me with profound respect for the epidemiologists and medical scientists on whose work it draws. If, through ignorance or hubris, I have misrepresented any of their findings, I apologise in advance.

John lliffe

Abbreviations

AAA	*Aids Analysis Africa*
Aids	Acquired immune deficiency syndrome
ANC	African National Congress (of South Africa)
ARHR	*Aids Research and Human Retroviruses*
ART	Antiretroviral treatment
ARV	Antiretroviral
ATICC	Aids training, information and counselling centre
AZT	Azidothymidine
BMJ	*British Medical Journal*
CAR	Central African Republic
CHEP	Copperbelt Health Education Project
CRF	Circulating recombinant form
DNA	Deoxiribonucleic acid
EJHD	*Ethiopian Journal of Health Development*
FACT	Family Aids Caring Trust
FAO	Food and Agriculture Organisation
HAART	Highly active antiretroviral therapy
HIV	Human immunodeficiency virus
HSV	Herpes simplex virus
HTR	*Health Transition Review*
IDS	Institute of Development Studies
IDU	Injecting drug user
IFORD	Institut de Formation et de Recherche Démographiques
IJSA	*International Journal of STDs and Aids*
JAMA	*Journal of the American Medical Association*
MRC	Medical Research Council
MONGOs	My Own NGOs
NACOSA	National Aids Convention of South Africa
NACWOLA	National Community of Women Living with Aids
NAPWA	National Association of People with Aids
NEJM	*New England Journal of Medicine*
NGO	Non-governmental organisation

NS	New series
OCEAC	Organisation de Coordination pour la Lutte contre les Endémies en Afrique Centrale
PEPFAR	Presidential Emergency Programme for Aids Relief
PHC	Primary health care
PLWA	People living with Aids
PLWHA	People living with HIV/Aids
RNA	Ribonucleic acid
SAMJ	*South African Medical Journal*
SSM	*Social Science and Medicine*
STD	Sexually transmitted disease
STI	Sexually transmitted infection
SWAA	Society for Women and Aids in Africa
TAC	Treatment Action Campaign
TASO	The Aids Support Organisation
THETA	Traditional Healers and Therapies Against Aids
TRSTMH	*Transactions of the Royal Society of Tropical Medicine and Hygiene*
UMOH	Uganda Ministry of Health
UNAIDS	Joint United Nations Programme on Aids
UNDP	United Nations Development Programme
UNGASS	United Nations General Assembly Special Session
UNICEF	United Nations Children's Fund
UNIRIN	United Nations Integrated Regional Information Network
USAID	United States Aid for International Development
UWESO	Uganda Women's Effort to Save Orphans
VCT	Voluntary Counselling and Testing
WAMATA	People Struggling Against Aids in Tanzania (Swahili)
WHO	World Health Organisation
WHO:GPA	World Health Organisation: Global Programme on Aids

1
Intentions

This book has a modest purpose. Many history students interested in Africa wish to study the HIV/Aids epidemic but are hampered by the lack of an introduction to the detailed literature. This book is intended as an introduction, for students and other readers.

The book is not a work of research. A thorough history of the epidemic during its first thirty years would demand fieldwork in affected communities, interviews with those involved, and study of unpublished records of international organisations, national governments, and private individuals. I have not attempted any of these, nor have I the necessary medical and anthropological skills. Instead, the book is a synthesis of the more important and accessible published material, put into a historical form.

A historical account offers four advantages. First, it suggests an answer to the question posed most provocatively by President Mbeki of South Africa: why has Africa had a uniquely terrible HIV/Aids epidemic?[1] Mbeki attributed this to poverty and exploitation. Some earlier analysts suggested that Africa had a distinctive sexual system.[2] This book, by contrast, stresses historical sequence: that Africa had the worst epidemic because it had the first epidemic established in the general population before anyone knew the disease existed. Other factors contributed, including poverty and gender relationships, but the fundamental answer to Mbeki's question was time. Like industrial revolutions or nationalist movements, Aids epidemics make sense only as a sequence.

Second, a historical approach highlights the evolution and role of the virus. Because HIV evolves with extraordinary speed and complexity, and because that evolution has taken place under the eyes of modern medical science, it is possible to write a history of the virus itself in a way that is probably unique among human epidemic diseases. At the same time, the distinctive character of the virus – mildly infectious, slow-acting, ineradicable, fatal – has shaped both the disease and human responses to it.

Third, many aspects of the epidemic come into focus only when seen in the longer context of African history. Although HIV/Aids was profoundly different from earlier African epidemics, it arose from the human penetration of the natural ecosystem that is the most continuous theme of the African past. That

1

the virus created a continental epidemic, however, was a consequence of Africa's massive demographic growth, urbanisation, and social change during the later twentieth century. Everywhere the epidemic took its shape from the structure of the commercial economy that had grown up during the colonial period. Human responses, in turn, became part of an ongoing interaction between inherited moral understandings of disease and the medical explanations propounded by international authorities and modern African doctors. Like all great epidemics, HIV/Aids became a catalyst of change, but in directions already set by longer historical processes.

Finally, the African epidemic has itself changed over time. It is still at an early stage: 'the end of the beginning', as the head of the UNAIDS organisation described it in 2001.[3] Yet in much of Africa the epidemic has already evolved from explosive expansion to maturity, while human responses have graduated from unwitting vulnerability to planned containment. In the process, many Africans have displayed the endurance common throughout their history. Their experience has taught the world much of what it knows about HIV/Aids. It is time to give that experience a historical shape.

2
Origins

The earliest convincing evidence of the human immunodeficiency virus (HIV) that causes the acquired immune deficiency syndrome (Aids) was gathered in 1959 amidst the collapse of European colonial rule in Africa. In January 1959 rioters briefly seized control of the African townships of Leopoldville, the capital of the Belgian Congo, shocking its rulers into frantic decolonisation. In the same year an American researcher studying malaria took blood specimens from patients in the city. When testing procedures for HIV became available during the mid 1980s, 672 of his frozen specimens from different parts of equatorial Africa were tested. Only one proved positive. It came from an unnamed African man in Leopoldville, now renamed Kinshasa. The test was confirmed by the Western Blot technique – generally considered the most reliable method – and by different procedures in three other laboratories.[1] Although nothing of this kind can be absolutely certain, there are strong grounds to believe that HIV existed at Kinshasa in 1959 and that it was rare.

One importance of the Kinshasa case is to establish a date by which HIV existed, but in itself the case does not imply that the Aids epidemic began in western equatorial Africa. If that unnamed African had been the first person ever infected with HIV, it would have been an incredible coincidence. Once Aids was recognised as a medical condition early in the 1980s, researchers found several early accounts of patients whose recorded symptoms had resembled it.[2] Luc Montagnier, whose laboratory first identified HIV, thought that the earliest case had been an American man who died in 1952 after suffering fever, malaise, and especially the *pneumocystis carinii* pneumonia that afflicted later American Aids patients,[3] but no blood had been stored for later testing and the symptoms demonstrated only suppression of the immune system, for which there could have been reasons other than HIV. The same was true of a Japanese Canadian who died in 1958 and a Haitian American in 1959. More convincing was the case of a fifteen-year-old, sexually active American youth who died in 1969 with multiple symptoms including an aggressive form of Kaposi's sarcoma, a tumour common in later Aids patients. His stored blood tested positive for HIV by Western Blot, but the finding was later questioned. Other possible early cases were found in western equatorial Africa. There was no stored blood by which to confirm a specialist's retrospective diagnosis of Aids in an African woman who was hospitalised at Lisala on the middle Congo in 1958 and died in Kinshasa four years later after suffering wasting and Kaposi's sarcoma. But a Norwegian seaman contracted HIV some time before 1966, possibly while visiting Douala on the coast of Cameroun in 1961–2, and later infected his wife and child; all three retrospectively tested HIV-positive, although with a form of the virus different from that found in Kinshasa in 1959.

These cases are intriguing and were the bases for early controversy about the origins of HIV, but they reveal little except that it existed but was rare in the 1950s. The real grounds for believing that the dominant form of the virus originated in western equatorial Africa, probably in the broad area of Cameroun and the Democratic Republic of Congo (DR Congo), lie in three other directions. One is that HIV clearly results from the transmission to human beings of the ancient and related simian immunodeficiency virus (SIV), an infection of African monkeys that had also spread to chimpanzees.[4] That such an animal disease should pass to humans is not surprising, because several major human infectious diseases are contracted from animals, notably plague, sleeping sickness, yellow fever, some forms of influenza, and, most recently, Creutzfeldt-Jakob's Disease.[5] How such a transmission took place with HIV will never be known, but one possibility may have been infection by blood in the course of hunting as men penetrated the equatorial forest. One study of 1,099 people engaged in hunting and butchering in Cameroun, published in 2004, found ten who had contracted simian viruses, although in this case not HIV.[6] Aids is a by-product of the human mastering of the natural environment that has been the core of African history.

SIV has been transmitted from animals to humans at least eleven times and probably many more. There are two forms of the human disease: HIV-1, which is responsible for the global Aids epidemic, and HIV-2, which is less virulent and infectious and is virtually confined to the West African coast between Senegal and Côte d'Ivoire. HIV-2, discussed in Chapter 6, is closely related to the SIV common in the sooty mangabey monkeys of that region. By 2005, HIV-2 infections had been divided into eight groups, each believed to have resulted from a separate transmission. Only two of these groups, lettered A and B, had established themselves as human epidemics, suggesting that many unsuccessful transmissions may also have taken place in the past.[7] By contrast, the animal virus most similar to (although still quite distant from) HIV-1 and probably ancestral to it is the SIV occasionally harboured by a species of chimpanzee (*Pan troglodytes troglodytes*) whose natural territory is the forest of Gabon, Equatorial Guinea, Central African Republic, Cameroun, and Congo-Brazzaville, somewhat north of Kinshasa. Three groups of HIV-1 have been identified and lettered M, N, and O. Each group must result from a separate transmission of SIV, because on a family tree of the virus they are separated by intervening SIV strains. Group M is responsible for the global epidemic that by 2005 had infected about 60 million people. Group O is equally virulent and may be at least equally old, having infected the Norwegian seaman during the 1960s, but it remained largely confined to the vicinity of Cameroun, even there causing fewer than 10 per cent of HIV cases in the early 2000s. Group N was probably a later transmission and remained very rare; in 2005 only seven cases were known, all in Cameroun.[8]

The fact that the likely viral ancestor of HIV-1 has been found only in the chimpanzees of western equatorial Africa is one of the three reasons for thinking that the virus originated there. The second reason is that only that region harboured not only all three groups of HIV-1 but all the subgroups of the dominant group M.[9] The significance of this point arises from the nature of the virus.[10] The human immunodeficiency virus is almost inconceivably small: one ten-thousandth of a millimetre in diameter. It consists of a package of genetic information (a genome) surrounded by a protein envelope, the whole containing nine genes, whereas a human being has 30,000–40,000. Like all viruses, HIV has no life of its own but is a parasite of cells, drawing its life from theirs. Transmitted from one body to another by blood, genital fluids, or human milk, the virus becomes attached to certain types of cells, the most important being the CD4 helper T-cells that activate the body's immune system. The virus enters a cell and integrates its genetic information into its host's, using the cell's life to reproduce itself, which is the sole function of a virus. In doing so the virus destroys the host cell – and hence ultimately the immune system – while producing an immense number of new viruses to attack further cells. The process from entry into a cell to the production of new viruses takes on average about two days, so that HIV passes through some 180 generations a year. Moreover, the reproduction process is prone to error, because HIV's genetic information is in the form of RNA (ribonucleic acid) and must be converted into the DNA (deoxiribonucleic acid) composing the cell's genome. The combination of speed and error in reproduction means that HIV mutates at about 1 per cent per year, or a million times faster than is normal in evolution.[11]

One consequence of this rapid mutation was that when the M group of HIV-1 was analysed during the 1980s and 1990s, it displayed great diversity. Using a range of specimens from Africa, North America, and Europe, researchers identified ten subgroups that differed from one another in their composition by up to 30 per cent. They were lettered A, B, C, D, Fl, F2, G, H, J, and K.[12] All subgroups were found only in western equatorial Africa, although it may be more accurate to say that the fullest range of diversity existed only there, because the viruses identified in the DR Congo, in particular, show as much diversity within supposed subgroups as between them. This suggests that HIV group M evolved and diversified in the broad Congo region before certain strains were carried elsewhere to create differentiated subgroups by what is called a founder effect.[13] At all events, there is a fundamental distinction between the great diversity of strains in western equatorial Africa and the domination of one or two subgroups (sometimes in combination) in every other region of the world: A and D in eastern Africa; a combination of A and G in West Africa; B in Europe and North America; C in southern Africa, Ethiopia, and India.[14]

Unlike many other viruses, such as influenza, HIV strains do not supplant one another at intervals but evolve and differentiate as they pass from one human body to another. Modern medical science can distinguish in great detail between these strains and reconstruct their genetic relationships. This makes it possible to write a history of HIV and its epidemic dispersal in a way that may be impossible for any other disease, using evidence from stored blood and living bodies. The first part of this book outlines such a history for the African continent. Moreover, medical science holds out at least the possibility of dating this history. It is plausible to argue that HIV mutates so extensively that its overall mutation is at a regular speed, which can be calculated from the evolutionary distance between classified specimens taken at known dates. This 'molecular clock' can then suggest dates for major events in the evolutionary sequence, such as the separation of one subgroup from another. One such calculation from 144 dated specimens was published in 2000, using massive computing capacity at Los Alamos. It suggested that the last common ancestor of HIV-1 group M – the point at which the subgroups of the global epidemic began to differentiate – lay around the year 1931, and with more confidence between 1915 and 1941. Since the researchers knew that the genes composing the HIV genome mutate at different speeds, they compared this calculation, based on the most mutable envelope gene, with a calculation from a less mutable gene, which suggested a 1934 date. The researchers checked their procedure further by independently dating the earliest HIV specimen taken at Kinshasa in 1959, which had been identified as an early version of the D subgroup shortly after its separation from the B subgroup. The computer dated it between 1957 and 1960.[15] In 2001 another research team published similar calculations based on different specimens; they dated the last common ancestor of group M to 1937 (by the envelope gene) or 1920 (by the least mutable gene). The second research team also suggested that HIV-1 group M separated from the strain of SIV ancestral to that in modern chimpanzees around 1675, or with more confidence between 1590 and 1761.[16] It would be unwise at this stage to attach too much importance to this date.

Among the many uncertainties surrounding these findings, the most relevant here is whether the notion of a molecular clock is invalidated by another feature of viral evolution known as recombination. A person can be infected by more than one strain of HIV. If that occurs, viruses of different subgroups may enter the same cell and, in the process of integrating their genetic material with the host's, may produce a new strain of virus combining elements from two or more subgroups. (SIV is subject to the same process and the original simian virus transmitted to humans as the ancestor of HIV-1 group M is itself believed to have been a recombinant form.)[17] Although the strain identified in 1959 appears not to have been a recombinant, one of the earliest recovered from the DR Congo in 1976 was, and it is even possible that supposedly discrete subgroups were products of recombination at a stage so early as to be no longer identifiable.[18] Recombinants can combine with other recombinants, creating immense genetic heterogeneity, especially in the western equatorial region where the epidemic is oldest and the diversity of subgroups is greatest. Certain recombinant forms, however, have been especially successful. By 2005, 16 had been classified as circulating recombinant forms (CRFs), for each of which at least three distinct specimens had been analysed. The most successful were CRF01_AE, the dominant form of HIV in South-East Asia, and CRF02_AG, responsible for at least two-thirds of West African HIV infections.[19] Recombination is probably at least as important as mutation in accelerating the evolution of HIV, but its implications for dating based on a molecular clock are complex and obscure. By blurring differences between subgroups it might make evolutionary events seem more recent than they really were, but by multiplying the number of strains it might make the events seem more ancient than they were. The two teams who estimated dates for the differentiation of the M group tried to exclude the effects of recombination, but geneticists feared that the problem was more difficult and that conclusions based on a molecular clock 'may be of very limited value'.[20]

However uncertain their findings, attempts to date the epidemic clarified several problems in its history. Together with the identification of the 1959 case in Kinshasa, they effectively ruled out the theory, propounded in Edward Hooper's fascinating book, *The River*, that the HIV-1 epidemic had been caused by a polio immunisation campaign in the Congo region during 1957–60 that allegedly used a vaccine bred on SIV-infected chimpanzee kidneys – a theory also contradicted by negative tests on surviving vaccine samples.[21] Instead, attempts at dating stimulated interest in the interwar period when the diversification of group M supposedly began. Noting that the earliest known HIV cases in Africa all occurred in francophone territories, researchers highlighted colonial innovations there that might have converted occasional viral transmissions into a disease capable of epidemic expansion: penetration of the forest for hunting, rubber collection, and logging; increased viral transmission through labour concentrations and vaccine campaigns against sleeping sickness and smallpox; and the adaptation of the virus to humans through rapid passaging by arm-to-arm inoculation that would have the effect of accelerating evolution.[22] No direct evidence linking these innovations to HIV had been published by 2005, but the problem of how a simian virus might become capable of causing a human epidemic attracted the attention of other researchers. HIV-1 group N and at least six transmissions of HIV-2 had not become sufficiently transmissable or infectious as to cause epidemics. These were the forms of HIV most similar to SIV, so it appeared that the mere transmission of SIV to humans was unlikely to cause widespread disease; the virus must have evolved from SIV to HIV within human bodies, and it must have done so for the first time and perhaps more or less simultaneously in two groups of HIV-1 and two of HIV-2. Preston Marx and others argued that the chance of this happening naturally was 'vanishingly small'. Instead, rejecting the 1931 date for the diversification of the M group but accepting 1959 as the first documented HIV case, they suggested that SIV had been converted into HIV by rapid passaging through African populations during the 1950s, owing to the introduction of supposedly disposable (but often in practice re-used) syringes to inject penicillin and other new medications. Between 1952 and 1960 annual world output of syringes increased from 8 million to something approaching 1,000 million.[23]

These theories remained theories, but they indicated the kinds of evolutionary stages that may have produced HIV: probably multiple transmissions of SIV from sooty mangabey monkeys in West Africa over a long period; perhaps less frequent transmissions of the rarer chimpanzee virus in western equatorial Africa; its evolution into HIV within human bodies, whether over some centuries or through the unintended effects of medical interventions; and its emergence by 1959 as a virus capable of causing a global human epidemic.

Yet a difficulty remained: there was no visible epidemic in 1959, nor for another twenty years. The likely reasons lay in three characteristics of the virus. First, as viruses go, HIV is difficult to transmit. Whereas influenza – 'the sickness of the air', as it was called in Ethiopia in 1918 – can be transmitted aerially to anyone close enough to inhale it, HIV can be contracted only by absorption of blood, genital fluids, or milk from an infected human body. In heterosexual intercourse – the chief means of transmission in Africa – the chance of infection in one sexual act between otherwise healthy partners has been variously estimated at between 1 in 10,000 and 1 in 500.[24] To create and sustain an epidemic, therefore, requires special circumstances, but the chance of transmission increases substantially if either partner has a sexually transmitted disease or if the already-infected partner is in a particularly infectious condition. This is the case shortly after infection, when a person is perhaps eight or ten times more infectious than usual, and in the last stages of the disease, when infectivity is even greater.[25]

The difficulty of transmitting HIV relates to the second likely reason for the slow emergence of a visible epidemic, which was the very gradual development of the disease within human bodies. For a few weeks after infection the virus has the advantage of surprise: viral load rises rapidly, lasting damage may be done to the immune system, and there may be feverish symptoms, perhaps often mistaken for malaria. Thereafter the immune system counter-attacks and an evenly matched war of attrition takes place in which HIV produces up to 10 billion new viral particles and destroys up to 2 billion CD4 helper T-cells each day. In HIV-1 this incubation period varies considerably but may last in adults for an average of nine or ten years – the period measured by a careful study in Uganda – before the immune system is so weakened that Aids supervenes. Death in untreated patients then follows almost invariably and relatively quickly, in an average of perhaps nine or ten months.[26] The infected person remains infectious throughout the disease. This long incubation period with only sporadic symptoms distinguishes HIV/Aids from previous epidemic diseases, renders it especially dangerous to human life, makes it difficult to check, ensures that it does not burn itself out, and, as will be seen, has given the Aids epidemic its unique character. As a comparison, the incubation period of influenza is not nine years but one to three days, while that of plague in Britain, considered unusually long and therefore dangerous, may have averaged about 30 days.[27] 'What is serious,' a West African villager said of HIV, 'is that this disease is silent, hypocritical, visible only when the damage is already irreparable.'[28]

There was a third reason why the potentially epidemic virus that existed in 1959 did not breed a visible epidemic for another twenty years. HIV/Aids does not kill but destroys the immune system's capacity to resist other opportunistic infections that are ultimately fatal. Some of these, notably tuberculosis, were infections already current in the region concerned, so that it may not have been easy to discern that a new disease was present. Retrospectively, however, these opportunistic infections are the signs that first reveal the emerging HIV epidemic. Their appearance in western equatorial Africa during the 1970s is the third reason – alongside the location of the simian ancestor and maximum diversity of subgroups – to believe that the HIV epidemic originated there.

3
Epidemic
in Western Equatorial Africa

HIV-1 first became epidemic during the 1970s in western equatorial Africa, its place of origin. It was at first a silent epidemic, unnoticed until established too firmly to be stopped. In this region, also, during the mid 1980s, the epidemiology of heterosexual HIV/Aids was first determined, exposing a pattern whose main features were to extend throughout sub-Saharan Africa but whose local peculiarities were also to limit epidemic growth within the western equatorial region itself. From this region, moreover, variants of the virus were carried to the rest of the continent.

Although HIV-1 had almost certainly existed in western equatorial Africa since at least the 1950s, it had hitherto struggled even to survive in a sparsely populated region of difficult, often forested environments and poor communications. This was clear from a group of villages at Yambuku in the north of the DR Congo. Blood taken from 659 villagers there in 1976, during one of the first outbreaks of Ebola virus, later revealed that five (0.8 per cent) were infected with HIV. When the villagers were tested again ten years later, HIV prevalence was still 0.8 per cent. Of blood samples collected across the border in southern Sudan in 1976, 0.9 per cent subsequently revealed HIV.[1] Such low levels of infection may well have existed in other rural areas of the equatorial region during the 1970s. They apparently existed also in Kinshasa. One of those testing positive at Yambuku had probably contracted the disease in the capital during the early 1970s. Of 805 blood specimens taken from pregnant women in Kinshasa in 1970, two later revealed HIV infection. So did blood taken there in 1972 from two of four patients with Kaposi's sarcoma.[2]

The conversion of this low-level infection into an expansive epidemic probably took place in the urban environment of Kinshasa during the 1970s. The key may well have been the exceptional infectivity of the newly infected, which meant that if the virus entered a network of sexual relationships in which partners were exchanged rapidly and extensively, it could build up a momentum of infection sufficient to reach epidemic levels. That is probably what happened in the United States, where HIV prevalence among homosexual men attending a sexually transmitted disease clinic in San Francisco

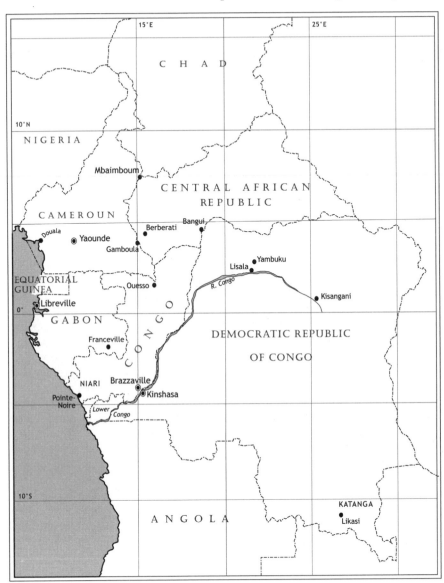

Map 1 *Western Equatorial Africa*

rose between 1978 and 1984 from 1 per cent to 65 per cent.[3] It happened at much the same period, although less explosively, among heterosexuals in the East African cities of Bujumbura, Kigali, and Nairobi, as also in rural south-western Uganda and in Abidjan in West Africa. The first occasion, however, was in Kinshasa, where HIV first encountered rapid partner exchange in urban sexual networks wider, although not necessarily much more promiscuous, than those of the countryside.

The first person to notice the change may well have been Dr Kapita Bila, the Congolese physician heading the internal medicine department at Kinshasa's huge, 2,000-bed Mama Yemo Hospital. 'Something dramatic happened in 1975,' he recalled a decade later, referring especially to a doubling of cases of Kaposi's sarcoma, a tumour that could take aggressive forms when the immune system was damaged and hence often became a conspicuous symptom of Aids. Other hospitals in the region observed this increase only in the later 1970s and early 1980s, but Kapita Bila dated it at Mama Yemo from 1975 and claimed that hospital records revealed cases at that time. The records also confirmed Congolese doctors' recollections that in the mid 1970s they had first noticed numerous cases of the severe wasting and diarrhoea that became the most common symptoms of Aids in African patients.[4] In the late 1970s doctors across the river in Brazzaville observed similar cases. Physicians in Kinshasa initially attributed these symptoms to tuberculosis, which spread epidemically in the region during the 1970s and 1980s, perhaps in synergy with HIV. By 1985, one-third of tuberculosis patients in Kinshasa's hospitals also had HIV.[5] A more distinctive indicator of Kinshasa's emerging HIV epidemic was cryptococcal meningitis, an agonising and commonly fatal infection of the brain. Hitherto generally confined to children, it spread in a distinctively urban form to adults with damaged immune systems and became increasingly common at Mama Yemo from the late 1970s.[6]

When blood taken in 1980–1 from antenatal clinic attenders in Kinshasa was later tested, it showed that HIV prevalence among them had grown during the 1970s from 0.2 per cent to 3 per cent.[7] The world's first HIV epidemic among a heterosexual population had begun before the existence of the virus was even suspected. That, more than anything else, was why Africa was to suffer so terribly during the following decades. Yet enlightenment now came quickly. In June 1981 American doctors published the first account of an epidemic of *pneumocystis carinii* pneumonia among American homosexuals. On reading it, physicians in Brussels and Paris realised that they had treated similar conditions since the mid 1970s, chiefly in Africans from the equatorial region or Europeans who had visited it. Of the first 96 recorded Aids patients seen in Europe, 54 were Africans, 40 of them from the DR Congo.[8] In contrast to infected Americans, however, they were heterosexuals in roughly equal numbers of men and women, they did not take drugs, and they had no obvious risk factor in common except their geographical origin. In October 1983 joint American and Belgian teams left for Kinshasa and Kigali.

At Mama Yemo, Kapita Bila showed the visitors the patients he suspected to be suffering from Aids. 'The moment I walked into the hospital in Kinshasa I realised something terrible was happening,' recalled Peter Piot, later the first head of UNAIDS.[9] 'Meningitis was only one manifestation of the disease,' wrote his colleague Joseph McCormick:

> Some developed such exquisitely sore mouths and tongues that they were unable to eat. Those who could manage a few bites of food were suddenly stricken by cramps and disgorged a copious amount of diarrhea. Their skin would break out in massive, generalised eruptions. Infected fungating masses would appear inside and outside their bodies. When the infection didn't consist of voracious yeast cells [as in cryptococcal meningitis], there were many other parasites ready to eat the brain alive. None of the victims could comprehend in any way what was happening to them or why. And we? All we could do was watch in horror, our roles as physicians reduced to scrupulous observers and accurate recorders of documentation. Our one hope was that if we could understand the processes we were observing, someone, somewhere, might find some solution.[10]

Diagnosing by symptoms, the team identified 38 Aids cases in Kinshasa's hospitals, 20 men and 18 women. Of these, 29 were from Kinshasa itself, but others came from all parts of the country, indicating how far the virus had spread. On 3 November the team presented its findings at a medical meeting at Mama Yemo, warning that the disease appeared to be sexually transmitted, incurable, and fatal. 'If there is a misfortune spreading terror in Kinshasa in the last few days, it is assuredly AIDS,' a local editor wrote five days later. 'It is spoken of in the most varied ways ... at the office, at the market, in bars, in families ... Never in my memory as a journalist have I seen such concentration on a subject as disagreeable as strongly feared.'[11] It was his last such comment, for President Mobutu's increasingly unpopular and insecure government banned the subject for the next four years. 'For the four million Kinois,' a foreign journalist wrote in 1986, 'the disease, for lack of any official information, still has no name. Signs, therefore, suspicions, often infantile beliefs. Aids all the same.'[12]

Reactions abroad to evidence that the disease was widespread in a heterosexual population were equally hostile. American medical journals rejected Piot's report and it took over a year to convince the American government. In the meantime the World Health Organisation cautiously endorsed the discovery by French scientists that Aids was caused by a retrovirus. McCormick persuaded the Centers for Disease Control in Atlanta to fund a research project in Kinshasa.[13]

Projet Sida, as it became known, began work in June 1984 and defined the epidemiology of the urban disease in a form that still dominated medical thought two decades later. A collaboration between American, Congolese, and Belgian specialists, initially led by an idealistic public health expert named Jonathan Mann, the Project had nearly 300 staff at its peak and the advantage of newly devised equipment to test blood for HIV. Its most important finding was that between 6 and 7 per cent of pregnant women at Kinshasa's antenatal clinics were already infected with HIV, whereas earlier estimates of the epidemic had observed only the much smaller numbers with advanced Aids. Mann warned in 1986 that 'one to several million Africans may already be infected'. He reckoned the annual incidence of new infections at between 0.5 and 1.5 per cent of hitherto uninfected people.[14] The Project also identified the means of transmission as sexual intercourse, exchange of blood by injection or transfusion, and infection from mother to child, excluding aerial transmission, insect vectors, and casual contact.[15] Sexual transmission was bidirectional, whereas the possibility of women infecting men had hitherto been uncertain. Among new infections, eleven were women to every ten men, although women in their twenties outnumbered men by three to one.[16] In other respects those infected did not have a strong social profile. The earliest observed cases had often been prosperous people who could afford multiple partners and medical treatment, but antenatal prevalence at Mama Yemo was somewhat higher than at a fee-paying hospital. The age profile, however, was distinctively bimodal, peaking in infants and young adults.[17] Perinatal transmission and pediatric Aids were among the Project's most novel findings. Mothers with HIV lost 24 per cent more of their babies in the first year of life than did those without it, the risk varying with the stage of the mother's disease.[18] Adult HIV was associated with tuberculosis and sexually transmitted diseases, the latter being one of several indications linking HIV to risky sexual behaviour. Some 27 per cent of Kinshasa's commercial sex workers had HIV.[19]

The Project also revealed an alarming connection between HIV transmission and blood transfusion, which had become common in large African hospitals since the Second World War. Mama Yemo gave about 80 transfusions a day, chiefly in childbirth or to severely anaemic children. The blood came from relatives or was bought from unemployed people recruited at the hospital gates. At least 5 per cent was infected with HIV. Since transfusion almost invariably transmitted the virus, the hospital was creating four new HIV cases each day. Of its patients aged 2–14 and too old to have been clearly infected perinatally, 11 per cent were HIV-positive and 60 per cent of these had received transfusions.[20] Injections with re-used and unhygienic needles were another alarming danger, for injections had been immensely popular among African patients since the 1920s. The Project found that one group of HIV-infected children under 24 months old with HIV-negative mothers had received an average of 44 injections (excluding vaccinations) during their lives. Among adults, HIV prevalence increased with the number of injections received. It was impossible to demonstrate causation, for patients may have needed injections because they were already ill, but Mann concluded that infected blood was a significant factor in HIV transmission, although, as the age profile suggested, sexual intercourse was more important.[21]

Projet Sida effectively ended in 1991 when rioting soldiers looted its premises and the expatriate staff withdrew, although Congolese doctors tried to continue the work. Meanwhile research had also revealed the extent of HIV elsewhere in the western equatorial region. Kinshasa's epidemic had spread up the river and into the neighbouring Lower Congo area, where estimated adult prevalence reached 4 per cent in semi-urban and 2.8 per cent in rural areas in 1989–90.[22] The distant mining towns of Katanga and their surrounding rural areas had similar prevalences at that time,[23] but little was known about the countryside outside the Lower Congo. Kinshasa's epidemic seems to have made only a limited impact on the immensity of the country at this period. Brazzaville, across the river, appears to have shared Kinshasa's epidemic pattern at a slower tempo. In the late 1970s it saw symptoms later characteristic of Aids and in 1983 it sent patients to France for positive investigation. The urban epidemic then grew quickly, reaching an adult prevalence of 8 per cent in 1991, while spreading at roughly half that level to Ouesso in the north, Pointe-Noire in the west, and the rural Niari region neighbouring the capital, although expansion into the sparsely-populated countryside elsewhere was slow.[24] By contrast, in Gabon, further to the north-west, an epidemic emerged more slowly. The first evidence of HIV there dated from 1983 and antenatal prevalence in the main towns of Libreville and Franceville rose only slowly to less than 2 per cent between 1986 and 1994, with even lower levels in the countryside.[25] Cameroun had a different but equally unspectacular experience. Perhaps because it was probably a site of early HIV evolution, the disease there remained scattered, much as it had been in the DR Congo until the later 1970s. Between 1986 and 1988 researchers in Cameroun found only 23 cases distributed among a dozen towns. This excluded the two main cities, Yaoundé and Douala, but neither played Kinshasa's role in breeding an epidemic. In 1992 each had an antenatal prevalence only slightly over 2 per cent. Instead, Cameroun's highest HIV concentrations at that time were on its eastern border with the Central African Republic.[26]

This was because the CAR experienced an epidemic more striking than Kinshasa's, expanding more rapidly both in the capital and to the rest of the country. Doctors in Bangui began to suspect Aids in 1982, confirmed it late in 1983, and came to think that they had seen it some years earlier in cases of cryptococcosis, tuberculosis, Kaposi's sarcoma, diarrhoea, and wasting. HIV must certainly have reached the region by the 1970s. Prevalence in Bangui's general population aged 15–45 rose from 2.3 per cent in 1985 to 7.8 per cent in 1987. By 1993 prevalence among antenatal women there had reached 16 per cent.[27] French doctors blamed the epidemic on sexual behaviour in a rapidly expanding town dominated by unmarried young people from a countryside with traditions of considerable sexual freedom. In 1987, 58 per cent of respondents aged 15–44 had had a child before the age of 20, 54 per cent reported extra-marital sex, 81 per cent had suffered a sexually transmitted disease, and only 34 per cent had used a condom. The epidemic was not primarily due to prostitution – not more than 21 per cent of Bangui's sex workers were HIV-positive during the later 1980s – but to rapid partner change, averaging between 20 and 40 partners a year according to a group of 56 men and 49 women examined in 1983–5, 60 per cent of whom were HIV-positive. Many poor young women engaged in sporadic subsistence sex. Multiple injections – eight a year on average for those with both HIV and tuberculosis in 1985–8 – added to the risk.[28]

From about 1985, when prevalence began to grow rapidly in Bangui, the epidemic also spread more widely. By 1990 some provincial towns in close communication with the capital had adult prevalence rates of 8 per cent. Two years later similar levels were recorded at Berberati and Gamboula, truck-stop towns near the Cameroun border with ties to diamond diggings that attracted many young people, while at Mbaimboum, where Cameroun, Chad, and the Central African Republic met, the prevalence among women in 1993 was 22.8 per cent. In parts of the DR Congo bordering the CAR Aids was known as 'Bangui'.[29]

This account of the epidemic's origins in western equatorial Africa has indicated distinctive circumstances that both enabled HIV-1 to establish itself as a human epidemic and constrained its growth within the region. Two circumstances were especially important. One was the mobility fostering the rapid spread of disease among young urban immigrants, truck drivers, alluvial miners, and their female partners, although constrained everywhere in the region by distance, insecurity, transport difficulties, and sparsity of population. The other was the rapid urbanisation that had begun in the later colonial period and escalated amidst postcolonial conflicts. Kinshasa had some 400,000 inhabitants when the earliest infected blood was collected there in 1959 and four times as many when indications of an epidemic first appeared in the mid 1970s. Once known as Kin la Belle (Kinshasa the Fair), it had become Kin la Poubelle (Kinshasa the Dustbin). Its decaying modern core was ringed by unserviced squatter settlements. The real value of its official minimum wage fell by 75 per cent during the first sixteen years after independence in 1960. Unemployment exceeded 40 per cent for men in 1980 and was much higher for women, who made up only 4 per cent of the country's formal urban labour force.[30] While the numbers of men and women in the city were roughly equal and nuclear families predominated, only 70 per cent of adult women were married in 1984, while their lack of economic opportunity other than petty trade, together with a formerly polygynous culture in which young unmarried people had much sexual freedom and gifts were a normal part of love-making, led a proportion of young women to depend on sexual relationships with men either for survival or for otherwise unobtainable goods.[31] Full-time prostitution was probably less important than in some eastern African cities where women did not trade and men heavily outnumbered them. In 1988 Kinshasa's sex workers averaged only 8.6 clients a week, compared with 35 among lower-class sex workers in Nairobi in 1987. Their 27 per cent HIV infection in 1985, although horrifying, contrasted with 61 per cent in Nairobi. It was estimated in 1988 that to eliminate all prostitution from Kinshasa would reduce HIV transmission by only 25 per cent.[32]

The bulk of transmission was rather among a minority of vulnerable individuals in wide networks of ephemeral sexual relationships in which the men were often significantly older and wealthier than the women. In an illuminating contrast with Rwanda that would have applied to the whole western equatorial region, Michel Caraël observed that 'Kinshasa, with its bars, its precocious, free, and joyous sexuality despite immense poverty, its litany of *bureaux* (concubines)' was 'light years away' from the 'austere Catholic town' of Kigali, where men had extra-marital relations chiefly with sex workers and then infected their wives, so that HIV was most common in the age range 25–35, whereas in Kinshasa the disease was more widespread among older men and younger women.[33] Kinshasa's sexual pattern raised HIV to epidemic proportions, but not the explosive proportion seen in Kigali. This was reinforced by the fact that over 90 per cent of men in the western equatorial region were circumcised, which probably provided some protection because the foreskin was especially liable to viral penetration, and that sexually transmitted diseases – although closely associated with HIV infection – were relatively rare, including the incurable genital ulcer disease caused by herpes simplex virus 2 (HSV-2) that was spreading throughout the world in synergy with HIV. A later comparison was to show that, thanks chiefly to these two advantages, Yaounde had significantly lower HIV prevalence than Kisumu in Kenya or Ndola in Zambia, despite high levels of extra-marital sex.[34]

These constraints help to explain the most remarkable feature of the HIV epidemic in western equatorial Africa: its failure to expand during the 1990s beyond the levels of prevalence reached early in the decade, although those levels were often at or above the threshold 3–5 per cent prevalence commonly thought to trigger exponential growth. In Brazzaville city, for example, prevalence at antenatal clinics fell between 1991 and 1996 from 8 to 5 per cent, suggesting, together with a peak prevalence in older age groups (men of 35–49 and women of 25–30), that this early epidemic had reached maturity at a modest prevalence.[35] The epidemic in Bangui, similarly, stabilised between 1993 and 1998, although at a level of 16 per cent that could be sustained only by a high incidence of new cases.[36] In Gabon and Cameroun, where the epidemic had begun later, there was more growth during the 1990s, but to adult levels below 7 per cent.[37] The most striking illustration was the DR Congo, often considered 'a risk environment *par excellence*',[38] where, however, the long-predicted epidemic explosion did not happen. In Kinshasa, for example, HIV prevalence among pregnant women declined between 1985–8 and 1992 from 6–7 per cent to 5 per cent and then remained at or below that level for the remainder of the decade.[39]

Analysts struggled to explain this surprising stability. Some suggested that the HIV strains evolved so early in this region might be less virulent than those elsewhere, but there was no hard evidence to support this. Others thought that poverty might have reduced the rate of sexual partner exchange.[40] More convincingly, it was pointed out that in Kinshasa, as in Bangui, the epidemic, having begun so early, had reached a stage of maturity at which a stable prevalence concealed a balance between deaths among older groups and a substantial incidence of new infections, chiefly among the young. Between 1986–7 and 1989–90 in Kinshasa, for example, prevalence among pregnant women under 25 nearly doubled, while among older women it fell slightly. The investigators estimated that the annual incidence of new infections in pregnant women aged 20–24 was almost 2 per cent, nearly twice that in the general population. 'A stable HIV seroprevalence in sentinel surveys,' they concluded, 'may be consistent with a dynamic epidemic.' The city's sex workers may have had a parallel experience, prevalence stabilising at about 35 per cent while annual incidence was 10 per cent.[41]

Both Kinshasa and the rest of DR Congo also enjoyed some protection against an explosive epidemic from the great distances between population concentrations and the difficulty of travel where transport had widely broken down and much violence and insecurity prevailed, these factors together preventing the linking of sexual networks that commonly fostered epidemics. The falsity of the common belief that 'war creates the perfect conditions for the spread of AIDS'[42] was also demonstrated at this time in neighbouring Angola, where national antenatal prevalence after nearly 40 years of warfare was found by a survey in 2004 to be only 2.8 per cent, with the lowest figures in central provinces 'that have been more protected by the effect of war,' as the Vice-Minister of Health put it.[43] By contrast, the two countries registering modest epidemic growth during the 1990s, Gabon and Cameroun, were the most peaceful in the region.

The limited capacity for expansion shown by the western equatorial epidemic during the 1990s had as its counterpart the survival there – perhaps especially in the countryside – of a diversity of HIV subtypes and recombinant forms far greater than anywhere else in the world. A more explosive epidemic might well have swamped this diversity by a single dominant strain more like those created by founder effects elsewhere. Yet it was from this region that the various forms of the virus were carried to the rest of the continent and the world. The most spectacular illustration was the transmission of the circulating recombinant form CRF01_AE from its hearth in the northern DR Congo and the neighbouring Central African Republic, where alone it was common early in the epidemic, to become the major strain of HIV in South-East Asia, although the means of this transmission are unknown.[44] A less dramatic example was the other major circulating recombinant, CRF02_AG, which provided 60 per cent of HIV-1 strains in Cameroun during the 1990s, especially in the north, and some 54 per cent in Gabon. Its ancestors probably lay in the DR Congo – one of them was a virus collected at Yambuku in 1976 – but CRF02_AG itself was rare in both Congos during the 1990s and appears therefore to have taken shape in the Cameroun–Gabon region, whence it was carried northwards to become the dominant form of the virus throughout West Africa.[45] By contrast, the subtypes (as distinct from CRFs) of HIV-1 transmitted to other parts of the continent appear to have been carried directly from the DR Congo. Subtype A was the most common form there, especially in the north, and was carried into East Africa, where it shared predominance with subtype D, itself rare elsewhere except in the DR Congo.[46] Less certainly, subtype C, which came to dominate southern Africa (and Ethiopia), was common only in the south of the DR Congo, whence it may have been carried southwards.[47] The history of this radiation from the equatorial region is the next issue to consider.

4
The Drive to the East

Eastern Africa was probably the first region to which HIV was carried from its western equatorial origin, along several different routes that cannot now be traced in detail. The virus entered a region divided historically into two contrasting natural and social environments: the well-watered, densely peopled kingdoms around Lake Victoria and on the Ethiopian plateau, and the less centralised societies in the drier savanna country where population clustered only on highland outcrops, in colonial cities along transport routes, and on the Indian Ocean coast. This framework gave HIV/Aids in eastern Africa its distinctive contrast between explosive epidemics in the Lake Victoria basin and the capital cities, on the one hand, and slow penetration into the remainder of the region, on the other. Varying relationships between cities and countryside were especially important in the process, as were the mobile groups linking them together and the factors – widespread labour migration, male predominance in urban populations, low status of women, lack of circumcision, and prevalence of sexually transmitted diseases – that bred higher levels of infection than in western equatorial Africa.

The virus first entered the Lake Victoria basin bordering the DR Congo. Patients from Rwanda and Burundi were seen alongside Congolese in European hospitals during the late 1970s and early 1980s. They not only led expatriate researchers to visit Kigali as well as Kinshasa in 1983 but encouraged observers of the epidemic to believe that Rwanda, Burundi, and perhaps even Uganda had been simultaneous or even earlier places of origin alongside western equatorial Africa. The location of the chimpanzee host makes this unlikely, however, as does the distribution of HIV-1 subtypes, for there is no indication in the Lake Victoria basin of the diversity of strains found in the DR Congo. Until well into the epidemic, the A and D subtypes dominated the region.[1]

In Rwanda the first probable case recorded was a mother who displayed characteristic opportunistic infections in 1977 and subsequently tested positive for HIV along with her husband and three children.[2] A retrospective study found that by 1982 some 12 per cent of blood donors in Kigali were infected.

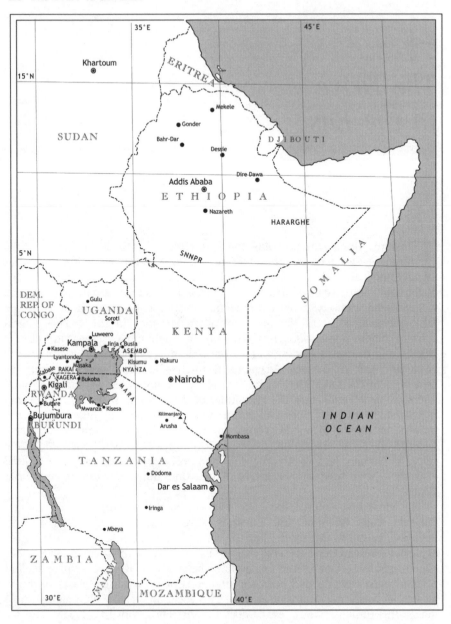

Map 2 *Eastern Africa*

The team visiting the hospital there a year later identified symptoms of Aids in 26 patients.[3] The virus had apparently established itself during the 1970s and reached epidemic proportions by the early 1980s. The evidence from Burundi is even stronger, for 658 blood specimens taken during a study of haemorrhagic fever there in 1980–1 later revealed an HIV prevalence of 4.4 per cent, reaching 7.6 per cent in Bujumbura and 2.8 per cent in the countryside, at a time when Kinshasa's antenatal prevalence was only 3 per cent. During 1983 cryptococcal meningitis, Kaposi's sarcoma, tuberculosis, and other opportunistic infections became increasingly common in Bujumbura and doctors suspected Aids, which was confirmed serologically in 1984.[4]

Bujumbura's epidemic grew remarkably fast during the early 1980s. By 1986 some 16.3 per cent of women tested at antenatal clinics were infected. Thereafter growth slowed temporarily, rising only to an urban prevalence of 18.3 per cent in 1992, which nevertheless implied a high incidence of new cases.[5] One reason for the epidemic's virulence may have been its close association with tuberculosis, long prevalent in Burundi. In 1986, 55 per cent of tuberculosis cases treated in Bujumbura were HIV-positive, while tuberculosis cases in Burundi as a whole increased between 1985 and 1991 by 140 per cent. The epidemic's most striking feature, however, was its urban concentration. While urban antenatal prevalence in 1992 was 18.3 per cent, it was only 5.2 per cent in semi-urban and 1.9 per cent in rural areas.[6] Rwanda's first rough sample survey of people of all ages in 1986 showed a similar contrast between 17.8 per cent prevalence in towns and only 1.3 per cent in the countryside. The highest rates among pregnant women were in Kigali, where they rose even more quickly than in Bujumbura, reaching 33 per cent in 1993.[7]

The rapid infection of Kigali and Bujumbura took place in countries where sexual behaviour among the overwhelmingly Christian general population was remarkably strict. In a survey conducted during the late 1980s, only 10 per cent of men and 3 per cent of women aged 15–19 in Burundi reported sexual intercourse during the last twelve months, compared with 51 per cent and 30 per cent respectively in the Central African Republic.[8] The result was a different epidemic pattern, dominated not by widespread partner exchange but by commercial sex. Sex workers had long been Africa's urban witches, blamed for all manner of social ills, so that there is a danger of stereotyping their role in the epidemic. Yet everywhere in eastern Africa, except Uganda, they were the first focus of infection. In 1984 a study of 33 sex workers in Butare, Rwanda's second town and home to a military base and university, found 29 infected with HIV, along with 28 per cent of their clients, who frequented a median number of 31 sex workers a year. Of 300 Aids patients in Bujumbura in 1987–9, 106 of the 184 men had frequented sex workers and 21 of the 116 women had themselves been sex workers.[9] Both countries were overwhelmingly monogamous, with exceptional numbers of unmarried women. In the early 1990s Kigali had 50 per cent more men than women aged 20–39. Fifteen years earlier the city also had an estimated minimum of 2,000 *femmes libres*, many of them uprooted by the destruction of Tutsi power since the revolution of 1961.[10] On average, men in Kigali made their sexual debut at 18 but married at 24–28; in the meantime, since other young women in this 'austere Catholic town' were carefully protected, they frequented sex workers and often continued to do so after marriage. Circumcision was rare, condoms despised, sexually transmitted diseases widespread, sexual coercion common, and women depended overwhelmingly on a male partner for income.[11] Although epidemics in both countries initially focused around sex workers, therefore, their clients quickly spread the disease to their regular partners. In the late 1980s, 80 per cent of infected women and 76 per cent of infected men in Kigali had an infected partner.[12]

On the eve of the genocide of 1994, antenatal prevalence in the Rwandan countryside – 'in the hills', as they said in Kigali – remained less than 5 per cent. In rural Burundi it was even lower.[13] The contrast with the relatively equal urban–rural prevalence that will be seen in Central Africa is difficult to explain in small countries with excellent transport systems, dense rural populations, and large income differentials between town and country. The towns did spread infection to their rural environs. A study in the Butare region in 1989–91 showed no association between HIV prevalence among rural women and the frequency with which they visited the town, but a significant association if their regular partner visited it daily.[14] Yet these were small towns. The largest, Kigali, had only 220,000 inhabitants in 1986, only some 3 per cent of Rwanda's population. They had no industry to attract the long-staying migrant workers who were probably most responsible for spreading infection to Central African villages. Whatever the reason, Aids in Rwanda and Burundi began and remained until the mid 1990s essentially an urban disease.

The contrast elsewhere in the Lake Victoria region was remarkable. In the lakeshore districts of Masaka and Rakai in south-western Uganda and the Kagera region of north-western Tanzania, Africa experienced its first rural-based Aids epidemic, a product of a prosperous peasant society at a moment of profound crisis. In East Africa during the 1970s the post-independence order was beginning to unravel. General Amin seized power in Uganda in 1971, precipitating eight years of violence and a *magendo* economy of illegality and self-help until the Tanzanian invasion overthrew him in 1979. Tanzania, although politically more stable, suffered severe economic decline as a result of the socialist strategy adopted in 1967, a decline accentuating Kagera's long-standing problems of isolation, land scarcity, and agricultural decay. In Kenya, too, the prosperous era of Jomo Kenyatta gave way from 1978 to growing stringency and corruption under Daniel arap Moi.

HIV penetrated first into the borderland between Uganda and Tanzania west of Lake Victoria. Some have believed that the virus had been present in Uganda since the late 1950s or 1960s, pointing especially to occasional cases of the aggressive form of Kaposi's sarcoma later found in some Aids patients. This is possible, but aggressive Kaposi's sarcoma was a consequence of immune suppression rather than necessarily of HIV; nobody at the time noticed any change in the epidemiology of the disease, as they did in the early 1980s, and no stored blood from the region prior to the late 1970s has shown HIV antibodies.[15] Without stronger evidence it seems more in accord with the continental pattern of the epidemic to think that Aids first appeared on the Uganda–Tanzania border in the late 1970s and HIV a few years earlier.

Its arrival cannot now be identified exactly. According to Uganda's chief epidemiologist, symptoms later characteristic of Aids were first reported late in 1982,

> when several businessmen died at Kasensero, an isolated small fishing village on Lake Victoria. This small town was also known for smuggling and illicit trade, and when these deaths occurred fellow traders shrugged it off as witchcraft. Others thought it was natural justice against those who had cheated. The only common characteristic the victims had was that they were all young and sexually active and stayed away from home for several days chasing wealth and presumably using it generously for their recreation and merriment.[16]

Across the border in Tanzania the first three Aids cases in Kagera region entered hospital in 1983. Retrospectively, however, medical workers believed that they had seen earlier cases. Kitovu Mission Hospital in Masaka district of Uganda was later said to have recorded 84 during 1982 alone. An African doctor in Rakai district believed that his uncle had died of the disease in 1980. The leading expatriate specialist later thought he had seen the corpses of Aids victims in Kampala in 1979 or 1980. Taken as a whole, the evidence suggests that HIV entered the region during the 1970s and became epidemic in the early 1980s.[17]

Local people called the new disease 'Slim' because wasting was commonly its most visible symptom. 'In the first six months,' Dr Anthony Lwegaba reported from Rakai in 1984,

> the patient experiences general malaise, and on-and-off 'fevers'. For which he may be treated 'self' or otherwise with Aspirin, chloroquine and chloramphenicol etc. In due course, the patient develops gradual loss of appetite.
>
> II. In the next six months, diarrhoea appears on-and-off. There is gradual weight loss and the patient is pale. Most patients at this point in time will rely on traditional healers, as the disease to many is attributed to witchcraft.
>
> III. After one year, the patient develops a skin disease ... which is very itchy. Apparently it is all over the body. The skin becomes ugly with hyperpigmented scars. There may be a cough usually dry but other times productive.
>
> IV. Earlier on after a year, the patient may be so weak that even when taken to hospital (not much can be done due to late reporting), goes into chronicity and death.[18]

Like the local people, Lwegaba blamed Slim on the young fishermen and smugglers who had flocked to the lakeshore to exploit the Nile perch fisheries and the *magendo* economy. 'Since perch-fishing began,' an investigator noted,

> temporary fishing camps of grass huts and sheds have grown up seasonally on the lakeshore, with predominantly male populations. Male labour relies, for food, drink and sexual services, on cafés, teashops, and bars, largely run by women. Each camp is associated with particular farming communities, which may be at a distance of up to 15 kilometres from the shore.[19]

It was probably in these fishing camps and neighbouring villages that partner exchange reached the frequency required to raise HIV to the epidemic levels elsewhere found only in the urban environments of Kinshasa or Kigali. Fifteen years later researchers studied such a fishing community in Masaka district. Its men had on average one new sexual partner every twelve days. Some 41 per cent of their partners were regular and 59 per cent casual; 85 per cent were contacts within the village, 8 per cent in other fishing villages, and 6 per cent in the nearby trading town. The village women, in turn, had 90 per cent of their sexual contacts with other villagers and 42 per cent with casual, paying clients. Such promiscuity was highly localised, so that HIV prevalence in different parishes of the district in the mid 1990s was to range from 4 per cent to 20 per cent. 'It is our mating patterns that are finishing us off,' a researcher was told.[20]

Although this epidemic began in the countryside, the difficulty of transmitting HIV makes it likely that it would have died away if it had not been carried to more open sexual networks in trading centres, the capital, and eventually the entire East African region. The researchers in Masaka found surprisingly little sexual exchange between village and town, but they did find that sexual activity varied enormously between individuals.[21] It was perhaps hyperactive and mobile individuals who transmitted HIV to the main-road trading centres where it next flourished. In the Kagera region, for example, the virus appears to have been carried from border trading posts to inland commercial centres like Kamachumu, long a focus of coffee marketing and politics. Thence it spread to the regional capital, Bukoba. By 1987 prevalence among those aged 15–24 was 24.2 per cent in Bukoba town (reaching 42 per cent in its lowest-status section) and 10 per cent in the neighbouring Bukoba and Muleba rural districts.[22] Once the virus was established in trading towns, workers carried it back to hitherto unaffected villages. In the Kagera village studied by Gabriel Rugalema, for example, Aids was introduced in 1987 by 'a woman with an unstable marriage who worked part-time as a commercial sex worker in Rwamishenye (a suburb of Bukoba town). She came back to the village after she had been weakened by infections and died a few weeks later.' Another 18 women and 41 men died there during the next nine years:

> A majority of the men who died were involved in off-farm income generation, particularly those who had worked as itinerant traders. Others included carpenters, masons, and casual labourers ... Only six of the deceased men could be strictly classified as full-time farmers.... As for the women, the majority of the deceased were, as may be expected, full-time farmers.[23]

In Rakai district, similarly, a computer simulation suggests that the annual incidence of new infections among people aged 15–24 peaked in 1987 at about 8.3 per cent.[24] Two years later, prevalence among men and women aged over 13 varied from 26 and 47 per cent respectively in main-road trading centres to 22 and 29 per cent in local trading village and 8 and 9 per cent in agricultural villages. In 1990–2, 31 per cent of all households in Rakai district contained an infected member. The worst impact was in the truck-stop towns along the trans-African highway between Kampala and Kigali, notably

Lyantonde, where HIV was found in 67 per cent of the bar girls tested in 1986 and in 53 per cent of the entire adult population in 1989.[25]

The prominence of the trans-African highway was one indication that the epidemic had by the mid 1980s spread far beyond the west lake region. Three categories of mobile men appear especially to have carried it. One was the military: General Amin's soldiers retreating from the infected border region in 1978–9, Tanzanian troops pursuing them through western and northern Uganda, and Ugandan forces seeking to repress rebellion in the north and east during the 1980s. The northern Gulu district, the chief source of Amin's troops, recorded 15 per cent prevalence among pregnant women in 1987 and probably became the main route by which HIV entered the southern Sudan and was carried northwards by soldiers and refugees to Khartoum, where in 1998–9 nearly half of those infected had the D subtype found in Uganda and DR Congo.[26] The western Ugandan districts of Kabale, Kasese, and Kabarole, prominent in early Aids returns, may also have been infected initially by rival armies. Military actions during the 1980s in Luweero and Soroti districts, further east, were probably important in spreading the disease there.[27]

A second group carrying the virus were long-distance drivers who infected or were infected by bar girls at their overnight stops in towns like Lyantonde. One study of 68 drivers in Kampala in 1986 reported that 35 per cent already had HIV.[28] The third occupational group, with a more diffuse and less certain impact, were migrant labourers carrying the disease to rural homes. 'With the AIDS pandemic,' a hospital in the remote south-west of Uganda reported in 1991, 'it is still the returnees to Bufumbira that introduce this deadly disease into the population which otherwise knows no promiscuity. Among the returnees are also counted the taxi drivers and the long-distance truck drivers.'[29]

Kampala held a special position. In retrospect, its main prison may have held cases as early as 1979 or 1980, when patients with aggressive Kaposi's sarcoma also appeared in the main Mulago Hospital, soon followed by others with the chronic diarrhoea and wasting of Slim disease.[30] Nobody linked these infections to the emerging Aids epidemic elsewhere in the world until late in 1984, by which time HIV was already entrenched in the city and spreading rapidly. 'It all started as a rumour,' the chief epidemiologist later reflected. 'Then we found we were dealing with a disease. Then we realised that it was an epidemic. And, now we have accepted it as a tragedy.'[31] Studies of prevalence among pregnant women in Kampala showed 11 per cent in 1985, 14 per cent in 1986, 24 per cent in 1987 – then the highest figure in the world outside Kigali – and a peak of over 30 per cent in 1989.[32] Notably, however, Kampala's epidemic was not focused on a core group of sex workers and their clients, in contrast to other East African cities. There was little association between HIV infection and commercial sex, which was unorganised, diverse, illegal, and impossible to distinguish from other sexual relationships involving gifts.[33] Instead, Kampala's sexual pattern was closer to Kinshasa's, with more young women than young men, sexual debut at an average age of fourteen in Uganda generally in 1989, 69 per cent of men and 74 per cent of women aged 15–19 having sexual experience, a rising age at marriage, and many young women whose dependence on gifts from male lovers had been accentuated by the economic disorder of the 1970s and 1980s.[34] It was a pattern vulnerable to HIV but capable of change.

Although reports of a novel disease in Rakai reached the authorities in 1982–3, Uganda was then in the midst of civil war and no action was taken until Lwegaba's report coincided late in 1984 with laboratory evidence that patients at Mulago Hospital with Kaposi's sarcoma were infected with HIV. Milton Obote's government, then in power, ordered an investigation. A team visited Masaka, conducted examinations at Mulago, and concluded that Slim was 'part of the spectrum' of Aids, although with opportunistic symptoms specific to East Africa. Ruling out transmission by casual or indirect means, the researchers blamed heterosexual promiscuity, perinatal transmission, and blood transfusion, estimating that Mulago Hospital might be creating two new cases each day. HIV-positive patients at Mulago reported on average twice as many sexual partners as HIV-negative patients. Another risk factor was a sexually transmitted infection, especially genital ulcer disease.[35]

Uganda's HIV epidemic appears to have peaked in 1991, when 21.1 per cent of women attending antenatal clinics tested positive and some 1,200,000 people were thought to be infected.[36] By then the virus had reached almost all parts of East Africa. In Tanzania, the area first affected after Kagera was probably Dar es Salaam. An expatriate may have contracted the disease there as early as 1980, but the first firm evidence was a prevalence of nearly 2 per cent in stored blood collected from pregnant women and blood donors in 1984–5. Thereafter antenatal prevalence in the city rose to 8.9 per cent in 1989 and 14.8 per cent in 1997.[37] The disease was probably introduced from Kagera, perhaps by returning soldiers but more probably by Haya sex workers and bar girls from the region, who had been prominent throughout East Africa since the interwar period, driven perhaps by male control of land and income in a highly commercialised region. By 1986, 29 per cent of Dar es Salaam's bar girls had HIV, with a prevalence of 35 per cent among the 33 per cent of them who came from Kagera. Two years later, 60 per cent of notified Aids patients in Dar es Salaam originated from Kagera, many of them no doubt people seeking treatment. Of Tanzania's first 212 notified Aids cases, 60 per cent of males and 46 per cent of females said that they were heterosexually promiscuous.[38] Yet this initial social profile was soon obliterated by the epidemic's expansion. When women at family planning clinics in Dar es Salaam were surveyed in 1991–2, there was still a positive association between HIV infection and number of sexual partners, but even infected women had a median of only two partners within the previous five years, while married women claiming fidelity to husbands had a significantly greater risk of infection if the husband had not been faithful, a risk that increased with the woman's own education and her partner's.[39]

Dar es Salaam was a thousand kilometres from Kagera and almost as remote from Tanzania's other borders, yet by August 1986, less than two years after HIV was recognised in the capital, its main hospital had admitted cases from each of mainland Tanzania's twenty regions. Some were probably infected from Dar es Salaam. In 1988 the highest prevalence, after Kagera, was in Iringa region on the Tanzam road linking the capital to Zambia.[40] Other areas, by contrast, acquired HIV by cross-border contact. In the south-western Mbeya region, for example, an explosive HIV and tuberculosis epidemic between 1986 and 1994 was caused by the C subtype of HIV-1, probably introduced from Zambia to the south and most prevalent at the border and in urban and roadside locations.[41] Mwanza region, south of Lake Victoria, was probably infected from Kagera, but Mara region, on the eastern shore of the lake, appears to have shared the severe epidemic in the neighbouring Nyanza province of Kenya. In the Kilimanjaro and Arusha regions of northern Tanzania the disease was blamed on young, mobile traders returning from Kagera, Dar es Salaam, and Kenya. As everywhere in the continent, the epidemic there took its shape from the structure of the commercial economy, with a focus among urban bar girls and sex workers, high infection among young adults driven from fertile mountainsides by land scarcity, and prevalence declining as the disease radiated out into the countryside. In Arusha region in 1992, for example, adult infection was 10.7 per cent in the poorer parts of the regional capital, 5.2 per cent in the wealthier parts, 2.2 per cent in semi-urban areas, and 1.6 per cent in the countryside, where at this time the disease was still seen as a complaint of despised urban aliens.[42] Because HIV entered Tanzania from all directions, the country had an unusual diversity of subtypes and unique recombinant forms.[43] Twenty-five years after its first appearance in Kagera the disease was still spreading into remote parts of the country.

While the link from the west lake epidemic to Dar es Salaam was strong, that to Nairobi and the Kenyan epidemic is no more than probable. Kenya's first Aids cases were concentrated in three locations: Mombasa on the coast, Nairobi in the centre, and the Nyanza province on the eastern shore of Lake Victoria. Any of these may have infected the others, or each may have been infected separately. If HIV reached the two cities directly from west of the lake, the main link, as in Dar es Salaam, was probably women from Kagera prominent in low-status sex work in Kenya since the interwar period. Of 418 women of this kind studied in Nairobi in 1985, 358 were Tanzanians and 37 Ugandans.[44] Blood specimens tested retrospectively showed that even in 1981 some 4 per cent of the city's sex workers were infected, a proportion that grew exponentially to more than 85 per cent in 1986. Of men with genital ulcer disease attending a Nairobi clinic, 3 per cent had HIV in 1981 and 15 per cent in 1985, leaving doubt whether women or men were first infected. In 1985, 2 per cent of women at antenatal clinics also tested positive, showing that infection was spreading to the general population.[45] That was the year when the Kenyan authorities belatedly admitted that the disease was present.

For epidemiologists, HIV in Nairobi was a classic example of an epidemic rapidly transmitted within a core group and then passed on by a bridging group – the sex workers' clients – to the general population. This happened in Nairobi, as not in Kampala, partly because the Ugandan epidemic began in the countryside and partly because of differences between the cities. In 1979 Nairobi's 827,775 people included 138 males for every 100 females, with an even larger imbalance among adults. At least half its employed men had no wife in the city.[46] Wealth and poverty were sharply juxtaposed and women with little education seldom found formal jobs. The result was an exceptionally overt, mercenary style of commercial sex, especially in the Pumwani red-light district, where a community of over a thousand sex workers, many from Kagera, sat outside their rooms waiting for brief encounters with working men at a price of 30–50 US cents. Each averaged nearly a thousand partners a year, working only by day because the night was too dangerous. Some 42 per cent had genital ulcer disease.[47] Study of their clients in 1986–7, when the epidemic peaked, found that 8 per cent contracted HIV from them and that 96 per cent of infected clients were either uncircumcised or had genital ulcer disease or both. Five years later, 76 per cent of women in Nairobi seeking treatment for a sexually transmitted disease reported only one partner during the previous three months and had presumably been infected by him, indicating the potential for transmission to the general population. HIV prevalence at Nairobi's antenatal clinics may have peaked in 1994 at about 17 per cent. Four years later over 40 per cent of Kenya's new HIV infections were thought to come through commercial sex.[48]

The sex workers themselves suffered terribly. Nearly half of those hitherto uninfected contracted HIV each year. They then generally developed Aids within about half the normal time, perhaps owing to multiple infection or other sexually transmitted diseases.[49] Their danger was discovered almost accidentally in 1985 during a preliminary survey of sexually transmitted diseases. When astonished researchers told sex workers that two-thirds of the 60 tested had HIV, they met 'stunned silence'. Only five wanted to know their personal status, although most quickly adopted the free condoms pressed upon them. 'When one gets beyond the initial prejudices and stereotypes,' the organisers wrote, 'one finds the prostitute knowingly risking AIDS, sacrificing her own hopes for the sake of her children or brothers and sisters.'[50]

The explosive epidemic in Nairobi almost monopolised attention in Kenya, so that little is known of HIV elsewhere during its first decade. Perhaps mis-leadingly, the coast region reported three times as many Aids cases as Nairobi in 1991, the great majority no doubt in Mombasa, where 54 per cent of 3,628 sex workers tested positive between 1993 and 1997 and adult prevalence in 2000 was 10.8 per cent.[51] Elsewhere prevalence during the early 1990s was relatively low, except in towns along the trans-African highway between Nairobi and the Ugandan border. In 1993 both Nakuru and Busia reported higher antenatal prevalence than either Nairobi or Mombasa. From the mid 1990s there was also rapid growth in the Central and Eastern provinces around Nairobi. Kenya's adult infection rate probably peaked around 1998, officially at 13.9 per cent although the true mark may have been substantially lower.[52]

Kenya's anomaly was the Nyanza province bordering Lake Victoria, which experienced an explosive epidemic that is perhaps the least understood in Africa. The earliest infections may have come across the lake soon after the epidemic began on its western shore, for between 1986 and 1993 Nyanza reported 15,605 Aids cases – 31 per cent of all Kenya's cases – implying widespread HIV prevalence in the early 1980s at least. By 1993, prevalence at antenatal clinics in Kisumu, the regional capital, was 20 per cent and rising quickly.[53] In the absence of detailed analysis, the best explanation of this epidemic suggests a combination of circumstances fostering disease elsewhere but seldom joined in one place. One was participation in lakeshore fishing culture. 'The beaches attract a continual inflow of people,' it was reported: 'young men in pursuit of an easy cash income and women following the men. They live outside the traditional social structure and subsistence farming households, and drinking, casual sex, theft, HIV/AIDS and high death rates among young men are common.' Nearly half the adults in these areas may have been infected by the early 2000s.[54] Equally vulnerable were young people with casual jobs on sugar plantations and especially on the fringes of the transport industry, for Nyanza straddled the trans-African highway and had its own motor transport network. Its dense rural population, closely linked to the urban focus of infection in Kisumu, bred rural prevalence levels among adults reaching 30 or 40 per cent in the early 2000s, while scarcity of land and lack of rural opportunity perpetuated migration to Kampala, Nairobi, and workplaces throughout Kenya, where Nyanza people often had exceptionally high rates of HIV.[55]

The social organisation of the Luo people also contributed to the epidemic. One study attributed over half their infection to the fact that some 90 per cent of Luo men, unlike most Kenyans, were not circumcised.[56] Their society was strongly patriarchal. In interviews at clinics in Kisumu in 2000, with Luo forming 81 per cent of those questioned, men reported unprotected sex with an average of 11.2 partners, women with 2.5. It is not clear whether these women included sex workers, but they numbered an estimated 1,400 in Kisumu in 1997–8 and 75 per cent of them were HIV-positive.[57] Many were probably divorced or separated women with few other opportunities in Luo society. Luo themselves saw the epidemic as only the culmination of a century of economic decline and social disintegration, focusing particular attention on their custom of inheriting widows (and hence, supposedly, the virus that killed their husbands) and on alleged youthful promiscuity. One study in the rural Asembo area in 2004 showed that 33 per cent of boys and 22 per cent of girls under fourteen years of age claimed sexual experience, which had probably been common among youths in the past but had taken non-penetrative forms. A survey of women in Kisumu in the late 1990s found HIV infection only among those who had engaged in premarital sex.[58] Female prevalence there rose from 8 per cent at age 15 to 29 per cent at age 17, at which age only 2 per cent of men were infected. Of every five people with HIV, three were women.[59] The connection between gender inequality, sexual behaviour, and vulnerability could scarcely have been stronger.

Except, perhaps, in Ethiopia. In its origins the Ethiopian epidemic differed from those elsewhere in eastern Africa, but in most other respects it was, despite the country's distinctive history, surprisingly similar, especially in the unsuspected early spread of heterosexual infection arising from sexual exploitation of women. The problem in Ethiopia, however, is not, as in Nyanza, why an extensive epidemic took place, but rather, as in pre-genocide Rwanda, why the epidemic was not more extensive. This may seem paradoxical, for in the early 2000s about 1,500,000 Ethiopians had HIV. Yet that implied a prevalence in those aged 15–49 of 4.4 per cent, only half the proportion in Tanzania and two-thirds of that in Kenya.[60]

One reason restricting the epidemic was that HIV reached Ethiopia somewhat later than the other eastern African countries. The first two cases were diagnosed in Addis Ababa in 1986. Retrospective tests on stored blood revealed one case in 1984 and another in 1985, but none in earlier specimens. Analysis of the diversification of the virus suggested that it had arrived in 1983. The virus itself, introduced at least twice, was subtype C of HIV-1, in contrast to the A and D subtypes dominant in East Africa. How the subtype mainly found in southern Africa and India also reached Ethiopia is unknown, but its complete domination of the epidemic – in contrast to the diversity of subtypes in Tanzania – suggests not only Ethiopia's isolation but a rapid saturation of a core group of vulnerable people from whom the infection spread to the wider population.[61]

The core group were the sex workers of Addis Ababa and other major towns, together with their habitual clients. Founded in 1886 on the model of a military camp, the capital was a sprawling jumble of permanent buildings and the squatter shacks in which over four-fifths of its nearly two million people lived. Women were a majority of the population, especially in the younger age ranges, for Ethiopian women married very young, divorce was common, and there was little place for unmarried women in the countryside. In the town, such women survived chiefly by informal activities, of which commercial sex was one of the most important. In 1973–4 an Ethiopian sociologist reckoned that some 27,000 women worked in bars, the chief meeting places for the city's men. An official survey in 1982 identified 15,900 full-time sex workers in the city. A less official one, seven years later, estimated 24,825, excluding streetwalkers and women working from their own rooms, adding that 55 per cent had only one or fewer partners per week.[62] Divorce, disagreement with parents, and lack of money to continue schooling were reasons often given for entering commercial sex. Major provincial towns had smaller but similar groups of sex workers.

Commercial sex had a role in Ethiopian urban culture similar to that in Kigali. Female virginity at marriage was vital to respectable families, if perhaps less so to their daughters than in the past, partly because marriage ages were rising with education. Men, by contrast, suffered little inhibition on sexual experimentation and on average (in 2000) married seven years later than their wives. Given this imbalance, as in Kigali, young men commonly had their first experience with sex workers and up to half continued to frequent them thereafter. Early in the epidemic most of these sexual encounters were unprotected, for Ethiopians were unfamiliar with condoms and hostile to them.[63] Sexually transmitted diseases liable to facilitate HIV transmission were common, especially among sex workers. A study in Addis Ababa in the early 1990s found that only 9 per cent of women in their first marriage and 1 per cent of sex workers had no serological evidence of such a disease, while 33 per cent and 46 per cent, respectively, were infected with HSV-2, which caused genital ulcers and particular susceptibility to HIV. Moreover, Ethiopia's health services were slender even by African standards, taking only 0.4 per cent of the national budget in 1999 and providing fewer than 20 per cent of pregnant women with antenatal care, as against an average of over 60 per cent in sub-Saharan Africa.[64]

HIV first became established in Addis Ababa among sex workers during an explosive epidemic in the late 1980s. In 1987, 5.9 per cent of them tested positive; by 1990 the figure had risen to 54.2 per cent. Prevalence was especially high in city centre brothels. By contrast, in 1989 only 4.6 per cent of the capital's pregnant women were infected.[65] Other places of very high prevalence among sex workers at this date were the trucking towns of Dessie, Nazareth, Mekele, Bahr-Dar, and Gonder on roads radiating outwards from Addis Ababa. In the far north, however, the disease was still rare, although it had penetrated to all parts of the country. Study of 23 towns in 1988 showed an average prevalence of 17 per cent among sex workers, 13 per cent among long-distance truck drivers, but only 3.7 per cent among blood donors (who broadly represented the general population).[66] Among the latter, rapid epidemic growth began three or four years later than among sex workers, the annual incidence of new urban infections peaking in 1991 at about 2.7 per cent. Prevalence among antenatal women in Addis Ababa rose from 4.6 per cent in 1989 to 11.2 per cent in 1992–3, reaching its likely peak of 21.2 per cent in 1995.[67]

At the same time, the ratio of infected men to infected women in the capital fell from 3.7:1 in 1988 to 1.5:1 in 1994, suggesting that an epidemic that had begun among a core group had spread to the general population. In a study of 2,526 factory and estate workers in and around Addis Ababa in 1994, HIV infection in men was strongly associated with reported sexual behaviour and past history of syphilis, but in women it was associated with socio-demographic characteristics (low income, low education, and living alone) rather than sexual behaviour. Moreover, the burden fell increasingly on young women. In 1995, antenatal prevalence in Addis Ababa was 23.7 per cent among women aged 15–24, 17.7 per cent among those of 25–34, and 11.1 per cent among older women. In Dire Dawa, a railway town east of the capital, 57 per cent of all infected women in 1999 were aged 15–24.[68]

Ethiopia's urban epidemic ceased to expand during the mid 1990s, although numerous new infections continued to compensate for the rising number of deaths. The missing element in the story, however, was expansion to the countryside, for the remarkable point about Ethiopia – in contrast, say, to Nyanza – was how little impact the disease had made in rural areas, where estimated adult prevalence was 0.3 per cent in 1990 and 0.8 per cent in 1995. This was partly misleading, for such was the predominance of the countryside in Ethiopia – 83 per cent of the population in 1999 – that rural infections overtook urban from 1997. Yet rural prevalence in 2000 was still only an estimated 1.9 per cent. It was highest in the central Amhara region, but in the remote Southern Nations Nationalities and Peoples Region, at that date, only 37 per cent of women had even heard of Aids, although the impact grew rapidly thereafter.[69] Rural people, there and elsewhere, blamed townsmen and foreigners for the disease: 'We Hamar don't have cars with which to reach America. We don't go to England, to *gal* [highland] country, to Germany, and going there, we don't come back bringing illness. It comes to us by foot.'[70]

As in Rwanda and Burundi, it is difficult to explain the weakness of urban–rural transmission of HIV in Ethiopia during the 1990s. One element may have been the dispersed pattern of rural settlement that limited interaction. Studies of the extent to which farmers frequented sex workers in market towns found inexplicably varied proportions.[71] As in Rwanda, occasional visits might do little to spread a virus so difficult to transmit, especially in a culture with near-universal male circumcision. The most detailed rural study, of a Muslim area in eastern Hararghe, concluded that it was protected from infection by its Muslim social order and its lack of exposure to high-prevalence urban groups.[72] Perhaps this last point was the most important. The HIV/Aids epidemic throughout eastern Africa had been shaped by the network of communication provided by commercial economies. Vigorous around Lake Victoria and along the trans-African highway, they were less integrated in Rwanda and Burundi or the emptiness of central Tanzania. The particular weakness of its commercial economy had shaped much of Ethiopia's modern history, notably its uncompleted revolution. Now the same circumstances helped to protect its countryside against infection.

5
The Conquest
of the South

The countries of southern Africa, although infected with HIV slightly later than those further north, nevertheless overtook eastern Africa's levels of prevalence during the mid 1990s and then experienced the world's most terrible epidemic. By 2004 the region had 2 per cent of the world's population and nearly 30 per cent of its HIV cases, with no evidence of overall decline in any national prevalence, which in several countries exceeded 30 per cent of the sexually active population. The chief issue in southern Africa is therefore to explain the speed and scale of epidemic growth. The obvious explanation is the region's history of white domination and the dramatic economic change and social inequality it had wrought. The view here is that this is true, but the connections were not always obvious, while, as everywhere in Africa, the scale of the epidemic was chiefly due to the long incubation period that enabled it to spread silently beyond hope of rapid suppression.

By chance, both the earliest definite indication of HIV in southern Africa and the best evidence of the silent epidemic anywhere in the continent come from the remote rural Karonga district of northern Malawi, bordering Tanzania and Zambia. Karonga's people, famed in colonial times for their education received from Scottish missionaries, had migrated as clerks and craftsmen throughout the industrial centres of southern Africa. This may first have exposed them to HIV. The virus's arrival in Karonga can be traced because the district experienced a mass campaign against leprosy and tuberculosis that included two total population surveys, in 1981–4 and 1987–9, each of which took and stored blood specimens from everyone in two sections of the district. All 44,150 specimens have been tested retrospectively for HIV, although only those from people aged 15–49 are included in the calculations. The results give a uniquely detailed picture of the dynamics of a local epidemic.[1]

In the first round of investigation, none of the 1,041 specimens taken in 1981 had HIV. Four infected specimens were taken in 1982, one in 1983, and six in 1984, making a total of eleven in 12,979 specimens, or less than 0.1 per cent. Four were men and seven women. Eight were recent arrivals in

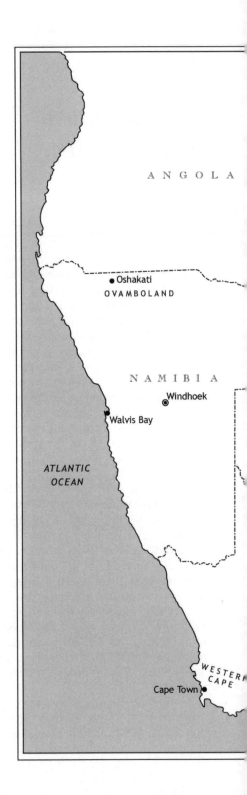

Map 3 *Southern Africa*

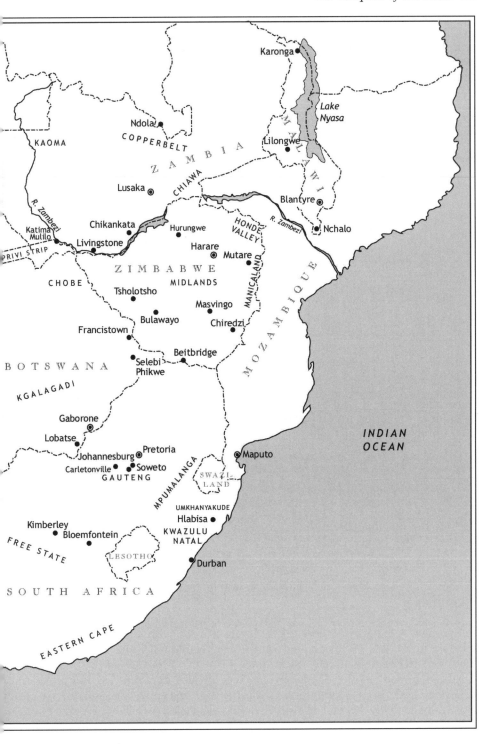

the district: four from other parts of Malawi (including the main city, Blantyre), two from Tanzania, and two from Zambia. Not only was the disease brought from several outside sources almost simultaneously, but several different subtypes were introduced. The two arrivals from Tanzania brought subtypes A and D, the two forms dominant in East Africa. Of the other nine specimens from this period, six were later identified as subtype C, while the other three could not be positively identified but were closest to subtype C and possibly an extinct variety of it.

Of the six individuals definitely identified with subtype C, one came from Zambia, two had been born in Zambia but had lived in Blantyre, two had come from elsewhere in Malawi, and one was a long-term resident of Karonga. Subtype C was to dominate the southern African epidemic, causing some 94 per cent of infections there in 2001.[2] It may have originated in the southern DR Congo,[3] which had many links with neighbouring Zambia, especially through the mining towns of Katanga and the Zambian Copperbelt. A possible reconstruction, compatible with evidence of early infection elsewhere in Malawi and Zambia that will be quoted later, is that elements of the East African epidemic (subtypes A and D) spread across the border into rural Karonga, but that the bulk of infection (subtype C) was carried from the southern DR Congo into Zambia, probably first to the Copperbelt, spread to other urban centres (including Blantyre) by 1983, and was carried from these centres into Karonga. Something can even be known of the process of infection. Of the six specimens with subtype C, four were so closely related genetically as to form a single cluster (cluster 1) with a single origin. One of the four was the long-term resident of Karonga. The other three had come from other parts of Malawi. The most likely scenario is that one person introduced the strain from elsewhere in Malawi and infected the other three after arriving in Karonga, although this cannot be certain.

Cluster 1 becomes central when attention shifts to the second round of blood collection in 1987–9. This revealed not 11 but 189 HIV-positive specimens, a prevalence of 2 per cent. Of the 168 specimens that could be analysed by subtype, 152 (90 per cent) belonged to subtype C, 6 to D, 3 to A, 3 were unclassified, and 4 were recombinants. Not only had subtype C established itself as the dominant form, but so had cluster 1: 40 per cent of those with subtype C (61 people) were infected with variants of that strain, probably introduced no more than five or ten years earlier by a single individual. Nothing could illustrate more vividly the explosive potential of a virus whose existence in their bodies was almost certainly unknown to most of those harbouring it.

The data collected in 1987–9 reveal much more about HIV epidemiology in Karonga. A majority of those infected were women, with an especially rapid increase in the late 1980s among women aged between 15 and 24, whereas men with HIV were generally older. Some 87 of the 189 infected people had not been present in the district in 1981–4, divided between 48 returning absentees and 39 new immigrants. Clearly the epidemic was still driven chiefly by mobility beyond the district. Prevalence increased with years of schooling and was most common among traders, salaried employees, casual labourers, and generally those who were not peasant farmers. Those with the best and the worst housing had higher prevalence than those with houses of intermediate quality. Of eighteen couples in which both partners were infected, only twelve were infected with closely related viral strains. Most intriguing was the dominance of subtype C, for one unanswered question about the epidemic is whether this subtype, which by the 2000s was responsible for more than half the world's HIV infections, had greater evolutionary fitness than other subtypes. Despite much research and several detailed differences in its mode of operation, no conclusive evidence of this had emerged by 2005, although one study had shown that viral concentrations were more than three times as high in the blood and semen of Malawian men, over 90 per cent of them with subtype C, than in Americans with subtype B.[4]

Although the data from Karonga are uniquely detailed, it was clearly not the first part of Malawi to experience HIV infection. Study of stored blood taken in southern Africa before 1974 has revealed no evidence of HIV, but the first 17 Aids cases were reported from Malawi's health facilities in l985, some with aggressive Kaposi's sarcoma, and a year later nearly 4 per cent of Malawian mineworkers in South Africa were HIV-positive, the only national group from Central Africa significantly infected. Given the long incubation period before the appearance of symptomatic Aids, and given the wide extent of HIV infection evident by the mid 1980s, Malawi's silent epidemic probably began before 1980, or only slightly after HIV can be discerned around Lake Victoria. Census data show that mortality in Malawi increased significantly between 1977 and l987, but chiefly among children, who commonly died of Aids more quickly than adults.[5]

The virus may have reached Zambia slightly earlier than Malawi, although the evidence is indirect. In 1983 Anne Bayley, a surgeon in Lusaka, found herself treating unprecedented numbers of young adults afflicted with aggressive Kaposi's sarcoma. When tested in 1984, 91 per cent of these were found HIV-positive. Bayley later thought that the first case might date back to 1980 and that HIV had probably reached Zambia in the mid 1970s, initially spreading slowly. She added – a conclusion presumably reached by retrospective testing – that in 1981 fewer than 1 per cent of women at Lusaka's antenatal clinics were HIV-infected.[6] Many early patients in Lusaka with Kaposi's sarcoma had associations with the Copperbelt, where tuberculosis cases suddenly multiplied from 1984 and the first small HIV tests in the general population of mining communities in 1985 showed 13.5 per cent prevalence in males and 21 per cent in females. Of deaths from Aids reported from Zambia between March and July 1987, 46 per cent were from the Copperbelt and 18 per cent from Lusaka.[7] Yet the situation in the capital was alarming enough, for tests there in 1985 showed that 8 per cent of pregnant women were infected. In February 1986 Aids patients were also dying in Livingstone on Zambia's southern border with Zimbabwe.[8]

In reality, the silent epidemic had penetrated Zimbabwe some time before, although perhaps three or four years later than Zambia and Malawi as the virus was carried southwards. The first cases of Aids and aggressive Kaposi's sarcoma were diagnosed in 1983. Alarm arose only when blood was first screened in 1985 and it was revealed that over 2 per cent of donors had HIV. Infection then concentrated in the northern city of Harare, with only 0.05 per cent of donors testing positive in Bulawayo, further south. Thereafter, however, expansion became general and rapid. At the district hospital at Hurungwe in Mashonaland West, the annual number of patients diagnosed with HIV rose between 1986 and 1988 from 16 to 292. In Manicaland province, on Zimbabwe's eastern border, all districts recorded increased mortality from the late 1980s. By 1990 national antenatal prevalence was 12.9 per cent.[9]

Botswana was invaded next, slightly later than Zimbabwe and just as stealthily. Over 200 blood specimens collected in the north during 1984 showed no HIV. 'It's not a problem in Botswana,' an official declared, 'AIDS is primarily a disease of homosexuals and there is no homosexual in Botswana.' The first case reported at that time was indeed a white homo-sexual.[10] When the first Tswana tested positive a year later, the Minister of Health 'allayed fears by mentioning that the modes of transmission of the disease means that it could not become a big epidemic'. Within another year, however, he was speaking of 'a scourge that could decimate a large portion of the human race' and recommending 'a stable, faithful relationship with another uninfected person'. By then Botswana had 30 known HIV cases and feared that the real number might be more like 3,000. In 1990 tests showed that 5–7 per cent of blood donors in towns and 1–2 per cent in the country-side were infected.[11]

During the 1990s these four countries of Central Africa overtook East Africa as the chief focus of the global epidemic. Malawi experienced rapid growth of infection during the later 1980s in the major towns, led by Blantyre where infection rates at the hospital antenatal clinic rose from 2.0 per cent in 1985 to 25.9 per cent in 1991 and a peak of 32.8 per cent in 1996. A small study there in 1990–5 suggested an annual incidence of new infections among women of 4.21 per cent, or perhaps four times the rate during the Kinshasa epidemic. During that period, however, prevalence probably grew even faster in the countryside, narrowing the hitherto wide urban–rural differential. In 1996 adult prevalence was 23 per cent in urban, 18 per cent in semi-urban, and 12 per cent in rural areas. Given that only 12 per cent of Malawians lived in towns, most infections were rural.[12]

By the mid 1990s Zambia's prevalence had overtaken Malawi's. According to a later estimate, adult infection peaked in 1994–5 at about 17 per cent. As in Blantyre, the growth of the epidemic in the late 1980s was especially rapid in Lusaka, where antenatal prevalence rose to a roughly stable 22–27 per cent at different clinics in 1990–3. The difference was that 50 per cent of Zambians were urban and that overall prevalence in Copperbelt province almost equalled that in the capital.[13]

Yet Zambia, too, was soon overtaken. Zimbabwe's prevalence figures are especially difficult to interpret, with wide variations between those quoted by national and international authorities and even wider fluctuations at individual sentinel sites. The most reliable data are probably for antenatal clinic attenders in Harare. Prevalence among them was 10 per cent in 1989 and 18 per cent in 1991, both figures substantially less than in the main cities of Malawi and Zambia, but it grew further to a peak of 32 per cent in 1995 and then fluctuated around that level. Yet only 28 per cent of Zimbabwe's people were urban.[14] The distinctive feature of its experience during the 1990s was the high level of prevalence outside the main cities, often so high that the statistics must be treated with caution. Three kinds of areas were worst affected. One contained towns on main roads close to borders, where truck drivers might socialise for several days while negotiating their way across the frontier. Beitbridge, on the South African border, recorded 59 per cent HIV prevalence in 1996, while the figure at Mutare, near the frontier with Mozambique, reached 37 per cent in 1997.[15] Second, the trucking routes contributed to high prevalence in provinces and districts through which they passed. Masvingo province, which registered a barely credible provincial figure of 49.4 per cent among pregnant women in 2000, was bisected by the road from Harare to South Africa, while Midlands province, with a reported 45.1 per cent prevalence in 2000, straddled the route from Harare to Bulawayo.[16] Yet this devastating provincial infection that distinguished Zimbabwe was not confined to transport routes but existed even in remote rural areas. In 1993–4 overall adult prevalence was already 24 per cent in the Honde valley, a fairly isolated part of Manicaland. Shortly thereafter, 22 per cent of pregnant women tested HIV-positive even at Tsholotsho in arid northern Matabeleland.[17] As will be seen later, both its excellent transport system and its high levels of oscillating migration between country and town made rural Zimbabwe especially vulnerable to infection.

Those characteristics operated even more powerfully in Botswana. From only 2 or 3 per cent in 1990 its national adult prevalence soared to 23 per cent in 1995 and either 28 per cent (according to the government) or 36 per cent (according to UNAIDS) in 2000, the latter figure being the highest in the world.[18] As the epidemic spread south, its momentum seemed to accelerate, suggesting the possibility that rapid passage of the virus from person to person might be increasing its virulence, although there was no hard evidence of this. The acceleration in Botswana was noticed first not at the capital, Gaborone, but at Francistown, where the main road crossed into Zimbabwe and antenatal prevalence reached 24 per cent in 1992 and 34 per cent in 1993. Gaborone soon followed, as did the mining town of Selebi Phikwe; in 2000 these three towns registered antenatal prevalences of 44, 36, and 50 per cent respectively.[19] Yet this initial urban predominance was reversed as the epidemic grew. By 1999 prevalence among pregnant women was 22 per cent even in the Kgalagadi desert area, while the highest reported prevalence among them at that time was 51 per cent in the northern district of Chobe. Overall, according to the government, 'the 2002 survey reveals slightly higher rates in rural than in urban areas'. The annual incidence of new infections for the whole country at that time was estimated to be 6 per cent, roughly three-quarters of the level reached among young people at Rakai during the 1980s.[20]

An early attempt to explain the speed and scale of Botswana's epidemic highlighted three factors: 'the position of women in society, particularly their lack of power in negotiating sexual relationships; cultural attitudes to fertility; and social migration patterns'.[21] Gender inequality fostered the epidemic throughout Central Africa. Commercial sex, driven mainly by female poverty and lack of opportunity, has been little studied in Botswana, but elsewhere it was important especially in initial urban epidemics, although probably less central than in Nairobi or Kigali. Women held only 8 per cent of Zimbabwe's and 15 per cent of Zambia's formal sector jobs in the early-mid 1990s.[22] 'Divorce, rural poverty and superior earnings were the principal reasons cited' by sex workers in Harare in 1989; 70 per cent of them were divorced, probably with children to support, and nearly half came from drought-stricken southern Matabeleland. Six years later, 86 per cent of sex workers tested there had HIV, like 70 per cent of those working the main road between Zimbabwe and Zambia in 1987, 56 per cent in Blantyre in 1986, and 69 per cent in Ndola in 1997–8.[23] Although willing to use condoms, only about half of those in Harare in 1989 and one-quarter of those in Blantyre and Ndola in the mid 1990s could overcome their clients' opposition.[24] Studies of young male factory workers in Harare during the 1990s showed both their fecklessness and their difficulty in avoiding risk where HIV was so widespread. Their annual incidence of new infections was 2 per cent, meaning that half were likely to contract HIV during a normal working lifespan. Similar levels of infection existed among long-distance drivers.[25] A Malawian villager later recalled how passing tanker drivers infected local women:

> The wives were spreading the virus to their husbands, the unmarried women were infecting the young men, the young men making money from smuggling were going into Lilongwe and having sex there. People were behaving very freely and they had no idea that anything bad could happen to them.... By 1996, 12 years after the trucks first started arriving, the death rate in the village peaked at four a week.... Our neighbours from other villages would not come to help people who were sick or help at a funeral because of fear of contracting the disease.... We became completely isolated.[26]

More commonly, however, infection passed from promiscuous men to their wives. In one small enquiry in Lusaka, lasting a year, 26 per cent of HIV-positive husbands infected their wives, while only 8 per cent of HIV-positive wives infected their husbands. 'Men generally acquire infection first,' a careful study in Manicaland reported, 'frequently during spells of labour migration in towns or commercial areas, and then pass on the infection to their regular female partners based in rural areas.' By 1998 twice as many women as men there were infected, including four times as many among people aged 17–24, owing to the disparity of age between sexual partners.[27]

Nevertheless, women too could be 'movious', as Central Africans described it. Most were not: even the highest self-reported accounts of sexual behaviour suggest that only about 25 per cent of women had non-marital sex. Yet of those attending antenatal clinics in two areas of Manicaland in 1993–4, 16 per cent of married women, 43 per cent of single women, and 50 per cent of formerly married women were infected.[28] Among the many factors encouraging extra-marital sex, one of the most important was delayed marriage, due chiefly to education, labour migration, and the decline of polygyny. In Botswana in 2001, for example, the median age at first marriage or cohabitation was 28 for men and 23 for women. Consequently, in 1995 over 60 per cent of never-married women aged 20–24 there were mothers, while 41 per cent of boys and 15 per cent of girls aged 15–16 had sexual experience. In Lobatse and Francistown, with very high HIV prevalence, 47 per cent of men and 39 per cent of women aged 17–18 had a casual partner over a twelve-month period; 21 per cent and 16 per cent had at least two. Of teenage girls who bore children in the late 1980s, 40 per cent had them with men six or more years older than themselves. Young Tswana had adopted an experimental attitude towards sex – 'marketing themselves' as it was known – 'so that you can compare them and see who amongst them perfectly suits your life'.[29] Many women deliberately avoided marriage in order to maximise their freedom. It made them immensely vulnerable and created an exceptionally wide generation gap between young people and those raised under strong traditional or Christian influence.[30]

Botswana's late twentieth-century sexual order originated as an adaptation to education and labour migration.[31] It was one consequence of the mobility that drove the Central African epidemic, evident in the initial infection of Karonga, in the roles of long-distance drivers and dusty border towns like Beitbridge, and in the migration routes to the Copperbelt or the Nchalo sugar estate in southern Malawi, where the annual incidence of new infections is reported to have reached a brief peak of 17.1 per cent during 1994–5. In Zimbabwe, prevalence at antenatal clinics in 2000 ranged from 26.8 per cent in rural locations to 53.9 per cent in commercial (farming and mining) settings, peaking at 70.7 per cent in Chiredzi, another sugar plantation area.[32] HIV thus followed the pattern of the commercial economy, straddling the urban–rural divide that checked it in Ethiopia. In each Central African country there was a close relationship between patterns of infection and of oscillating labour migration. Botswana experienced rapid urbanisation – Gaborone's population multiplied more than ten times between 1971 and 1997 – but nevertheless had higher rural than urban prevalence of HIV because its people held to a long tradition of maintaining separate homes in towns and the countryside, between which they had in the past oscillated at different seasons, a practice now facilitated by motor transport. In Zimbabwe a similar oscillating pattern had grown up in the colonial period as men maintained land rights and families in the communal reserves while working in mines and cities. This, it has been argued, raised rural HIV prevalence close to urban levels.[33] Colonial Zambia had known a similar pattern of mobility, but its severe economic decline after 1974 made towns less attractive and travel to distant provinces more difficult, so that the urban–rural differential in HIV prevalence was wider than in Zimbabwe, although narrower than elsewhere. Malawi, a poorer country, initially had much higher levels of infection in Blantyre and Lilongwe than in the countryside, but the contrast narrowed during the 1990s, partly perhaps in the natural course of epidemic development but also because economic decline drove infected young people into the countryside.[34]

Botswana's epidemic was fuelled also by ethnic and cultural homogeneity, facilitating social interaction, and by its new-found diamond wealth, which gave it the world's highest economic growth rate during the last third of the twentieth century. Yet, as its citizens said, Botswana was 'a rich country of poor people', 47 per cent of them living below the poverty line in 1993–4. Such polarisation fostered both risk taking in the rich and vulnerability in the poor.[35] In Karonga those first infected had been the more prosperous and educated, but as the epidemic developed it focused increasingly on the poor. A survey of mining and industrial workers in Zambia, Botswana, and South Africa in 2000–1 showed HIV prevalence ranging from 4.5 per cent among managers to 10.5 per cent among skilled workers and 18.3 per cent among the unskilled.[36] In addition to driving women into vulnerable occupations, poverty fostered disease by weakening medical systems and putting treatment beyond the reach of the poor. Between 1980 and 2000 the number of notified tuberculosis cases in Zambia, Zimbabwe, and Malawi multiplied five times as a result of HIV infection and decaying health systems.[37] Although sexually transmitted diseases declined during the early years of the HIV epidemic, owing to wider use of condoms and greater emphasis on treatment, they were increasingly supplemented by HSV-2, which spread in synergy with HIV to infect 40 per cent of sexually active men and 61 per cent of sexually active women in Ndola in 1997. The lack of male circumcision in Central Africa added to the risk of HIV infection. In Botswana, ironically, circumcision had largely been abandoned during the twentieth century.[38]

While the epidemics in Malawi, Zambia, Zimbabwe, and Botswana reached maturity during the late 1990s, those in Mozambique and Namibia were still explosive. In both countries the warfare of the 1980s appears to have checked the spread of HIV by obstructing normal mobility. In Mozambique a study in ten provincial capitals in 1987 found average adult prevalence of 3.2 per cent, while in Maputo, isolated on the southern coast, antenatal prevalence was still less than 1 per cent in 1990.[39] In Namibia, similarly, only 4.2 per cent of pregnant women were infected in 1988–92, with one area of high prevalence (14 per cent) at Katima Mulilo in the Caprivi Strip, which was not only the headquarters of the South African army but a meeting point of long-distance transport routes from Angola, Zambia, Zimbabwe, Botswana, and Namibia, notorious for high levels of commercial sex. Once Namibia was assured independence in 1990, however, some 43,387 registered exiles returned, mostly from Angola and Zambia. Many may well have been infected, for in 1992–3 prevalence was 17.2 per cent among Namibian soldiers in the northern Ovamboland region, many of them previously based outside the country. During the mid 1990s Namibia suffered an explosive epidemic, antenatal prevalence rising from 4 per cent in 1992 to 21 per cent in 2001. The northern nuclei at Katima Mulilo and Oshakati (another transport focus) retained high levels, but so now did the capital at Windhoek and the main port at Walvis Bay. By 1996 Aids was Namibia's largest single cause of death. A relatively wealthy African country with great mobility, extreme income inequality, little female opportunity, and high levels of sexually transmitted diseases, it had many of the same conditions for epidemic expansion as Botswana.[40] Mozambique, by contrast, followed more the patterns of poor countries like Malawi and Tanzania, once its civil war ended in 1992. Many returning refugees were probably infected and especially high prevalence existed on the north-western border with Malawi and in the central region along the Zambezi valley, long garrisoned by heavily infected Zimbabwean and Mozambican troops. In Maputo, antenatal prevalence rose between 1994 and 2002 from 3 to 19 per cent.[41]

Meanwhile South Africa experienced the world's largest epidemic, with perhaps 5.3 million infected people in 2003.[42] Not only did the socio-economic structures of Apartheid make the country an almost perfect environment for HIV, but the beginning of the epidemic coincided with the township revolt of the mid 1980s and its peak took place a decade later during the transition to majority rule, which compelled ordinary people to concentrate on survival and distracted both the outgoing regime and its nationalist successor from making HIV their chief priority. Yet it would be naïve to think that even the most vigorous, stable, and popular government could have protected South Africa from a major epidemic. A contrast is sometimes drawn with Thailand, where an epidemic also became established during the early 1990s but was contained by 1999 at an adult prevalence of 2.2 per cent, whereas South Africa's was 19.9 per cent.[43] Yet this is to ignore the totally different ways in which HIV struck the two countries. Thailand was the first seriously affected country in South-East Asia, with no established epidemic on its borders and a disease that first took root among core groups of drug users, sex workers, and their clients, who could be targeted with impressive energy.[44] South Africa, by contrast, bordered a massive continental epidemic and, as will be seen, had no identifiable core group but a great diversity of cross-border contacts that can scarcely now be traced. Of course, better political leadership could have reduced the impact of HIV, but trying to prevent the extensive infection of South Africa would have been like sweeping back the ocean with a broom. Thanks to its uniquely long, asymptomatic incubation period, HIV-1 could probably never have been prevented from reaching epidemic proportions once established in a general heterosexual population. That happened not in South Africa but ten years earlier and 2,500 kilometres away in Kinshasa.

All this is clear from the way the South African epidemic began. The first diagnosed case, in 1982, was in a white, homosexual air steward who had probably contracted the disease in New York and died of the *Pneumocystis carinii* pneumonia common among American patients. 'Gay plague hits South Africa', the Johannesburg *Star* trumpeted.[45] Blood specimens from 200 homosexual men in Johannesburg in 1983 later showed that 32 were already infected. Although homosexuality was technically illegal in South Africa and a taboo subject among respectable Afrikaners, clinics were opened at major hospitals, injecting drug users were screened (and found negative), patients organised their own protection and care, and by 1990 the homosexual epidemic was already levelling off. Of 308 Aids cases reported in South Africa by January 1990, 207 had been in homosexuals, 195 of them white.[46] Their infection was not transferred to the general heterosexual population, for the strain of HIV-1 infecting American and South African homosexuals, subtype B, scarcely appeared among heterosexuals until the mid 1990s and then remained rare. By the early 2000s adult prevalence among whites was barely one-third of that among Africans.[47]

While the medical authorities concentrated on the epidemic among white homosexuals, more perceptive doctors realised that a more dangerous hetero-sexual epidemic threatened. The first African in South Africa definitely known to have suffered from HIV was a man from the DR Congo who apparently sought treatment early in 1985. During that year 522 blood specimens from Africans in Johannesburg were tested and all found negative.[48] The first serious alarm emerged in 1986, when tests on African mineworkers found only 0.02 per cent prevalence among South Africans but 3.76 per cent among men from Malawi. 'In the compounds and at work we were taunted and heckled,' the Malawians complained, '... they called us dying people.' The government ordered compulsory screening of migrant workers, but trade unions, medical officers, and the Malawian authorities all resisted until all recruiting there was abandoned.[49] Such Central African migrants certainly helped to introduce the disease. Two of the first black South Africans known to have contracted HIV were infected some time before 1986 by a Malawian mineworker. The only positive case among 240 African women tested in Johannesburg early in 1987 was a Malawian migrant. But none of the 94 'self-confessed promiscuous women' and 1,065 other women in mining areas tested in 1986 was infected and mineworkers did not become a core group spreading infection to the rest of the South African population, whose prevalence levels they generally shared.[50] Nor were sex workers an early focus of disease on the scale of Kigali, Nairobi, and Addis Ababa. By the late 1990s they were often heavily infected – 60 per cent in the Hillbrow area of Johannesburg, 56 per cent at truck stops in the Natal Midlands – but this was not the case earlier in the decade and professional sex workers were rare in African townships, where men seldom blamed infection on them.[51]

The lack of a core group is a striking feature of the initial infection of black South Africans. The infection was rapid: during 1987 blood screening suggested that HIV prevalence was already eight times higher among blacks than whites and was doubling every six months.[52] But it was infection by diffusion across a long, much-permeated northern frontier and through individual contacts in many sectors of a mobile, commercialised environment. One indication of this is that even by 1992 the strains of subtype C virus over-whelmingly dominant in the African population were drawn from all parts of Central Africa, with a large element from neighbouring Botswana, in contrast, for example, to the homogeneity of strains in Ethiopia. Among pregnant women who tested positive at Baragwanath Hospital in Soweto in 1991, 'A strong link was made with African countries to the north of South Africa or partners who travelled.'

Another indication of the complexity of transmission was that the highest HIV prevalence at that time was not in the industrial heartland of the Wit-watersrand but in KwaZulu-Natal.[53] Among the likely reasons for this predominance, which continued throughout the 1990s, were the region's dense rural population, the unusually close interaction between the country-side and the major city of Durban, high rates of mobility and migration, equally high levels of sexually transmitted diseases, and the fact that Zulu had abandoned circumcision two centuries before. Even in 1990 some of the province's highest prevalence rates, over 3 per cent of adults, were in rural areas crossed by truck routes to Swaziland and Mozambique, with concentrations among late teenage women and those who had recently shifted residence. A study there a decade later found that couples with a migrant male were nearly twice as likely to have one or more member infected with HIV than were couples without a migrant, but that in 29 per cent of couples with only one infected member, that member was the woman. Antenatal prevalence at that time in the northern Umkhanyakude rural district was 41 per cent, against 32.5 per cent for the province and 22.4 per cent for South Africa as a whole.[54] The current incidence of new infections among women aged 15–49 at Hlabisa, the region's main hospital, was 17 per cent a year, as high a figure as was recorded anywhere in Africa during the epidemic. The disease was closely associated with tuberculosis, which had been suppressed during the 1950s by chemotherapy but now became the chief opportunistic infection in HIV-positive patients. Tuberculosis cases at Hlabisa multiplied nearly six times between 1990 and 2001. 'The country,' wrote the doctor in charge, 'is busy burying its young.'[55]

The peak expansion of South Africa's HIV epidemic lasted from about 1993 to 1998, when the number of new cases began to decline.[56] Apart from KwaZulu-Natal, the worst-affected provinces were Gauteng, the Free State, and Mpumalanga, but perhaps the most severe impact was in the independent states of Lesotho and Swaziland, both tied to South Africa by labour migration. The mines were not initially major centres of infection and HIV only slowly penetrated Lesotho. Its statistics are particularly erratic, but prevalence appears to have been low until 1993, when a dramatic increase took place, reaching 31 per cent at urban antenatal sites in 2002. The carriers were returning mineworkers – 48 per cent were estimated to be infected in 2000 – who transmitted the virus to the women who in 2002 were 55 per cent of those infected.[57] Swaziland was less dependent on migration to South Africa, but there, too, rapid infection coincided with the acceleration of the South African epidemic around 1993. A year later, 16 per cent of antenatal clinic attenders were HIV-positive and the proportion increased continuously thereafter to nearly 39 per cent in 2003, a figure rivalled only in Botswana. Rural and urban prevalences were almost the same. This rapid, sustained, and widespread growth was probably driven chiefly by mobility within Swaziland and the particular subordination of young women.[58]

Within South Africa, similarly, high levels of mobility ensured that infection was relatively evenly distributed between town and country. In 2002 the first population survey found 12.4 per cent adult prevalence in African rural areas, 11.3 per cent on commercial farms, and 15.8 per cent in areas of formal urban housing, but a markedly higher prevalence (28.4 per cent) in 'informal urban areas', the squatter settlements ringing every town.[59] This was the most striking evidence anywhere in Africa that the epidemic had come to concentrate among the poor. One connection was the prevalence of sexually transmitted diseases which were roughly three times as common in informal housing areas as elsewhere. An intensive study in the Carletonville mining area of Gauteng in 1999 found that HSV-2, the main cause of genital ulcers, was the single best predictor of HIV, infecting 91 per cent of HIV-positive women and 65 per cent of HIV-positive men aged 14–24. Among men at an STD clinic in Durban, similarly, HIV prevalence increased between 1991 and 1998 from 5 to 64 per cent and HSV-2 prevalence rose from 10 to 41 per cent.[60]

A second connection between HIV and poverty concerned gender relationships. While commercial sex was relatively unimportant in the townships, widespread partner exchange like that in Kinshasa and Bangui was markedly more common among the young there than in other contexts.[61] Among men it was in part inherited from a polygynous tradition, but it was due also to the collapse of rural restraints on premarital sex (especially its restriction to non-penetrative intercourse), to artificial contraception that reduced the risk of unwanted pregnancy, to the disempowerment of poor young men who could not afford to marry and establish households, and to a reactive machismo that was further stimulated by the violence of the anti-Apartheid struggle.[62] Although observers overdramatised the 'lost generation' of the early 1990s, many young townsmen of the time aspired to be an *isoka*, the handsome, popular, and irresponsible hero who displayed his masculinity, in one of the few ways available in a township, by having penetrative sex with girlfriends whom he could not afford to marry. 'If I were to have many lovers,' one explained, 'people ... would think that I was a playboy, which is a very nice thing to be.'[63] Sexual debut came increasingly early, at a median of perhaps sixteen years. Condoms were despised as destroying both pleasure and trust. Many young men had little sense of their own danger: as late as 2003, 62 per cent of HIV-positive people aged 15–24 believed they were at little or no risk of infection. Others accepted the risk as one among many that they faced. 'We thought that with the new government we could relax, study, plan a future,' a man of twenty said in the mid 1990s. 'Now AIDS is here to give us no future, Well, we'll all just get it and that's life. We're cursed; we really are the lost generation.'[64]

For young township women, the danger could be more immediate. Of those aged 14–24 interviewed at Carletonville in 1999, 16 per cent had been forced to have sex against their will. Perhaps 2 per cent of women of childbearing age were raped each year. These were only the most blatant forms of coercion. More took the form of steady pressure rather than violence. Many men and women believed that a man who had given bridewealth for a woman, spent money on her, or received encouragement from her had a right to sex regardless of her wishes: 'Once you have kissed each other that means you are preparing for sex. If she refuses at that point you must just force her.'[65] Not all needed to be forced. For some poor young women, their sexuality might be their only means of survival or of acquiring coveted goods and other benefits. A study in Cape Town found that about 20 per cent of teenage women reported sex for money or presents. 'If he wants a woman like me, a man must pay,' one said. 'Forget about marriage ... that was something for our mothers and grannies, it's not for us.'[66] Yet even young women eager to be *regte*, steady girlfriends with hope of marriage, were equally at risk of infection, for it commonly implied unprotected sex. In the mid 1990s one-third of South Africa's teenage women bore a child. Ten per cent of these women had HIV. By the age of 25, one-quarter would be infected.[67]

In its silent origins, its rapid expansion, its association with mobility, its exploitation of gender inequality, and its growing concentration among the poor, South Africa's epidemic was an extreme version of a continental pattern, much as Apartheid had been an extreme version of a wider colonial order. The epidemic that had begun two decades earlier close to the equatorial forest had culminated at the southern extremity of the continent. From that extremity the counter-attack would eventually begin.

6

The Penetration of the West

The penetration of HIV-1 from the equatorial region into West Africa differed markedly from its expansion to the east and south. Except in Côte d'Ivoire, it was more gradual and less complete, reaching in the early 2000s prevalences only one-fifth or one-sixth of the highest elsewhere. The reasons for this are unclear but probably include obstacles to overland mobility from east to west, the wider economic opportunities open to West African women in towns, widespread male circumcision, relatively low HSV-2 prevalences, and the barriers to infection presented by Islamic moral and marital patterns. Another difference, of less certain relevance, was that when the HIV-1 virus entered West Africa, it found HIV-2 already established.

As a human disease, HIV-2 was probably older than HIV-1. It was closely related to the simian immunodeficiency virus found in sooty mangabey monkeys (SIVsm) living only in the West African forest region between the Casamance River in Senegal and the Sassandra River in Côte d'Ivoire, which was also the endemic location of the human virus. HIV-2 shared some 70 per cent of its genome with SIVsm but only about 42 per cent with HIV-1. Indeed, some of the eight groups of HIV-2 known in 2004 were more like SIVsm than they were like one another. This was because SIVsm was very widespread and diverse (although completely harmless) in sooty mangabey monkeys and because each HIV-2 group was probably the result of a separate transmission from a monkey.[1] Of the eight groups, six had failed to establish themselves in human beings, having infected only seven known cases between them. Of the two more successful, group A was the more common throughout the coastal region west of Côte d'Ivoire, while group B was found chiefly in Côte d'Ivoire and Ghana, although scattered cases of both existed elsewhere.[2] A study using molecular clock techniques estimated that the most recent common ancestor of group A existed in 1940±16 and of group B in 1945±14.[3] Yet, given the high prevalence of SIV among sooty mangabeys, their close interaction with human beings, and the frequency of twentieth-century transmissions, similar transmissions had probably taken place in earlier centuries.

This was more likely with HIV-2 than HIV-1 because HIV-2 was a less virulent and visible disease in human beings, possibly because its progenitor was so fully adapted to monkeys. HIV-2 was about three times more difficult than HIV-1 to transmit through sexual intercourse and at least ten times more difficult to pass from mother to child.[4] Mortality from HIV-2 may have been only about one-third of that from HIV-1, for viral loads were generally lower, those infected were often older, and progression to Aids might take on average as much as 25 years, so that many of those infected never reached that stage, although if they did the final illness was similar.[5] Given that the opportunistic infections fatal to Aids patients were often those common to the local disease environment, it was understandable that HIV-2 passed unnoticed until 1985, when researchers investigating the existence of HIV-1 in Senegal discovered the other virus almost by chance.[6] This probably explains why HIV-1 and HIV-2 appear to have emerged virtually simultaneously: the appearance is an optical illusion.

Once the discovery was made, retrospective testing of the earliest stored blood for HIV-2 antibodies revealed an intriguing pattern.[7] Apart from one obscure reference to an alleged case in Mali in 1957, the earliest may have been a Portuguese man who had lived in Guinea-Bissau between 1956 and 1966. Other infections there during the 1960s are also recorded. Five cases were found in Côte d'Ivoire during the 1960s. Stored blood taken in 1967 also revealed two cases each in Nigeria and Gabon, both outside the range of sooty mangabeys and presumably infected through travel. They were followed in the 1970s by infections from Mali, Senegal, and Angola, the last probably transmitted through the movement of Portuguese troops from Guinea-Bissau. By the 1980s scattered cases were reported from many parts of western Africa, often from the countryside, suggesting a low-intensity disease much like HIV-1 in its pre-epidemic days in western equatorial Africa. In Guinea-Bissau, however, the liberation war of 1960–74, the presence of Portuguese troops, the movement of refugees, and perhaps especially the widespread use of injections by Portuguese military doctors appear to have bred a localised and probably unique epidemic.[8] Hospitals in Portugal later treated many cases contracted in Guinea-Bissau at this time. A study in Bissau town in the late 1990s showed that levels of infection peaked among men in their sixties and women in their fifties who would have been sexually most active during the 1960s. Prevalence there among men who had served in the Portuguese army was 23 per cent; among the nineteen women who had had sex with white men it was 37 per cent. This wartime legacy gave Guinea-Bissau much the highest prevalence of HIV-2. In the mid 1980s, 26 per cent of paid blood donors there tested positive, as did 8.6 per cent of Bissau's pregnant women and 36.7 per cent of its sex workers in 1987.[9] Ten years later HIV-2 infected 13.5 per cent of people over 35 living on the outskirts of the town. High levels were also reported in rural areas and spilled over (largely through migrant sex workers) to southern Senegal and The Gambia.[10] Yet the epidemic never spread beyond this region. That would presumably have required a virus more infectious than HIV-2.

HIV-1 was such a virus. Its arrival in West Africa (as distinct from western equatorial Africa) is difficult to trace but possibly took place in about 1980, slightly after its appearance in East and Central Africa. A claim to have

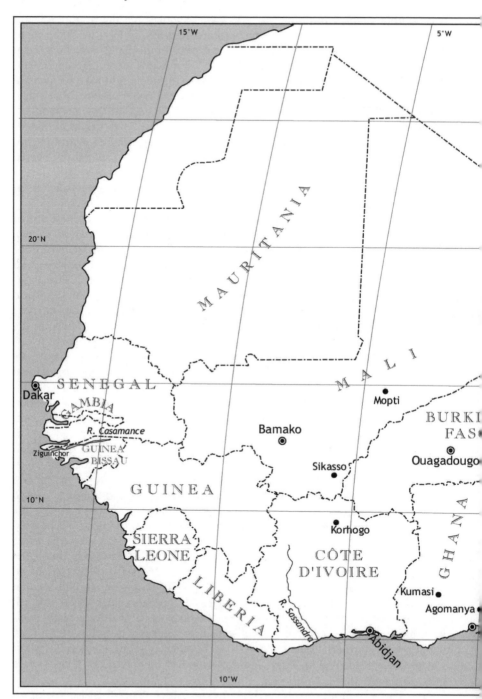

Map 4 *West Africa*

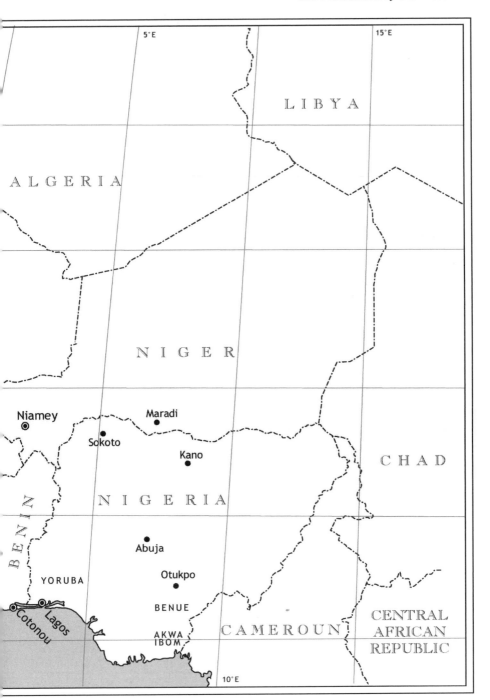

discovered one case in stored blood taken in Burkina in 1963 can almost certainly be dismissed. A Malian migrant who had never visited equatorial Africa died in Paris in 1983 with Aids-like symptoms, although this could as well have been HIV-2 as HIV-1. Ghanaian doctors came to believe that they had seen Aids cases as early as 1981, but no details are available and HIV-2 would again have been possible.[11] Otherwise, the earliest evidence comes from Côte d'Ivoire. Retrospective tests on stored blood taken there between 1970 and 1983 all proved negative. Adult mortality in Abidjan declined until 1985, the year when its first Aids cases were diagnosed, and then began to increase rapidly. In 1985, 38 of 79 sex workers were found to be infected there, together with 10 of 71 in the northern Ivoirian town of Korhogo. A year later HIV-1 prevalence was 3.0 per cent among pregnant women and 4.9 per cent among hospital staff in Abidjan. French researchers concluded that the first HIV infections there probably took place in about 1980.[12] Observers suggested at the time that the city's sex workers might have been infected by European tourists, but this is unlikely because the B subtype of HIV-1 prevalent in Europe did not become established in Abidjan or elsewhere in West Africa. Rather, the dominant strain came to be CRF02_AG, the circulating recombinant form rare in the DR Congo but common in Cameroun and Gabon, implying a northward diffusion comparable to the eastward diffusion of subtypes A and D into East Africa – a diffusion that in West Africa could have been carried in the first instance along the coast by sex workers and their clients moving between Libreville, Douala, and Abidjan. CRF02_AG became dominant among West Africa's coastal sex workers, throughout Côte d'Ivoire (where in the late 1990s it was responsible for over 90 per cent of HIV-1 infections), in southern Nigeria (causing 70 per cent of the entire country's infections), and in most coastal areas as far west as Senegal.[13] In some inland savanna regions, including northern Nigeria, another recombinant form, CRF06_cpx, was sometimes more common (cpx signifying a complex of more than two subtypes).[14]

There were several reasons why Abidjan and Côte d'Ivoire should have become the focus of West Africa's HIV-1 epidemic. Neglected until late in the colonial period but endowed with vast areas of virgin tropical forest, Côte d'Ivoire experienced rapid development during the first two decades of independence, with a 6.8 per cent annual growth rate of real Gross Domestic Product between 1965 and 1980.[15] Sparsely populated, its prosperity attracted immigrants both from economically faltering neighbours like Ghana and from the poorer savanna countries to the north. By the late 1980s some two million migrants from Burkina, over one million from Mali, and large numbers from Niger were present in Côte d'Ivoire at any time. Although many migrants worked in agriculture, over half lived in cities, especially in Abidjan, whose development as a major port increased its population between 1955 and 1984 from 120,000 to nearly 1,800,000. In 1975 some 40 per cent were non-Ivoirian immigrants. In older West African cities the control of retail trade by women fostered a rough equality of numbers between the sexes, but Abidjan, alone in West Africa, had the large male majority among adults that in East African cities like Nairobi led to highly commercialised sex, although in Abidjan it led also to more sophisticated forms of courtesanship, owing to the greater economic independence of women in West Africa and the region's less constrained sexual traditions.[16] Like Nairobi, Abidjan was a primate city on which the whole of Côte d'Ivoire's excellent transport system focused. And as Vinh-Kim Nguyen has shown,[17] two other features of Abidjan helped to make it an epicentre of HIV infection. One was an aspiration to modernity that bred individualistic choice, extreme differences of wealth, sexual adventurism – the median age of sexual debut was fifteen[18] – and complex, disassortative networks through which HIV could pass. In 1994, 51 per cent of Abidjan's men aged 20–24 said they had casual sex and 56 per cent never used a condom.[19] The other circumstance favouring an epidemic was the economic crisis that struck Côte d'Ivoire during the 1980s as the world economy faltered and the easy growth opportunities of the 1970s were exhausted. This bred unemployment, sexual commercialisation, weakened health services, and resort to Abidjan's 800 informal dispensaries 'that sprout like mushrooms after rain'.[20]

When HIV-1 prevalence was first measured in Abidjan in 1985, the city was on the verge of an epidemic more explosive than those in Kinshasa or even New York, with an annual incidence of new infections of over 3 per cent in 1989.[21] The core were the city's sex workers and their male clients. Between 1986 and 1993 HIV prevalence among sex workers rose from 38 to 86 per cent; at the latter date 50 per cent had HIV-1, 2 per cent HIV-2, and 34 per cent both. Studies showed that contact with sex workers was the chief risk factor for men, largely explaining why in 1988 men outnumbered women by nearly five to one among HIV-positive patients admitted to city hospitals and why 83 per cent of the 24,735 people estimated to have died of Aids-related diseases in the city between 1986 and 1992 were men. Deaths were most common among informal sector workers in the older working-class quarters.[22] By 1991, however, as the Minister of Health put it, the epidemic 'is in the process of passing from populations at risk to the general population,' as HIV-positive men infected their wives and other partners, creating a second peak of incidence. By 1993, the ratio of men to women infected had fallen to less than two to one.[23] Antenatal prevalence rose between 1986 and 1989 from 3.3 to 9 per cent. During the mid 1990s it fluctuated around 15 per cent. As in southern Africa, good transport and high levels of mobility ensured an unusually narrow difference between urban and rural prevalences. In 1994 an estimated 41 per cent of all West Africa's Aids cases were in Côte d'Ivoire.[24]

Abidjan was not only the place where HIV-1 and HIV-2 met, it was also the epicentre of infection for the entire eastern half of West Africa. This infection spread along two routes. One was the network of migrant sex workers who left their rural homes for a few years to work in the cities of neighbouring countries, seeking to bring home enough to set up a small business or finance their siblings' schooling, without revealing their occupation to their families or potential future husbands. Like sex workers everywhere in the continent, these women were invariably blamed for expanding the epidemic, although almost all must themselves have contracted the disease from infected men resident in the towns where they came to work. West African sex workers were extra-ordinarily mobile. Of those attending a clinic in Abidjan in 1992, 82 per cent were from Ghana, 9 per cent from Côte d'Ivoire, and 2 per cent from Nigeria, but by 1998 only 9 per cent were from Ghana, 29 per cent from Côte d'Ivoire, and 56 per cent from Nigeria. Recovery in the Ghanaian economy and recession in Côte d'Ivoire and Nigeria probably shared the explanation with numerous Aids deaths among Ghanaian women and violence towards the Ghanaian community in Abidjan following a soccer match in 1993.[25]

Ghana was the first country to which Abidjan's epidemic spread. Testing facilities became available there late in 1985 and were immediately deployed on sex workers. Of those tested in Accra early in 1986, only 5 of 236 were found HIV-positive, but when attention switched to women returning from Abidjan, 74 of 151 were found infected and many already gravely ill. At the end of 1987 the doctor in charge reported that Ghana had 276 known HIV cases, of whom 242 were women, 199 were sex workers returned from Côte d'Ivoire, and 145 came from Ghana's Eastern Region, where the patrilineal Krobo people allowed women no rights over land and young women had long been engaged in commercial sex. 'There is no work here,' a woman from the area explained at that time. 'In Abidjan I can earn 10,000 CFAs a day.... I have about 12 men a day. Since I heard about AIDS I always make them use condoms ... I don't know anyone who has it.'[26] Although Ghanaians habitually blamed HIV on these women, it was plainly an oversimplification, for they had been singled out for testing and their predominance among those with HIV demonstrated that they had seldom transmitted the virus, which many were probably too sick to do. Transmission was clearly more diffuse. Nevertheless, by 2001, as national adult prevalence hovered around 3 per cent, Eastern Region was still the most heavily infected area and commercial sex was still central to the epidemic. HIV prevalence in Accra at that time was 5.9 per cent among men who bought sex and 0.5 per cent among those who did not. Among men aged 15–19, 84 per cent of cases were attributable to commercial sex.[27]

This combination of relatively low general prevalence and high infection rates among mobile sex workers and their clients was widespread within the region of West Africa focused around Abidjan. In Benin, for example, HIV prevalence among pregnant women in Cotonou rose slowly from 0.4 per cent in 1990 to 3.4 per cent in 1997–8, while prevalence among the city's commercial sex workers rose from 3.3 per cent in 1986 to 58.0 per cent in 1997–8. It was calculated in the early 2000s that 76 per cent of male HIV infection in the city was contracted through commercial sex. Benin was unusual in that HIV prevalence in the general population was higher in some provinces than in the capital city, partly because commercial sex, a long-established practice there, was also widely dispersed, with a close correlation between infection in sex workers and in the general public.[28] The remarkable point, as in Ghana, was that high infection among commercial sex workers did not precipitate the explosive epidemic seen in Kigali, Nairobi, and Abidjan. One reason was probably the equal gender balance in West African cities other than Abidjan. Another was that condoms had come to be quite widely used in commercial sex: by 54 per cent of clients in Cotonou in 1997–8, so they claimed, and by 90 per cent in Accra in 2001. In Cotonou the age at first sex was relatively high and women in the general population reported few sexual partners. Most important, perhaps, were the two contrasts emphasised by a study in 1997–8 that compared Cotonou and Yaounde in western Africa with Kisumu and Ndola in the east: the high levels of male circumcision in West African cities (almost 100 per cent in Cotonou) and the relatively low levels of HSV-2 in the general population (12 per cent among men and 30 per cent among women in Cotonou).[29]

Away from the coast, in the savanna hinterland of Côte d'Ivoire, the network of commercial sex remained an important means for the diffusion of HIV, but it was supplemented by a second network of male migrant labour. The effects of migration were especially strong in Burkina, where Aids was often known as 'the Côte d'Ivoire disease', 'a disease of people who move around, who travel and cannot keep still', as an elder put it.[30] 'From Spring 1990 to Christmas 1992,' an anthropologist wrote of his village, 'a score of young-old migrants returned from Côte d'Ivoire, dreadfully bent, with their sticks, without bicycles or suitcases. They had simply come to die in Kampti and its environs.'[31] At first the national hospital in Ouagadougou admitted seven male cases for every female, but by October 1987 HIV prevalence among pregnant women in the city was 7.5 per cent and it appears to have hovered around that figure during the 1990s, although rising to 57 per cent among sex workers in 1994.[32]

Further north, in Niger and Mali, these patterns were repeated but at lower levels of disease and with larger proportions of locally born sex workers. In Niger, for example, 62 per cent of the first 40 Aids cases diagnosed at Niamey hospital were former migrants to the south; their risk factors were listed as 'prostitution, contact with prostitutes, blood transfusions and histories of visits to coastal countries'. Nearly three-quarters were men, a balance that shifted during the 1990s as infection spread more broadly, although still at relatively low levels. In 2003 adult prevalence was just over 1 per cent, but with 38 per cent among sex workers in Maradi.[33] Prevalence was somewhat higher in Mali, averaging 1.7 per cent in adults aged 15–49, according to a population survey in 2001, but with 30 per cent infection among sex workers and significant concentrations in Bamako and in towns like Sikasso and Mopti on migration routes to the south. Some 63 per cent of sex workers in Mali's four main towns at that time came from outside the country.[34] Low overall prevalence characterised other Sahelian regions like Mauritania and northern Chad, where, as in Sudan, levels of infection were higher in the south.[35]

The pattern suggests that the savanna region's Islamic social order may have limited the transmission of disease. In Niger, for example, a population survey in 2002 showed exceptionally low infection among young people, only about 0.3 per cent for men and 0.1 per cent for women. Women in this region married very young – a median age of sixteen in Mali – to men nine or ten years older. Often secluded, only 0.1 per cent of women in Niger reported more than one sexual partner in the last twelve months when surveyed in 1998. Most of the 11 per cent of men who reported paying for sex during that year were unmarried. Moreover, whereas women in West African coastal countries practised postpartum abstinence for 10–19 months, during which their husbands often sought other partners, in Mali and Niger the average was only

4–8 months.[36] The data suggest that in this Islamic region non-marital sex was to an unusual degree confined to commercial sex workers and young, unmarried, circumcised men, where it was least likely to spread infection to the general population. The same seems generally to have been true in North Africa, where, except in Sudan, official prevalence figures at age 15–49 were generally 0.1 per cent or less and about 100,000 people were thought to be infected in 2005. Although many of the earliest cases there were introduced from Europe by returning migrants, tourists, or injecting drug users, infection during the 1990s appears to have taken place mainly within indigenous but narrow sexual networks, both heterosexual and homosexual, with expansion into the general population confined by the Islamic marital and social order, although it was under increasing strain.[37]

The spread of HIV in Nigeria needs to be seen in this context. It was often described as a delayed epidemic, 'with a potential for rapid increase', but in fact it fitted logically into broader West African patterns. Nigeria experienced two infections by HIV-1, one in the south caused mainly by CRF02_AG and the other in the north caused by CRF06_cpx. Both revealed their first HIV cases in 1986, in sex workers, among whom and their partners much of the early proliferation took place.[38] In 1993 the first widespread sentinel survey showed prevalence of about 1.9 per cent among pregnant women. During the next six years it rose gradually to 5.4 per cent and the variation between different states widened, but those most affected were scattered broadly across the country. The highest prevalence (16.7 per cent in 1999) emerged in Benue state, in central Nigeria, where Aids was known as 'the Abuja disease'. 'No one suffers from this sickness in our village here,' it was said, 'but these women who go to Abuja [for commercial sex] suffer from it. They come home almost dead.' Of 40 people with Aids studied in that village, only one did not have a history of 'life abroad'. The next highest prevalence was 12.5 per cent in Akwa-Ibom state in the extreme south-east, where cross-border traffic coincided with great female independence and exceptionally high levels of commercial sex.[39]

Three reasons may help to explain why Nigeria did not suffer an explosive epidemic like that in Côte d'Ivoire. One was that Nigeria was too big and diverse, with many local epidemics but no primate city to transmit disease throughout the country. Rural prevalence was higher than urban in some states in the early 2000s. The second reason was that sex workers were mostly Nigerians and only marginally involved in the wider West African sex trade, at least until the later 1990s, so that even in 1994 only 13 per cent of sex workers in Lagos were infected. The third reason was the restraint imposed by the culture of the Muslim north, where women were commonly secluded and average HIV prevalence was significantly lower than in the centre and south-east.[40] It is more difficult to explain why prevalence was even lower in the south-west, where extra-marital sex had long been common among the Yoruba and had become increasingly so among the young in the course of the twentieth century, unless perhaps the very diffuseness of partnerships rather than their concentration around high-risk sex workers gave protection.[41] On the other hand, one factor encouraging the spread of disease was the mediocrity of Nigeria's health system, rated by the World Health Organisation as one of the worst in the world. In 1995 the Federal Ministry of Health estimated that 10 per cent of HIV transmission was by blood transfusion, a problem still unresolved ten years later.[42]

In 1995, also, Nigeria's health authorities estimated that at least 24 per cent of the country's HIV infections were by HIV-2, although the country lay well outside the range of the sooty mangabey.[43] The virus had probably entered Nigeria from the west at much the same time as HIV-1 was spreading from the east and south. Further west along the Guinea coast and in Senegambia, however, HIV-1 had to penetrate a region where HIV-2 was already endemic, if generally at low prevalence. The first search for HIV-1 in Senegal in 1985–6 chiefly revealed cases of HIV-2, both among sex workers in Dakar and especially in the southern Casamance region bordering the epicentre of the disease in Guinea-Bissau. Almost all were Senegalese who had never left the country, whereas the first HIV-1 cases identified were predominantly foreigners or Senegalese men who had travelled elsewhere in West or Equatorial Africa and often had histories of homosexuality or drug use. In 1990 Senegal's national prevalence of HIV-2 was reckoned to be nine times that of HIV-1, but the greater virulence of the latter enabled it to overtake HIV-2 in 1996–7. By 2004 HIV-1 in Senegal was sixteen times more prevalent than HIV-2, which was of equal importance only in the Ziguinchor region on the Guinea-Bissau border.[44] During the 1990s this reversal took place everywhere in the western coastal region except Guinea-Bissau, where the differential between the two infections narrowed but did not close, chiefly because of continuing (although declining) high levels of HIV-2 infection among older women.

Senegal gained international renown by limiting its national HIV prevalence at age 15–49 to little more than 1 per cent. Much of its infection was concentrated among the Jola people close to the southern border with Guinea-Bissau, where prevalence was two or three times the national average.[45] Young, infected Jola migrants began to return from Côte d'Ivoire during the late 1980s to die at home. Like the Yoruba and many other young people throughout the continent, they had during the twentieth century adopted risky patterns of pre-marital sex in response to the commercialisation of the economy, the need to migrate for urban employment, the declining status of women consequent on the spread of Islam, the increasing difficulty of marriage, the collapse of customary sexual restraints, the spread of sexually transmitted diseases, the marginalisation of the region within independent Senegal, the destructive impact of structural adjustment policies, and their continuing anxiety to bear children at the peak of fertility.[46] Elsewhere in Senegal, however, Muslim culture provided greater protection. There the median age of sexual debut was high, at about 19 years for both sexes during the late 1990s, levels of non-marital sex were low outside the capital, and condoms were quite widely used with casual partners. The government's important part in containing disease will be considered later, but Senegal's experience, like Nigeria's, fitted closely into the wider patterns of West Africa, where the great regional variations in HIV prevalence witnessed to an epidemic that had penetrated but not conquered.[47]

7
Causation:
A Synthesis

The HIV-1 epidemic that Kapita Bila had first glimpsed in Kinshasa in the mid-1970s had taken almost exactly ten years to spread and become visible among the African peoples at the three corners of the continent, appearing in Ethiopia, South Africa, and Senegal almost simultaneously in the mid-1980s. Having traced that expansion, it is time to return to President Mbeki's question: why has Africa had the world's most terrible HIV/Aids epidemic? An answer must bring together the nature of the virus, the historical sequence of its global expansion, and the circumstances into which it spread, giving particular weight among those circumstances to gender inequalities, sexual behaviour, and impoverishment. Many existing answers perhaps concentrate too exclusively on the circumstances, arguing for the primary importance of either sexual behaviour or poverty.[1]

The distinctive features of HIV as a virus were that it was relatively difficult to transmit, it killed almost all those it infected (unless kept alive by antiretroviral drugs), it killed them slowly after a long incubation period, it remained infectious throughout its course, it showed few symptoms until its later stages, and when symptoms appeared they were often those common to the local disease environment. This unique combination of features gave a unique character to the epidemic, 'a catastrophe in slow motion'[2] spreading silently for many years before anyone recognised its existence. One consequence was that whatever part of the world had the first such epidemic would suffer especially severely, for the epidemic would have time to establish itself, unseen, not only in many people over a large area but in the general heterosexual population, where it would be vastly more difficult to contain than in some limited high-risk group contracting the disease through the initial infection of individuals whose distinctive behaviour patterns had brought them into contact with it.

Thus the fundamental reason why Africa had the worst Aids epidemic was because it had the first Aids epidemic. Understandably, many Africans were initially unwilling to accept this, rejecting the notion that HIV evolved from SIV within Africa, despite the powerful evidence for it, because they felt that it was a racial slur – as indeed some commentators intended it to be. To deny the origin of the disease, however, was to deny oneself an understanding of the particular tragedy that had struck the continent.

One way of grasping the uniqueness of HIV/Aids is to contrast it with earlier epidemics in African history. These were of three types.[3] The most common were highly infectious diseases that swept briefly through large populations, swiftly killing susceptible people before burning out and becoming quiescent until the next epidemic. Smallpox, an ancient African disease, was of this type, as were cholera, an Asian disease that spread to Africa in several nineteenth-century epidemics, and the great influenza pandemic of 1918 – 'three-day flu', as it was known in South Africa – that killed between two and five per cent of the population in most parts of Africa. All these epidemics clearly differed from HIV/Aids in their greater infectiousness, their short incubation period, the speed with which they killed, and their brief but dramatic impact, which provoked equally dramatic human responses. Somewhat different were diseases with endemic reservoirs in African animals, from which they were transmitted to human beings by insect vectors, sometimes in epidemic proportions. This was true of plague, which especially infected North Africa from the fourteenth-century Black Death to the nineteenth century; malaria and yellow fever, both mosquito-borne diseases that became epidemic in specific natural conditions; and sleeping sickness, an endemic disease of wild game transmitted to human beings in epidemic form by tsetse flies as a result of disturbance of the natural environment during the early colonial period. HIV, too, had its natural reservoir, but was far more difficult to transmit as a human disease, was not carried by an insect vector, and consequently, once established in humans, was independent of the natural environment and free to spread throughout the continent. In that respect, HIV/Aids was more like two other diseases that also began as epidemics but became endemic, venereal syphilis and tuberculosis, both diseases of uncertain history that probably became widespread in inland regions of Africa only during the late nineteenth and twentieth centuries. They differed from HIV, however, in that they were easier to transmit, had more visible symptoms once established, but were less often fatal.

These contrasts demonstrate the distinctiveness of HIV/Aids as a disease, which shaped not only the progress of the epidemic but also, as will be seen, the ways in which Africans understood and reacted to it. Yet the comparison also reveals one common factor of all these epidemics (except perhaps plague once it was established in North Africa): that epidemics are intimately related to mobility, whether the clustering together of people in drought or famine that so often caused smallpox outbreaks, the human disturbance of the natural environment that precipitated epidemic sleeping sickness, the movement of returning soldiers along shipping lanes and railway lines that spread the great influenza, or the migration routes along which southern African mineworkers carried tuberculosis to their rural homes. In this respect the HIV epidemic was fully in the pattern of past epidemics.

A contrast with earlier African epidemics demonstrates the importance of HIV's distinctiveness as a virus. A contrast with other HIV epidemics demonstrates why it was so important for Africa that it had the first. During the

1990s it became clear that the epidemics that had begun in the United States and Europe during the late 1970s were unlikely to reach African dimensions. Once imported, both had taken root first among homosexuals and injecting drug users (IDUs), partly self-segregated groups quickly targeted by health services and bearing a stigma that helped to sensitise the general population to the danger of contracting HIV. The North American epidemic did spread among heterosexuals from poor urban minority groups, but they too were significantly differentiated from the bulk of the population, and in the meantime antiretroviral drugs had become available.[4] Latin American epidemics generally fell into the same pattern.[5] Greater international concern centred on the possibility that infections in Asia or Eastern Europe might expand into generalised heterosexual epidemics of the African type. All these, however, had begun among restricted groups of IDUs, homosexuals, commercial sex workers, or their clients. In Thailand and Kampuchea, early areas of concern, it proved possible to contain epidemics by targeting these groups, much as South Africa largely contained its initial epidemic among white homosexuals.[6] India, China, and Russia were seen as the danger points for a 'second wave' of HIV,[7] but sceptics pointed out that few antenatal clinics outside Africa (and Haiti) showed HIV prevalence of more than 1 per cent and that in Asia, at least, casual and intergenerational sex concentrated almost entirely on institutionalised commercial sex workers who could be targeted.[8] The important point, it was agreed, was for governments to intervene at the earliest stage of an epidemic.[9] This was the opportunity that Africa had not enjoyed.

Thus the origin and nature of the virus primarily determined the character of the African epidemic. But it was shaped also by the multitude of circumstances in which it took place, many of them with roots far back in the past. No one of these was decisive; all must be incorporated into an explanation. The most fundamental was the demographic context.[10] Before the twentieth century, Africa's hostile disease environment, harsh physical and climatic conditions, and history of exploitation had made it an underpopulated continent. During the twentieth century medical and other innovations had removed many of these constraints and population had grown at increasing pace, perhaps multiplying six or seven times in the course of the century. Growth peaked in the 1980s, when the population of sub-Saharan Africa grew at about 3.1 per cent per year, almost certainly the fastest natural increase over a long period for any large population in human history. It cannot have been entirely coincidental that HIV became epidemic at exactly the moment when demographic growth reached its peak. One long-term connection was the pressure that lay behind the penetration of the forest, exposing human beings to animal diseases of which SIV was only one. More immediately, population growth drove Africa's massive late-twentieth-century urbanisation – at about 5 per cent per year during the 1980s[11] – which created cities like Kinshasa and Abidjan, where networks of partner exchange were wide enough to raise HIV to epidemic levels. Later, in the 1990s, emerging areas of rural overpopulation and poverty, such as Malawi, would provide conditions for especially devastating epidemic impact. In both town and country, rapid demographic growth swelled in particular the numbers of young people who were especially vulnerable to HIV. In the mid 1990s, for example, one-third of all Tanzanians were aged between 10 and 24.[12] One reason why HIV spread more widely in Africa than elsewhere was this preponderance of young people.

The epidemic also came at a particular moment in Africa's medical history. The leading historian of HIV/Aids, Mirko Grmek, suggested that the epidemic was, paradoxically, in part a consequence of medical advance: that until medicine had reduced the prevalence of other infectious diseases such as tuberculosis and smallpox, death rates were too high to allow HIV to establish itself in sufficient numbers of people to reach epidemic proportions.[13] There is no obvious way to test this intriguing suggestion, which perhaps exaggerates the extent of medical advance in sub-Saharan Africa, where in the early 1990s communicable diseases still caused 71 per cent of morbidity.[14] Nevertheless, it is both true and disturbing that the epidemic followed immediately on the period of greatest medical improvement in the continent's history. Between 1965 and 1988, life expectancy at birth in sub-Saharan Africa rose from 45 to 51 years. Over the same period the ratio of doctors to population increased by about 50 per cent and the ratio of nurses to population more than doubled.[15] In 1974 the World Health Organisation launched its Expanded Programme on Immunisation, in 1977 it completed the eradication of smallpox, and in 1978 it adopted a global strategy of primary health care. Some have suggested that smallpox vaccination or polio immunisation may have spread HIV. Neither is likely, but it is possible that massive use of injections may have contributed to the HIV-2 epidemic in Guinea-Bissau and helped to adapt HIV-1 to human hosts, while blood transfusion was a significant factor in transmitting the virus early in the epidemic. On the other hand, medical advance – especially prior research into viral cancer – enabled scientists to identify HIV and its natural history with extraordinary speed and precision once the epidemic attracted attention. Had it occurred twenty years earlier, the response, as one specialist put it, might have been mere 'thrashing about'.[16]

In Grmek's analysis, the technology that identified HIV was, ironically, part of the same technology that enabled it to flourish.[17] He had in mind especially the advances in transport and human mobility that carried HIV to all parts of the African continent and the world. As with influenza and tuberculosis, mobile people spread HIV along their networks of communication and gave the epidemic the shape of the commercial economy, whether they were migrants taking the disease to rural Karonga, fishermen spreading it around the shores of Lake Victoria, long-distance drivers infecting Beitbridge and Berberati, or sex workers and labourers carrying the virus from Abidjan to savanna towns and villages. Everywhere infection concentrated along motor roads, which were especially central in Africa because its transport system largely postdated the age of railway building. Some have argued that HIV/Aids could not have become an epidemic disease before the existence of widespread motor transport, but that seems doubtful, for many diseases with shorter incubation periods spread their infection across continents in pre-modern times. Yet the high infection levels in Côte d'Ivoire and the association between oscillating migration and rural prevalence in Central Africa can leave no doubt of the importance of migrant labour and the regional inequalities underlying it in fuelling the epidemic.

Gender inequalities and sexual behaviour are among the most important and controversial of the circumstances shaping the epidemic. Early observers often attributed the scale of infection in Africa to high levels of sexual promiscuity. A survey in 1989–90 in eight mainland African states and three Asian countries (including Sri Lanka and Thailand) questioned this and suggested a more complicated situation.[18] It found that most African men had had sex during the previous year only with their regular partner and that only small percentages had had five or more casual partners. 'Non-marital sex,' the enquiry concluded, 'is a relatively rare event for a majority of men and women.'[19] The survey also showed that the difference in each country between rural and urban sexual behaviour was relatively small; a more important distinction may have been that urban sexual networks were wider. On the other hand, when compared with Sri Lanka, a country of severe restraint, African sexual behaviour was less inhibited; men and women began sex earlier, married earlier, had wider age differentials between husband and wife, and more often had pre-marital, casual, and commercial sex, a pattern that anthropologists attributed to the absence in Africa of the land scarcity that led Asian families to guard their women jealously, to Africa's polygynous traditions that encouraged men to seek multiple partners without linking sexual partnership to age,[20] and to the twentieth-century social changes – especially longer intervals between sexual debut and marriage – that encouraged pre-marital sex in areas as diverse as Kinshasa, Bangui, Kampala, Botswana, Soweto, Yorubaland, and southern Senegal.

When the survey compared African sexual behaviour with that in Thailand, however, a more complex picture emerged. Thailand shared Sri Lanka's restrictive sexual attitude towards most women but not towards men, so that Thai men were as sexually active as African men but concentrated their non-marital sex almost entirely on commercial sex workers. As has been seen, this was true in only a minority of African areas: in Rwanda, Burundi, urban Ethiopia and Senegal, and to some degree in cities with large male majorities like Nairobi. Moreover, Africa's entrepreneurial sex workers seldom worked in brothels, which made them more difficult to target with preventive measures than their counterparts in Thailand and elsewhere in Asia.

Four additional circumstances created opportunities for HIV infection in Africa. One was the widespread prevalence of sexually transmitted diseases, especially the global epidemic of HSV-2 that by the early 2000s doubled the risk of HIV infection for 70 per cent or more of the population in many regions.[21] Another – still unproven but strongly suspected – was the lack of male circumcision in large parts of eastern and southern Africa that helped to explain especially high HIV prevalence there.[22] The third, with a similar regional impact, was the lack of economic opportunities for women, especially in eastern and southern cities, which weakened their ability to protect themselves against infection. Added to that, a fourth circumstance was the frequent disparity of age between partners, resulting both from female poverty and polygynous traditions, which was of central importance in transmitting disease between age groups.[23] Ironically, a major feature of precolonial African societies, the rarity of endogenous social strata, made them especially vulnerable to HIV.[24] Thus although African sexual behaviour was far from the generalised promiscuity of Western myth, it contributed in important ways to the scale of the epidemic. The best proof of this would be the role that behavioural change would later play in reducing infection.

Poverty was the other major circumstance shaping the epidemic, but again its impact was far from simple. HIV/Aids was not in any sense a 'quintessential disease of poverty'.[25] Africa did not have a more terrible epidemic than India because it was poorer but because it was infected first. At the national level, HIV did not target the poorest countries, as high prevalence in Botswana and other parts of southern Africa demonstrated. At the social level, the most striking point was the wide range of people infected. 'HIV affects ordinary people,' wrote Noerine Kaleeba, founder of The Aids Support Organisation in Uganda. 'It does not only affect "the poor". It does not only affect "the affluent". It affects a cross-section of people.'[26] One indication of this was that blame for the epidemic was seldom allocated on grounds of economic class. The pattern seen in Karonga, where infection was associated with mobility, education, and off-farm employment, was common early in the epidemic, but not universal. At Kabarole in western Uganda in 1991–3, for example, people aged 15–24 with secondary schooling were more than twice as likely to be infected than the uneducated, but the first attempt in Masaka to relate infection to categories of wealth, measured by household property ownership, found that 'both male and female heads of the poorest households were most likely to be HIV positive'.[27]

A nuanced picture emerged from the most careful study, in Kisumu in western Kenya in 1996, using a composite index of education, occupation, and household possessions to define socio-economic status. It found that among men over 25 there was no association between this status and HIV prevalence, among men aged 15–24 and women over 25 higher socio-economic status was associated with somewhat higher HIV prevalence, but among women aged 15–24 prevalence was highest among those with low socio-economic status. The poorer women had wider age differentials from their husbands, were less likely to use condoms, and had higher rates of HSV-2.[28] Poverty, it appeared, did not give birth to HIV, but it was an effective incubator.

South Africa's population survey of 2002 found a strong concentration of the disease in informal urban locations but no statistically significant association between infection and household poverty, suggesting that social environment was more important than mere income.[29] One connection was probably the prevalence of other sexually transmitted diseases, as in Kisumu. A second was the greater poverty of women. Others may have been malnutrition and parasite infestation that increased susceptibility to disease and the likelihood of perinatal transmission, although research in this field was still at an early stage.[30] More visible were the effects of poverty in making progress from Aids to death so much faster in Africa than in developed countries, owing to greater exposure to opportunistic infections and less access to medical remedies – especially, after 1996, to antiretroviral drugs.[31] Most visible and distressing of all was that poverty accentuated the suffering of Aids patients bereft of the most elementary palliative care.

This was the point where Africa's poverty added so greatly to the scale of the epidemic. After significant economic growth and medical advance in most regions for thirty years after the Second World War, the global depression of the late 1970s that reversed Africa's fortunes coincided exactly with the transformation of HIV into an epidemic disease. The depression exposed African regimes that were over-extended, over-staffed, and over-borrowed. Between 1965 and 1980 sub-Saharan Africa's real Gross Domestic Product had grown at 4.2 per cent a year; between 1980 and 1990 it grew at only 2.1 per cent a year, or only two-thirds of the rate of population growth.[32] During the 1980s per capita health spending more than halved in the poorest countries.[33] Heavily indebted regimes seeking international support had to accept structural adjustment programmes demanding still further economy on services, including user fees at medical institutions that did less to raise money than to deter the poor from using them. In Zambia utilisation of urban health centres fell by 80 per cent.[34] Instead patients turned to indigenous healers, while biomedical doctors and their wealthier patients retreated to private practice. This was the context within which Africans and their governments faced the first and worst of HIV epidemics.

8
Responses from Above

Although it is unlikely that the world's first HIV epidemic in a general heterosexual population could have been prevented from causing terrible suffering, it is also true that the measures taken by national and international authorities during the 1980s and 1990s were generally considered inadequate. Most African governments were slow to grasp the scale of the crisis, because many were weak regimes faced with more immediate problems, the crisis was itself so novel, and they perceived a threat to the national dignity that they had so recently asserted. Consequently, the first epidemic did not produce the first response. When African regimes did eventually react, they found that the Western powers dominating international affairs had already defined strategies designed to tackle their own less threatening epidemics. These strategies, propagated by the World Health Organisation in one of the most striking modern examples of globalisation, proved less effective in Africa. Whether any other strategy could have been more effective, especially in the earlier stages of the epidemic, remains uncertain.

The Western strategy was designed to counter epidemics in stigmatised but articulate minorities of homosexuals and injecting drug users. The crux was to avoid demonising and isolating these minorities, win their voluntary cooperation, persuade them individually to abandon high-risk behaviour, collaborate with them in caring for the infected, and educate the wider public to avoid infection. HIV was not to be treated like the epidemic diseases of the past, which Western societies had not experienced for sixty years, but like the dominant degenerative diseases of the time, such as cancer. This strategy fitted smoothly into the liberal, doctor-dominated health and sexual policies of Britain and France.[1] It worked less smoothly in the United States, where doctors had less control over public policy, the Reagan administration did not conceal its distaste for deviant minorities, and militant homosexual groups defended their interests in the name of human rights.[2] The effect, however, was largely the same: by 1986–7 Western Aids policies were firmly voluntaristic and sensitive to the rights of the individual patient, with a relative unconcern for the protection of the uninfected because infection was concentrated among

65

minorities and easy to avoid. In Africa a balance between individual freedom and the public good had to be sought in quite different circumstances.

One circumstance was that Africa in the 1980s still had both vivid memories of past epidemics and major current infections to control. Mass immunisation against measles, polio, and other infectious diseases was the chief medical preoccupation of the decade. The last smallpox case had occurred in 1977. A new strain of cholera was spreading across the continent, causing over 5,000 deaths in Tanzania alone.[3] Most countries still had leprosy programmes and many had handicapped former patients begging in the streets; in 1972–3 the President of Mali had ordered the removal of this 'human garbage' from his capital.[4] Four years later the first Ebola epidemics terrified even experienced health workers. The likelihood that HIV would meet stigma and repression was therefore strong. Hospital staff often isolated and neglected the first Aids patients as if their mere proximity was infectious. Staff at Baragwanath Hospital in Soweto burned the first patients' clothes, attended them in gowns, masks, and theatre boots, and refused to open body bags to enable relatives to identify corpses. 'I wouldn't touch him if I were you,' a nurse at Mulago Hospital in Kampala warned. 'He has AIDS. We don't touch him, we only show his mother what to do.'[5] Early in the epidemic there were many demands for the sterilisation of those infected.[6] One HIV-positive woman addressing a meeting of chiefs in Botswana 'was asked why the government "hadn't responded to AIDS with the same commitment that it had to the foot and mouth epidemic?" That is by quickly slaughtering all the infected cattle to prevent further infections.'[7] Nearly 80 per cent of surveyed women in Botswana and Zimbabwe in 1988 wanted people with HIV/Aids to be quarantined. A year later President Moi of Kenya is reported to have ordered this, but his instructions were 'quietly ignored'.[8] Although quarantine might be effective in an island like Cuba, it would have been utterly impracticable in Africa by the time the disease was recognised. In practice, organised discrimination was rare, despite popular demands. One reason was the good sense of the senior doctors who controlled medical policy in most African states, men such as Aaron Chiduo, Tanzania's Minister of Health, who insisted that 'Law can never succeed to control the disease. We must concentrate on persuasion.'[9] Another reason was probably that governments lacked the capacity to implement large-scale discrimination.

Most African regimes sought rather to distance themselves and their countries from the epidemic. The suggestion that HIV had originated from African monkeys was regarded as a particularly insulting form of racism by nationalist politicians and many African physicians. Even Samuel Okware, Uganda's cool-minded epidemiologist, rejoiced when in 1987 'We managed to out-argue the theories about the Monkey origin' and oblige the WHO, for the sake of harmony, to describe Aids as 'caused by one or more naturally occurring retroviruses of undetermined origin'.[10] For political leaders, moreover, HIV/Aids was a profoundly distasteful subject to mention in public. It questioned their competence because they had no remedy, it threatened to raise demands for assistance that they could not afford to give, it distracted them from more pressing anxieties, it was potentially divisive, its victims had as yet no political voice, and it might damage their country's image and tourist industry, as it had already damaged Haiti's.[11] Public denial was therefore the norm. Mobutu silenced the Congolese press for four years after the first announcement of the epidemic's presence. Kapita Bila narrowly escaped imprisonment after addressing an Aids conference without official permission.[12] Zimbabwe's doctors were initially instructed not to mention Aids on death certificates. Senior figures like Houphouët-Boigny in Côte d'Ivoire, Hastings Banda in Malawi, and Moi in Kenya ignored the subject entirely or denounced the Western press for 'a new form of hate campaign'.[13] Even Nelson Mandela, after a bold speech in 1991 had angered a rural audience, retreated into silence during his presidency, later explaining that in the 1994 election 'I wanted to win and I didn't talk about AIDS' and then 'had not time to concentrate on the issue' while President.[14] The most positive responses came from Museveni in Uganda and Abdou Diouf in Senegal, two young and highly intelligent leaders with the backing of skilled medical advisers. 'To not be open about AIDS is just ignorant,' Museveni told a journalist. 'This is an epidemic. You can only stop it by talking about it – loudly, so that everybody is aware and scared, and they stop the type of behaviour that encourages the spread of the disease.'[15]

Initial pressure for action came chiefly from senior doctors. In January 1983 South Africa's Department of Health responded to the first homosexual deaths by appointing working groups to trace contacts, conduct tests, and survey those at risk, adding a more formal Advisory Group on Aids early in 1985. During 1984 Kinshasa's Ministry of Health collaborated in Projet Sida, while Brazzaville's doctors spent nearly two years pressing their government to abandon its insistence on secrecy until in December 1985 it finally set up a national committee charged to organise blood screening, data collection, prevention, diagnosis, and care. In Cameroun, similarly, doctors at the University Hospital took the lead in forming a national committee, although with slender resources.[16] Zimbabwe was the first Third World country to adopt a policy of screening all blood before transfusion, in July 1985. At the same moment the staff at the University Teaching Hospital in Lusaka reported growing numbers of Aids cases to the chief medical officer, who promptly ordered a press blackout, a national surveillance campaign, and acquisition of blood-testing equipment. The lead in eastern Africa fell to Rwanda, where the investigation in 1983–4 stimulated an awareness campaign and blood-screening in l985, followed by a national committee and epidemiological survey in 1986.[17] Tanzania, Kenya, and Ethiopia all formed national Aids committees during 1985, Ethiopia even before an Aids case had been reported. In Uganda, where evidence of an epidemic had existed since 1982–3, civil war and the chaotic state of the Ministry of Health prevented action until Museveni's National Resistance Army took Kampala in January 1986, when officials briefed the new minister and a committee headed by Okware began to organise public education, condom supply, and blood screening. Museveni threw his weight behind the programme in September 1986, apparently alarmed especially by the prevalence of infection in the army. Since his Health Ministry's budget, in real terms, had fallen by 93 per cent since 1970, Uganda sought aid from the World Health Organisation.[18]

The WHO had been slow to respond to the HIV epidemic. Created at the end of the Second World War to coordinate international health measures and advise member governments, it had come to concentrate its limited resources on preventive medicine in Third World countries. HIV/Aids, by contrast, 'is being very well taken care of by some of the richest countries in the world ... where most of the patients are to be found,' as a WHO memorandum stated in 1983.[19] Its first meeting on the subject in November 1983, although attended by Kapita Bila, listed the chief priorities as safeguarding blood supplies and alerting homosexuals. WHO's priority for the Third World at this time was primary health care, launched in 1978 with the passionate commitment of the Danish Director-General, Halfdan Mahler, who dismissed HIV/Aids in September 1985 as a dangerous diversion:

> Dr Halfdan Mahler said in Lusaka yesterday that if African countries continued to make AIDS a 'front-page' issue, the objectives of health for all programmes by the year 2000 would be lost....
>
> 'AIDS is not spreading like a bush fire in Africa. It is malaria and other tropical diseases that are killing millions of children every day,' he said....
>
> However, Dr Mahler said he expected the WHO with the help of other governments and non-governmental agencies to mobilise resources and draw up a strategy to fight the syndrome.[20]

This belief that HIV/Aids obscured Africa's real health problems was to survive vigorously into the next century. Yet even before Mahler spoke, the first Aids Conferences in Atlanta and Brussels in 1985 had given global publicity to the heterosexual epidemic, hearing alarming (and sometimes unreliable) reports of prevalence in several parts of Africa.[21] In January 1986 WHO's Executive Board recognised HIV/Aids as 'becoming a major public health concern' and urged the Director-General to 'cooperate with Member States in the development of national programmes'. Two months later a meeting of the organisation's African members in Brazzaville recommended each state to create a national Aids committee, conduct an epidemiological assessment, establish a surveillance system, expand its laboratory facilities, and launch a public education programme. In May 1986 the annual World Health Assembly urged the creation of an organisation to coordinate WHO assistance. As African countries like Uganda increasingly sought aid, Mahler established a Special (later, Global) Programme on Aids headed by the American director of Projet Sida, Jonathan Mann.[22]

Mann was the most important figure in the history of the Aids epidemic. Aged 39 and trained in public health, he brought into the Global Programme the American Aids activists' hatred of discrimination, driving administrative ability, impatience of WHO bureaucracy, experience of suffering in the wards at Mama Yemo, and an idealism that entranced international audiences.[23] 'The danger of AIDS brings with it an historic opportunity,' he told a conference in 1988, '... through AIDS and our common fight we are led onwards, irresistibly, towards a new vision of the possible – a new paradigm of health – expressing a universal message out of the special circumstances and insights of our time.'[24] In four years he raised the Global Programme's annual budget from less than one million to over one hundred million dollars.

The programme had four initial priorities. The most urgent was to screen blood supplies in poor countries so that medical systems no longer created new infections. This was expensive – in the early 1990s it absorbed about half the anti-Aids budgets of several African countries – and never fully effective: in 2004 the WHO estimated that transfusions might still cause 5–10 per cent of worldwide transmissions, or 700–1,400 a day.[25] The second priority was to train medical staff, first in the clinical management of Aids and then in the counselling of those tested for HIV. The third objective was public education, which, in the absence of a vaccine or cure, was the only means available to check the epidemic. Mann insisted on its efficacy:

> We have had proof of it in many regions of the world … that when one informs and educates individuals in a language that they understand and in a manner appropriate to their needs, when sanitary and social services exist, and when the social climate is favourable and not discriminatory, then information and education can effectively bring about a modification of behaviour.[26]

To prevent discrimination was the fourth and, for Mann himself, probably the most important element in the Global Programme. Against the many who urged the compulsory testing of job applicants, hospital patients, and international travellers, or the isolation of those found HIV-positive, he insisted passionately that this would not only breach their human rights but would deter people from seeking medical care, endanger the healthy, and accelerate the epidemic:

> The public health rationale for preventing discrimination against HIV-infected persons is cogent and practical. If HIV infection, or suspicion of HIV infection, leads to stigmatisation and discrimination – such as loss of employment or forced separation from family – then those already HIV-infected and those who are concerned they might be infected will take steps to avoid detection and will avoid contact with health and social services. Those most needing information, education, counselling or other support services would be driven away and this would seriously jeopardise efforts to prevent HIV infections. Stigmatisation and discrimination – these are threats to public health.[27]

This logic convinced the WHO. In 1992 its World Health Assembly resolved 'that there is no public health rationale for any measures that limit the rights of the individual, notably measures establishing mandatory screening'. Mann saw this as his greatest achievement. 'For the first time in history,' he wrote, 'preventing discrimination against infected people became an integral part of a strategy to control an epidemic of infectious disease.'[28]

Whether Mann was right is one of the most important questions about the African Aids epidemic. For it can be argued against him that his strategy did not work; the epidemic spread despite or even because of it; the principles were unrealistic; his human rights were in reality the rights only of patients with no concern for the rights of others; the emphasis on individual rights propounded by America's homosexual minority was irrelevant to a mass heterosexual epidemic; and no Western government faced with an epidemic on the African scale would have dreamed of maintaining such a policy. Mann's strategy, in fact, could be seen – and later in the epidemic sometimes was seen – as an example of intellectual imperialism, of globalisation at its most arrogant.[29] Yet that was later in the epidemic, when treatment was available to attract the infected to seek medical care and when familiarity with the disease had somewhat reduced the stigma surrounding it. Mann, earlier in the epidemic, pointed to opinion surveys showing wide support for discrimination and clearly feared its potential cruelty.[30] His strategy may have restricted that cruelty while the danger was greatest.

From 1986 to 1990 Mann's Global Programme ruled. Because the WHO could intervene in a member country's medical affairs only at its request, states were encouraged to invite WHO assistance in devising short-term plans to control HIV/Aids while medium-term plans were prepared. By June 1988, 151 countries had sought WHO assistance – usually in the form of two or three expatriate public health experts – and 106 had formulated short-term plans. As Mann justifiably declared, 'There is simply no precedent in the history of global health for the speed, intensity, or scope of this global mobilisation against AIDS.'[31] The plans generally provided for a national Aids committee with a small executive staff within the Ministry of Health, equipment to screen blood before transfusion and test potential patients, laboratory support, a programme of staff training and public education, a preliminary assessment of HIV prevalence, measures to outlaw discrimination, a WHO grant to cover the six to eighteen months of the plan, arrangements to draft a medium-term programme covering three to five years, and WHO support for a donors' conference to mobilise funds for that programme. All these activities were supposed to operate through the field agents of the existing primary health care system, rather than creating a new vertical structure.[32]

The first medium-term plans, mostly covering the late 1980s and early 1990s, provided for more representative national Aids councils, introduced sentinel surveillance of HIV prevalence to be measured when taking blood specimens from women at antenatal clinics, and targeted the high-risk groups who at this time were seen as the main drivers of the epidemic. For the last of these strategies the model was the programme in Nairobi providing STD treatment and free condoms for commercial sex workers, which gained their warm support, reduced the annual incidence of new infections among them from 47 per cent in 1986–7 to 7 per cent in 1991–2, and was claimed to prevent between 6,000 and 10,000 HIV cases each year.[33] Similar campaigns followed in Kinshasa, Abidjan, Bulawayo, Cotonou, and other cities, although this approach proved less effective in Africa than in Asia because extra-marital sex in Africa was less concentrated on sex workers, who were themselves individualistic and unorganised. There was less attention at this stage to their male clients, although several programmes targeted mobile groups like truck drivers. Mass distribution of condoms, often financed by USAID and supplied through social marketing techniques, was another common feature of medium-term plans. Between 1990 and 1998 the number supplied to sub-Saharan Africa by this means rose from 18 million to 236 million.[34]

Medium-term plans paid less attention to STD treatment, although some outside observers thought it the most effective means of controlling HIV.

The most successful of these early Aids programmes were in Senegal and Uganda. Senegal was arguably the only country in sub-Saharan Africa to prevent a generalised HIV/Aids epidemic, its adult prevalence never rising much above 1 per cent. One of its advantages was that initial infection was with the less virulent HIV-2, while the first HIV-1 case was not observed until 1986. An unusually effective STD programme operating since 1978 offered a model for action against HIV. Licensing and inspection of sex workers, inherited from the French, provided greater control than existed elsewhere in sub-Saharan Africa. Male circumcision was universal. Sexual activity was restrained in the countryside by Islamic morality and in towns by widespread condom use with casual partners. With President Diouf's support, Senegal's doctors were especially quick to institute control of the blood supply, mount public education, mobilise community leaders, and encourage non-governmental organisations. Success bred success: Senegal's containment of HIV became a matter of national pride and a lever to secure generous external aid.[35]

Uganda's situation was different, but its leaders too responded vigorously. When its Aids Control Programme formulated a five-year plan with WHO assistance in 1987, it faced the worst HIV epidemic in the world, with 24 per cent adult prevalence in the capital and annual incidence of 8.3 per cent among young people in Rakai. Uganda's representatives had astonished the World Health Assembly in May 1986 by frankly announcing the scale of their crisis. The Global Programme rewarded their candour by declaring the plan a model for Africa and arranging a meeting in May 1987 at which donors pledged more than the US$20 million needed to fund it. Its principles, Okware explained, were frankness and health education, 'the only way at the moment to prevent AIDS'.[36] The effective local government system was mobilised for this purpose and Museveni instructed officials to speak about the disease at all public meetings. In 1987 the school syllabus incorporated HIV instruction, with end-of-year exams. Blood screening, sentinel surveillance, epidemiological research, and patient care were further points in the programme, but condom distribution, originally included, was deferred when Museveni doubted its acceptability. It was only cautiously reintroduced in later years.[37] By 1989 Uganda was training health officials from other African countries. But prevalence continued to grow, while control over the funds flowing into the programme provoked rivalry within the Ministry of Health, between the Ministry and other branches of government, and among the various donors. Arguing that HIV/Aids was not only a medical problem and that all branches of government must be mobilised against it, the World Bank persuaded the government in 1990 to move control out of the Ministry of Health to a multi-sectoral Uganda Aids Commission. This created such bureaucratic confusion, rivalry, and extravagance that by 1995 even the Bank was channeling its funds back to the Ministry. Beneath the surface, however, the original programme continued. Museveni and the doctors exploited the donors with considerable skill, a host of official and non-governmental agencies were encouraged to contribute, and young Ugandans in particular began to change their behaviour to avoid infection.[38]

All African governments followed the Global Programme's procedures, but few with the energy displayed in Senegal and Uganda. Some launched their plans late: The Gambia in 1992, Chad in 1994. Several programmes, as in Ethiopia and Nigeria, were interrupted by civil conflict or military intervention. Others suffered long intervals between one plan and the next – four years (1993–7) between Botswana's first and second medium-term plans, for example, at the time when the epidemic was spreading most quickly. Several experienced the 'lack of a strong political will and commitment on the part of the Government' of which Tanzania's planners complained in 1998. Whereas Senegal benefited from continuity of medical leadership, Cameroun's Aids Council had eight directors between 1985 and 1999.[39] All programmes were severely short of funds after the donors' initial enthusiasm waned. In Congo-Brazzaville, for example, 'the peripheral care structures no longer received any funds from the state' between 1992 and 1997, all donor funds being retained in the capital or allocated directly to NGOs, so that the Aids programme, like Cameroun's, was said to resemble the earlier partition of the country between concessionary companies.[40] Even in relatively wealthy Côte d'Ivoire, the extreme concentration of medical services in Abidjan hamstrung the initial programme. In poorer countries like Tanzania or Malawi the problem was rather a lack of resources and administrative capacity. At Kisesa in northern Tanzania in 1994–8, 'The district budget for AIDS control activities was ... barely sufficient to pay one Ministry of Health staff member with a motorbike to supply condoms and provide AIDS education at government health facilities in a district of more than 300,000 people, including an estimated 10,000 infected adults.'[41] The most disastrous failure of policy at this period, however, was in Nigeria. When Aids was first reported there, the able Minister of Health, Dr Olikoye Ransome-Kuti, developed an elaborate federal programme. But donors were unwilling to subsidise an oil-rich country with military rulers who took no interest in the subject. In 1996, when the programme's sixth director resigned, federal spending on Aids was about 5 per cent of Uganda's, which had only half as many people with HIV. Three years earlier only one of the country's 589 local government areas had submitted the Aids report required from it. In 1997 the government published a policy statement first contemplated in 1991.[42]

The power and limitations of international orthodoxy in Aids policy were best displayed in South Africa. Expelled from the WHO, its white regime did not participate in the planning fervour of the late 1980s, when its main concern was the small homosexual epidemic and its models were American and European. When Aids Training, Information and Counselling Centres (ATICCs) were established in major cities from 1988, they were located in white areas and initially had a largely white clientele. Only in 1989 did officials begin to take seriously the danger of a large-scale heterosexual epidemic among the black population. Even then action was inhibited by a health system divided between 17 autonomous regional bodies, the indifference of political leaders preoccupied with preserving white supremacy, and a conservative prudery that vetoed an Aids education programme in schools.[43]

Instead, and uniquely, South Africa's HIV/Aids programme was formulated from below, and here the WHO orthodoxy proved powerful. African National Congress (ANC) leaders in exile in tropical Africa became aware of the emerging epidemic during the late 1980s. Once the party was legalised in February 1990, contacts were made with the Department of Health and activists in South Africa, leading to a conference in April at Maputo where it was agreed to establish a task force to prepare an HIV/Aids programme.[44] Amid recurrent political conflict, a National Aids Convention of South Africa (NACOSA) was created during 1992 embracing the ANC, government health bodies, and representatives of trade unions, business, churches, and NGOs, charged with developing a national strategy. Its drafting committee included the two ANC leaders mainly concerned with health, Drs Nkosazana Zuma and Manto Tshabalala-Msimang, and drew on the expertise of doctors, ATICC staff, and activists. The plan they presented to the new ANC government in July 1994 was drafted with WHO assistance and embodied all the current international priorities. A multisectoral National Aids Control Programme was to be established in the President's Office and implement schemes covering education, prevention, counselling, care of all kinds, welfare, research, human rights, and law reform, all integrated into the primary health care programme and involving participation by people living with HIV/Aids. The annual cost was estimated at 256 million rand, against a current public health expenditure on HIV/Aids of 31–36 million rand. Appended to the 231-page document was a 4-page 'Priority Programme of Action' for the first year, to be met from the Department of Health budget, embracing only prevention activities, strengthening the primary health care system, and tackling discriminatory practices with respect to HIV/Aids.[45] This was the real plan, trimmed to accord with the ANC's larger health programme, which concentrated on creating a single and equitable national health system 'based on the Primary Health Care approach'. Like governments in tropical Africa eight years earlier, the Department of Health, to which Aids was in fact entrusted, then prepared a short-term plan for 1995–6 'with a view for expansion into a medium-term plan'.[46] The lines were drawn for ten years of conflict that would focus international attention on South Africa and obloquy on President Mbeki, a conflict between, on the one side, people with Aids and their idealistic sympathisers, and, on the other, politicians determined to rectify centuries of racial injustice.

The HIV/Aids plans of the late 1980s and 1990s were largely devised by doctors. Medical workers faced many difficult issues posed by the epidemic. The most immediate was their own safety. Although careful studies found that HIV prevalence among medical staff was similar to that in the general population, doctors and nurses often worked without protective equipment and felt themselves at great risk. The average health worker at hospitals in Mwanza in northern Tanzania in 1993 was pricked five times and splashed with body fluids nine times each year.[47] Midwives felt especially vulnerable, as did surgeons, who, as elsewhere in the world, demanded to know the HIV status of patients before operating. One displayed a notice stating, 'No test, no operation'. Medical authorities denounced attempts to impose mandatory testing, but many hospitals in francophone Africa tested all patients without their knowledge or consent.[48] Although discrimination generally lessened as the disease became more familiar, UNAIDS stated in 2004 that in four Nigerian states,

> One in ten providers reported refusing to care for HIV-positive patients, and 10 per cent reported refusing them admission to a hospital. Furthermore, 65 per cent reported seeing other health-care workers refusing to care for an HIV or AIDS patient. Some 20 per cent felt that many people living with HIV had behaved immorally and deserved to be infected.[49]

Compulsory testing was anathema to the human rights principles of the WHO, which supplied testing reagents 'under very clear agreement of only using them for surveillance and blood transfusion purposes'.[50] In reality many companies and institutions tested applicants for jobs or scholarships, including American embassies (during the 1990s), over one-third of major companies in Kenya, South African Airways and the Electricity Supply Company (until South Africa outlawed this in 1999), several church bodies in Central Africa, and Botswana's overseas scholarships board. Many insurance companies demanded HIV tests, especially for larger policies. Numerous churches and some Muslim leaders refused to conduct marriages without prior testing and a number denied marriage to people with HIV. Senegal was one of the first countries to test military recruits, a procedure adopted widely as HIV prevalence among soldiers reached alarming proportions. Doctors who objected that compulsory testing breached a patient's right to confidentiality and exposed him to discrimination also opposed compulsory notification of HIV cases to the medical authorities. This was required in Angola and Kenya and was several times contemplated in South Africa but rejected because it would serve little purpose and might deter patients from seeking medical advice.[51]

Perhaps the most difficult decision facing medical staff was whether to disclose the result of a positive HIV test. Both indigenous and colonial practitioners had opposed giving a patient what was in effect a death sentence. 'How do you expect me to feel when you tell me that I am going to die?' one woman complained to her doctor, '... I want you to tell me that I am going to live.' Moreover, as Okware asked, 'What will we do with him?'[52] Some, he feared, might suffer shock, commit suicide, or deliberately spread their infection. Others might be abandoned by their families. Early in the epidemic, therefore, the most common practice was to withhold the result. Of 28 doctors questioned in the Central African Republic during the early 1990s, six never told patients the result, eighteen did so perhaps once a quarter, and four about once a week; the general practice was not to tell asymptomatic or advanced cases, but only those suffering early symptoms, and then by using euphemisms to avoid the dreaded word Aids while hinting strongly enough to enable the patient to decide whether or not to accept the truth.[53] Increasingly, however, doctors – especially young doctors – rebelled against the dishonesty this implied and the danger it caused. Many insisted that patients must be informed so that they could avoid infecting others. By the late 1980s the medical authorities in Kenya, Uganda, and Tanzania had all concluded that patients should normally be told their condition.[54] Gradually this became more common, although far from universal.

Other dilemmas were even more difficult. For those committed to the human rights perspective, a fundamental principle was that a patient's HIV status must not be revealed to anyone else without his or her consent. 'Confidentiality must be respected at all times and is non-negotiable,' the NACOSA plan proclaimed.[55] In Kenya, Uganda, and Botswana the medical regulations in force early in the epidemic all incorporated this dogma. Without it, many doctors insisted, patients would not tell them the truth. Yet if a doctor knew that a patient's infection threatened the sexual partner, should not the partner be warned? Ideally, the patient should give the warning, but if the patient feared or refused to do so, as was often the case, was the doctor justified in breaking confidence and perhaps exposing the infected partner to revenge? Would the law support the doctor? Would it condemn him if he did not give warning? A WHO consultation observed unhelpfully that the doctor 'will be required to make a decision consistent with medical ethics and relevant law'. The South African Medical Association, after much discussion, set out careful procedures, as did Tanzania.[56] Asked in the mid 1990s whether they would inform a partner under these circumstances, six doctors in Cape Coast, Ghana, said yes, five said no, and two said no, but....[57] Zimbabwe and Botswana contemplated legislation to compel infected people to inform a partner before having sex, but opponents urged that this would discourage people from being tested.

If it was proper to inform a partner, the next question was whether it was proper to tell anyone else. Nurses were especially hostile to enforced confidentiality, not only because of the risk to themselves but because it prevented them from giving appropriate care and threatened to spread the disease. 'It is Eurocentric – perhaps it is good for white people,' they complained. 'But we Africans are different – we care about others, we care about our neighbours .... This *secrecy* is killing us.'[58] In practice they were often told the situation or could guess it, but the problem was greater for lay caregivers, who often – in 90 per cent of cases in one Zambian study – did not know whether their patients had an infectious and lethal disease.[59] Observers complained that this not only endangered the carer and violated her human rights but threatened the patient with unsuitable care or, more seriously, with neglect by those fearful of an unknown condition. During the late 1990s several regimes in southern Africa met these dilemmas by adopting a notion of 'shared confidentiality' first devised at the Salvation Army Hospital at Chikankata in Zambia. As formulated by the authorities in KwaZulu, South Africa, 'Confidentiality in this context means confining the knowledge of a patient's HIV/AIDS status to as small a number as possible of specified people.'[60] The Aids Support Organisation in Uganda had pioneered a similar approach less formally. It was said to accord with the widespread African custom of entrusting a patient's treatment to a family grouping.

Doctors had to decide not only who should be informed but who should give the information. Many were unwilling to do so themselves, not only from natural distaste for a painful task but because they simply had no time for what was often a lengthy process of explanation and reassurance, taking at least 45 minutes, according to one specialist. As a young physician put it, 'We doctors should concern ourselves with the tough medical tasks which other people cannot do. Counselling is not a technical job, anybody can do it.'[61] Initially it was commonly delegated to nurses, often with little preparation, but soon it was realised that counselling was a skilled task needing training and unusual gifts. The Aids Support Organisation was a pioneer in this field and its methods became the model for many parts of the continent. Given in the wrong way, the test result could be devastating: 'One elderly doctor scolded her: "Now your baby might die." An orderly hissed: "Look at you. You've got AIDS."'[62] Many nurses, often from stern Christian families and sterner training schools, had little sympathy for Aids patients. In one study of nurses and laboratory technicians in Lagos state, Nigeria, in 1999, 'Some (55.9 per cent) of the health workers felt that PLWHAs are responsible for their illness, while 35.4 per cent felt that they deserve the punishment for their sexual mis-behaviours.'[63] Among frightened, uneducated patients, nurses had 'a reputa-tion for rudeness and even cruelty'. 'I think they can't handle all the dying and maybe that is why they are angry,' one patient conjectured.[64] The strain was immense. At Kitovu Hospital, in the heart of the western Ugandan epidemic,

> Hospital personnel are caring for increasing numbers of terminally ill patients.... Staff who are trained to cure find it difficult to see so many patients fail to respond....
>
> Many lack even the attendants who normally care for inpatients; they come because they have no one else to care for them. This puts an added stress on the hospital and the staff.
>
> Staff of the Complex are also falling ill with AIDS.... They are weak, have dimin-ished ability to concentrate, and are anxious that they will lose their jobs....
>
> Staff have many family burdens and worries. Many are trying to support in-creasing numbers of orphans. Many of them have sick and dying family members.... It ... means that staff come on duty already heavily burdened and anxious.[65]

For hospital doctors, too, the flooding of the wards with Aids patients devalued medicine. 'Death no longer becomes a very serious affair,' one at the Kenyatta National Hospital in Nairobi commented. Medicine lost much of its intellectual interest, for 'the diagnosis is obvious'.[66] Doctors who could no longer cure lost their hitherto high prestige and self-confidence. 'It pains me to care for an AIDS patient. It really pains me,' a physician in Kagera complained. 'Because whatever I give I know it is not helping the patient.... I would like a disease which kills quicker. This one is too slow in killing.'[67] Often, moreover, there was nothing to give because reduced health budgets could not provide the drugs that doctors knew could at least palliate their patients' sufferings:

> These patients are desperate. They move from hospital to hospital. We may see a patient who has visited five, six, seven hospitals....

You treat their opportunistic infections, but the first time they come in they are 60 kg, then the next time they are 50 kg and then they are 40 kg. You see these patients deteriorate over time and you run out of things to tell them. They go to different hospitals and in the end they come back. They are really just looking for something nobody can give them.[68]

Many doctors and nurses found no answer to their situation but to abandon their professional principles in the medical strikes recurrent throughout the continent. A study of registrars – the resident ward doctors – at Kenyatta National Hospital in 1997–9 found that 82 per cent were suffering some degree of the moral and emotional exhaustion known as burn-out, 'as a result of working in an environment characterised by poor communication among hospital staff as well as a lack of resources and high numbers of patients with HIV/AIDS'. 'Regarding HIV/AIDS,' one said,

it is impossible to go home and forget about it. Even the simplest opportunistic infections we have no drugs for. Even if we do there is only enough for a short course.... Just because of the numbers I am afraid of going to see the patients. You are afraid of the risk of infection, diarrhea, urine, vomit, blood.... Just walking in a room you think you will get TB. It is frightening to think about returning.[69]

Amidst this widespread collapse of morale, devoted physicians shone all the more brightly. One, who must stand for them all, was Elly Katabira, who opened the first specialised Aids clinic at Mulago Hospital in Kampala in 1987 and worked there for the next two decades. 'Health workers knew there was no cure for AIDS,' he recalled, 'so they assumed that people with AIDS didn't warrant any medical care. We started the AIDS clinic to show what could be done. We had to demonstrate to patients and health workers alike that people with AIDS who come in very sick can leave the hospital walking.'[70] Katabira insisted that 'all mentally competent people should be informed of their [test] results':

It is not easy to tell any one that he or she has got AIDS and that he is going to die in the next few months. Yet some of the patients need to know and some ask to be told. This is not the type of news you can pass on in a hurry. You need to be prepared to explain the gravity of the news and be able to offer comfort and support to the patient, and be able to answer some of the questions which are likely to be asked, related to the fate of the victim.

This is counselling and it starts with the one who breaks the ice, who is usually the doctor.[71]

He coped with the strain by blocking out everything except 'that patient sitting in front of me':

What I think is most important ... is support – counselling and reassurance that, yes, you are sick, but there are a lot of things you can do to improve your living without medicine. Simple things, like reducing your alcohol intake and going to the doctor as soon as you feel sick. And dealing with dependants. A parent will never get better if she's worried about her children. These things are considered second-rate, but I think they're very important....

Many people think that because I'm in the field of AIDS, I look at it as something special. No.... The problem is wider. I go to the pediatric ward, and kids are dying because there is no amoxicillin [a basic antibiotic]. I could have walked away in protest, but I must do each and every thing possible to get my patient through the next day. Use what you have.[72]

Despite such dedication, it was increasingly clear in the early 1990s that the response coordinated by the WHO was having little effect in checking the epidemic. Some thought, indeed, that the coordination itself was partly to blame, that national Aids plans, 'hatched like chickens by groups of inter-national consultants', sought to impose identical structures – hierarchy, medicalisation, verticality, dependence – smothering the local initiatives emerging before the WHO intervened. This judgment was too sweeping, but it was true that all but the most successful programmes escaped the ownership of the communities whose energy they needed for success. In Kenya and Tanzania, for example, the programmes were seen essentially as WHO agencies to which national governments refused to contribute even the small sums they had promised.[73] By the mid 1990s governments in sub-Saharan Africa were providing about 9 per cent of public HIV/Aids spending in their countries. In an extreme but not unique case, between 1987 and 1995 nearly 98 per cent of Burkina's expenditure in this field came as foreign aid. The figures are misleading, for most of the epidemic's cost fell on private individuals.[74] They are misleading, too, because the total sums contributed in foreign assistance were relatively small. In 1990 some 93 per cent of global expenditure on HIV/Aids took place in developed countries. As the number of infected Africans grew, expenditure per infection peaked in 1988 before roughly halving during the 1990s. In 1991 international funding for the Global Programme declined for the first time.[75]

By then Mann had quit his post as the Programme's director, following conflict with other WHO personnel and open disagreement with the Japanese Director-General, who, with the support of many African countries, wanted to decentralise the Programme and its 200 staff to regional offices – which Mann had deliberately bypassed – and reduce what he considered its tendency to overshadow primary health care.[76] Mann was frustrated, too, by what he saw as 'growing complacency, persistent denial, and resurgent discrimination'. Like other activists, he felt that the initial stress on public education and the targeting of high-risk groups like sex workers had failed, partly because the African epidemic had spread into the general population, partly because experience had shown that 'by itself information is insufficient to change behaviour'. Behavioural change and risk avoidance required a degree of personal autonomy that many people – women, the young, the poor – often lacked. The problem was not risk but vulnerability, to which the only answer was empowerment, and that required change at the social and ultimately the global level.[77] This thinking was beginning to enter WHO strategy. In 1989 the World Health Assembly urged member states to expand the role of NGOs and of people living with HIV/Aids, whose previous lack of activism – in contrast to their agitation in the United States or Brazil – illustrated Africa's depoliticisation since independence. A year later the Assembly urged states 'to strengthen the involvement of women by including in national AIDS committees a representative of women's organisations'. Under pressure from feminist organisations, the World Aids Conference of 1992 for the first time gave the position of women a central place in Aids strategy.[78]

The whole structure of the Global Programme was also under attack. Many national programmes had lost direction. One survey found that Aids committees had not met during 1991 in 14 of 27 African countries. Donors grew increasingly impatient. In 1995 USAID channelled 87 per cent of its aid for Kenya's HIV programme to NGOs and the private sector, avoiding the corruption and incompetence of the government. By then impatience had extended beyond the WHO's clients to the organisation itself. In the early 1990s several international agencies – World Bank, UNICEF, UNDP, European Union, and others – established their own Aids policies and programmes, bypassing what they saw as the WHO's ineffectiveness. In 1992 an external review of the Global Programme suggested that responsibility should be shifted away from the WHO and the narrowly medical perspectives through which it worked.[79]

The first half of the 1990s was the time of deepest disillusionment in the African Aids epidemic. The virus was still expanding at accelerating pace, especially in southern Africa, with no indication as yet of reaching a plateau, much less declining. Early hopes of a vaccine or cure had come to nothing. Annual international conferences were occasions for collective gloom, un-relieved by new ideas or new remedies. National programmes were enmeshed in bureaucracy and ineffectiveness. The WHO was losing its leadership role. Beneath this surface, it is true, some of the forces that would eventually reactivate resistance to the epidemic were appearing in the new emphasis on NGOs, women, people with HIV/Aids, and the vulnerable generally – the impetus from below that the initial Global Programme had lacked. But these were only the first signs of change. For the present, as of 1995, the ordinary people of Africa, infected or affected, had to oppose their own resources against the epidemic.

9

Views
from Below

The chief reasons for the failure of international Aids policies in Africa during the late twentieth century were that they came too late to check an expanding epidemic and had no effective medical remedy with which to do so, but another reason was that the medical thinking underlying international policies often conflicted with the ways in which most Africans perceived the crisis. Their responses were diverse, as is commonly true in epidemics, but this was particularly so with HIV because its long incubation period and lack of distinctive symptoms bred confusion and encouraged denial. At an individual level, as a Ugandan woman said, 'Everybody suffers from *silimu* differently.'[1] At the collective level, understandings were set within the context of a long dialogue between indigenous notions of causation, which were chiefly moralistic, and the medical explanations propagated by governments and Western-trained doctors. Similar debates surrounding cholera epidemics in nineteenth-century Europe and America had resulted in victory for medical explanations because they worked, but in late twentieth-century Africa the doctors had no effective remedy and moralism remained powerful. Yet this moralism was not merely traditionalist, for it had blended with the imported moralism of world religions. The result was a hybrid, a popular response to the epidemic that was at once stigmatising, caring, and capable of motivating behavioural change.

The initial response to HIV/Aids was commonly to blame Others. Indignant at suggestions that the virus had originated in Africa, intellectuals insisted that it was rather 'the white man's burden', a disease of American and European homosexuals, imported, it was said in Kinshasa, in canned food threatening both health and authenticity. Villagers in Burkina held that HIV originated when a white man paid a woman to have sex with a chimpanzee.[2] The ANC's periodical suspected 'the laboratories of many imperialist countries'. Other black South Africans saw it as an Apartheid device, spread perhaps by teargas, designed to decimate the black population – an outcome described by one white extremist as 'like Father Christmas'.[3] Immigrants and refugees from other African countries were widely held responsible. Villagers blamed townsmen. Elders blamed the young. Men and women blamed one another. Everyone blamed sex workers, 'the main route of AIDS', as Museveni described them in 1990.[4] Seldom, however, did rich and poor hold one another responsible.

Initial government warnings instilled fear and prejudice, Of the three emphasised in Zimbabwe, 'AIDS kills' was understood to mean imminent death, 'AIDS cannot be cured' encouraged hopelessness, and 'AIDS is spread in promiscuous sex' signified that all HIV-positive people were promiscuous.[5] The initial fear was commonly fear of the unknown, for people with visible Aids were rare and many complaints were construed as possible symptoms. Perhaps because infection spread slowly and silently, there was little panic – although the first case to appear in Kumasi caused a traffic jam[6] – but much rumour, one of many ways in which the epidemic was shaped by the largely oral character of African societies. Suspicion focused especially on infected men alleged to spread the disease deliberately, 'so as not to die alone'. A mob in western Uganda beat to death a man suspected of infection who boasted of having had sex with over thirty women. Several governments contemplated legislation to criminalise deliberate infection, although doctors insisted that it would be almost impossible to prove.[7] Rumour helped to create the pervasive uncertainty of the late 1980s, a period known in Kagera as *patashika*, 'confusion'. 'They are all simply bewildered, as in the period of war which they have survived,' a health worker said of infected people in Uganda.[8] Some relapsed into resignation. At Kasensero, in 1987,

> One old man of about 80 had lost son, daughter and five grandchildren, all apparently from Slim, since 1985 and only one grandchild survived to tend the seven graves among the *matoke* [banana] trees; 'everything is in the hands of God,' the old man said. Another grandfather testified that in the last two years five of his eight children had died of 'diarrhoea and coughing'; 'God must have his reasons,' he said quietly.[9]

Others took refuge in the denial that oral cultures facilitated. It was the predominant response in Kinshasa in 1987. 'I just don't want to think about AIDS,' a Cabinet minister explained, while younger men disparaged SIDA (the French acronym) as Imaginary Syndrome to Discourage Lovers (*Syndrome Imaginaire pour Décourager les Amoureux*), Invented Syndrome to Hide Abuses (*Syndrome Inventé pour Dissimuler les Abus*), or Insufficient Salaries for Years (*Salaires Insuffisants Depuis des Années*).[10] Denial was to survive far into the epidemic. In 2002 an anthropologist found it dominant in a South African village that had nine funerals in a single weekend. It was a coping device by which to preserve dignity in unspeakable circumstances.[11]

Among the best-known denialists was the Nigerian musician, Fela Anikulapo-Kuti, who denied the existence of HIV, slept with hundreds of women, and died of Aids in 1997.[12] Others, by contrast, used music and song – as occurs widely in postcolonial Africa – to highlight issues closed to ordinary discussion. Luambo Makiadi 'Franco', himself HIV-positive, alerted Kinshasa youths in 1987:

> Aids has divided the nations,
> Aids has destroyed my marriage,

Aids has divided my family.
They ate and drank with me,
And now they are fleeing me,
It is said that because I have Aids
All my friends have deserted me.[13]

In Kagera, songs of the 1980s blamed HIV on witchcraft, dishonest young traders, or sex workers, but with time the mood shifted to emphasise the 'flooding river', the scale of the catastrophe, and then to expressions of either exhaustion or resilience.[14] In Dr Banda's repressive Malawi, similarly, early songs warned that 'Aids has come', often blaming the (usually female) sufferer, while 'The tribe is finished' of 1988 captured the mood of dejection, but 'We are all at war with Aids' expressed a new determination associated with Banda's fall in 1994.[15] Most poignant was 'Alone', by the dying Ugandan musician, Philly Lutaaya:

Out there somewhere
Alone and frightened
Of the darkness
The days are long
Life of hiding
No more making new contact
No more loving arms
Thrown around my neck.[16]

By the early 1990s knowledge of the epidemic and its fatal consequences was widespread, although with much surviving confusion. In a poor country like Tanzania, for example, a survey in 1991–2 found that 98 per cent of men and 93 per cent of women knew of HIV/Aids, whereas in 1993 only 17 per cent of India's women had that knowledge and even as late as 2001 only 82 per cent of Indian men and 70 per cent of women had heard of the disease.[17] In Kagera, one of the first areas affected, awareness arose first in 1982–3 among men aged less than 35 and spread in turn to older men, younger women, and older women, becoming universal by 1989. That was probably a common pattern, but with marked regional differences. In Nigeria in 1999, awareness among women ranged from 88 per cent in towns to 69 per cent in the countryside, and from 91 per cent in the south-east to 50 per cent in the north-east and 47 per cent in the north-west, both strongly Islamic regions where women were often secluded.[18] The main source of information there was the radio, as was generally true throughout the continent. The chief exceptions were Ethiopia, where relatively few households had radios and the main channels of communication were meetings of peasant associations and urban wards, and Uganda, where more people (70 per cent of men and 82 per cent of women in 1995) listed friends and relatives among their chief sources of information.[19] Alongside knowledge, however, there was much confusion. In Tanzania, as late as 1999, 46 per cent of women believed that HIV could be transmitted by insect bites, a widespread misconception presumably inherited from colonial propaganda against malaria, while 42 per cent thought that HIV could be contracted by sharing food, probably a memory of precautions against leprosy or tuberculosis. This confusion of HIV with other diseases added immensely to fear and stigma, as did a general over-estimation of the transmissibility of the virus, sometimes thought to be an inevitable consequence of intercourse with an infected person. At the same time, however, confusion with other medical messages led Kinshasa factory workers to believe that HIV could be transmitted only to someone of the same blood group and fostered notions that infection could be prevented by insect repellant or by taking antibiotics or birth control pills before sex.[20]

Awareness that Aids existed and was fatal did not necessarily breed a sense of personal risk. 'If people do not know of anyone who has the disease,' it was reported from Lesotho, 'then they do not feel at risk even though they may know that their behaviour places them at risk.' During the 1990s that personal contact with infected people increased, but most unevenly. In Ethiopia, in 2000, only 28 per cent of people knew someone infected by or dead of HIV/Aids, as against 91 per cent in Uganda. 'The way I had seen him suffering,' a Malawian recalled, 'that's when I came to my senses.'[21]

Before antiretroviral drugs became available in Africa, the period from the inception of Aids to death averaged some nine or ten months, although with much variation. The patient was not normally bedridden throughout; intervals of relief and relative activity were interspersed with progressively more frequent and lengthy attacks of opportunistic diseases. At this point poverty was the problem most frequently quoted by patients and caregivers because it denied them the food, medicines, and other necessities to prolong life and reduce suffering. 'I have got many complaints,' a 23-year-old Malawian patient explained:

> Hunger is my problem. The selling of my bicycle has worsened my problems. I am unable to go to hospital. I don't have transport, I lack soap for bathing and for washing clothing. I don't have trousers. The trousers which I had, I sold them, I lack clothing. Another complaint is the wound which is not healing. I have a lot of pain. If only I had medicine for pain reliefs. Because of all these problems I will die soon.[22]

The most frequent symptoms reported by patients in Uganda were 'fever (60 per cent), followed by cough (45.5 per cent), continuous diarrhoea (32 per cent), sores on the inside of the mouth (18 per cent), weight loss (14 per cent), swellings on the side of the mouth (10 per cent), and *herpes zoster* (6 per cent)'. In addition, many patients – 58 of 100 in one study at Bloemfontein Hospital – suffered psychiatric morbidity. The combination of diarrhoea, wasting, and infections of the mouth made feeding of patients especially difficult for the poor. 'Sometimes when my son tells me "I want such and such a thing" I cry after I fail to think how I can find the things that he wants,' a caregiver explained.[23] Many opportunistic conditions could be relieved by an inexpensive drug, cotrimoxazole, which was widely used in Europe for twenty years before it was recommended for use in Africa in 2000.[24] In the final stages of disease, the policy of leaving sufferers to die at home commonly prevented effective palliation of the terminal pain that was perhaps the most terrible aspect of the epidemic:

I can't even begin to describe the kind of pain he was in. He had this terrible headache, which lasted for five days. He never lost consciousness.... I had known all along that Chris was going to die, but I wasn't prepared for the way that he died. Such undignified pain and suffering.[25]

As people became more familiar with the disease, they became if anything less willing to be tested for HIV infection.[26] Knowledge of their HIV status might help them to protect others but was of little advantage to themselves when no remedy existed. 'I'll do the HIV test when there is a cure for AIDS,' one said. 'I don't want to make myself miserable.'[27] As late as 2000, only an estimated 5 per cent of infected people in the developing world were aware of their condition.[28] Those who did seek testing during the 1990s were less often those most at risk than those worried by poor health or planning marriage or conception.[29] Reactions to a positive test result varied. 'Some people display no emotions,' a counsellor in Natal explained, 'others become violent and abusive. Some patients take a long time to absorb the shock and reach acceptance while others are pragmatic and feel that they will die some day anyway so what difference does having AIDS make.' Shock followed by verbal and physical distress were naturally the most common initial reactions. 'Hearing this news shattered me to pieces,' one remembered, 'it was like reading out my death sentence.'[30] Some assumed that they had only days to live. In one Tanzanian study, 19 per cent of those tested positive contemplated suicide. Research there and in South Africa suggested that young people with HIV were 35–40 times more likely to attempt suicide than those without it. A few killed their dependants as well as themselves.[31] More lapsed into despair:

I felt that I am a person that is dying any minute. I'm just dying, I will soon leave this world. I had a few important things that I really liked. I decided, well, I'm dying, so I sold them all and the others I decided just to give out to my relatives, as I wanted to remain just as myself.[32]

By contrast, some of those tested positive retained equanimity by flatly denying the diagnosis. A counsellor in Ethiopia found that uneducated people had difficulty in understanding the test and seldom appeared disturbed by the result, while educated people initially reacted negatively, often appearing shocked, bursting into tears, or expressing denial, before asking practical questions about how to behave in order to live longer.[33] It was the counsellor's task to bring the applicant to this state of acceptance. 'I became very emotional and found myself at a complete loss as to what to do about my situation,' Azariah Ndonji recalled. 'I wanted to kill myself. But I had a wife and two small daughters.' His counsellor talked him out of suicide:

Since then I have never thought about anything other than living positively. It has not always been easy. My 25-year-old wife has been confirmed HIV positive and both she and one of my daughters have been ill. I do wish my wife had not fallen into this situation. If God could have prevented her being forced to face this death too, I would have been so relieved. But it was not to be.

... I have accepted my fate for what it is. it makes me bitter that I have to spend so much time worrying about my health. I find myself watching over my health almost daily. Every small itch, skin irritation or abnormal cough makes me wonder whether the hour of my death is about to arrive. But, so far, I have recovered my health each time. I can reassure myself that I am going to live a little longer and in a positive way.[34]

'An HIV diagnosis is life changing,' another recalled, 'it brings about such feelings of fear, shame and isolation, it makes people feel dirty, abnormal, frightened. The first challenge is to regain a sense of self worth, self-confidence and dignity.'[35] Many claimed that those who responded most positively also survived longest.

As Ndonji's testimony suggests, positive HIV tests were often interpreted as much in terms of the family as of the individual. Heterosexual Aids in Africa, unlike homosexual Aids in the West, was above all a family disease. 'When I inform a person tested that she is carrying HIV,' a doctor wrote, 'she cries immediately: "My children, Oh, my children!"'[36] Another shared this experience:

> I am often struck ... to observe that young unmarried seropositives are more affected morally by the impossibility of creating a family or being a support to their parents than by the fact of knowing their expectation of life to be limited. For those who already have a parental responsibility, what will become of the couple and the children is their principal concern.[37]

This care could stimulate positive responses. TASO in Uganda found that some people, on testing positive, abandoned long-term plans and focused all their remaining energy on providing for their children. But concern for the family could also encourage concealment. Many were less worried about having HIV than about informing their partner. Women 'fear being beaten up, losing the roof over their head, their partner, everything,' explained a South African township worker.[38] Several studies found that only a minority of infected women told their partners. When they did so, most received a more supportive response than they expected, but in a typical instance in Dar es Salaam in 1999, although 49 per cent of husbands were supportive and 16 per cent undertook to be tested themselves, another 16 per cent blamed their partners, 4 per cent assaulted them, and 4 per cent abandoned them.[39] Some drove wives away:

> Makhalemale found out she was HIV-positive in 1993. When she told her husband, he shoved her into a pot of water boiling on the stove, scalding her arm. She went to her job selling shoes 'as if everything was okay'. But her husband showed up telling her to go back home, get her things and leave him, because how could he live with someone infected with HIV? That was at 10.00 in the morning. At 3.00 that afternoon she was fired from her job.[40]

Conflict was especially likely when, as was often the case, the first member of a family found infected was a baby, for then husband and wife might blame one another and the husband's family might insist on expelling the wife lest she infect him. Yet HIV-positive men were generally even less willing to inform their partners – in Botswana in 2001, 29 per cent of men and 36 per cent of women shared their results[41] – despite the fact that they could normally rely upon a wife to care for them, from both affection and interest. An Ethiopian explained:

> She tells me that she will always be by my side up to the end of my life.... This is because she suspects that she could have the virus in her body too.... Her fear lies in the fact that if I die of this disease, she may be left alone. She is afraid that her parents and relatives may not want to support her if she is sick. She fears the stigma that other people may show against her as a widow who lost her husband due to AIDS.[42]

Evidence from Malawi, however, showed that the proportion of women thinking it legitimate for a woman to divorce a husband suspected of infection increased as the epidemic progressed.[43]

Rather than inform their partner, infected people often told their mother, especially in West Africa where this was the closest relationship and the one most likely to yield care. Others informed siblings of the same gender or close friends. Women often had particular difficulty in telling their children, because of the pain it would cause them and the possibility that they might reject their parents. Failure to disclose infection, of course, endangered an uninfected partner, for it was virtually impossible to change behaviour for a long period – say, by insisting on using condoms – without arousing suspicion. Secrecy obliged the infected partner to live in fear of detection and perhaps to forego care and support. It ran counter to the custom of sharing health problems with family members. To maintain silence in these circumstances witnessed to the intense fear of stigmatisation, not only of the individual but of the entire family.[44]

The Aids epidemic accentuated the gender inequalities and tensions on which it fed. Adultery, now mortally dangerous, bred fear and distrust in marriage systems with polygynous traditions and double standards. During the 1990s fear reduced partner exchange in many regions, angering men for whom prowess no longer brought prestige. For women, commonly obliged to rely on men for economic support, casual relationships were increasingly dangerous and marriage seemed to offer even greater security than before. Yet it was in reality a danger, for probably 50 per cent, and perhaps 80 per cent, of women with HIV had been infected by their husbands.[45] Despite the danger, the preservation of the relationship was often the first priority, for the divorcee or widow was likely to lose access to property and perhaps control of children, whose fate in an Aids-infected world was commonly her chief concern. Women were generally more willing than men to protect themselves against HIV. Some were sufficiently strong to live with an infected husband without contracting the disease:

> When he first learned he has HIV, he asked me to stay with him, to stay by him. And because God gave me a soft heart, I stayed....
>
> We don't sleep together, because he won't use condoms. I told him, 'My body is my body, please don't abuse it.' ...
>
> My children are all I think about. They are what I live for.[46]

Yoruba women, with unusual economic independence, were able to insist on using condoms with infected husbands, but many women feared even to suggest it. Moreover, some preferred unprotected sex because they wanted children, perhaps all the more urgently if they had already lost a child to Aids or feared early death. A study of infected European and African women in a Parisian hospital found that 29 per cent of the Europeans but 61 per cent of the Africans would have wished to carry a pregnancy to birth.[47]

These considerations make it easier to understand the silence surrounding the epidemic. These were honour cultures in which public display or discussion of sex, except in closely defined circumstances, was shameful not only for the individual but for the family. 'In our society,' a young Congolese graduate explained,

> we do not learn to speak the truth. People would rather hide the truth if it is unpleasant....
>
> To say you have AIDS! That would be a terrible shame; the family would never support you! If a man is known as a good man, he will have many people depending on him; he cannot now say he is sick, that will destroy them. It is a question of honour, and the medical information is in conflict with this system of honour.[48]

Concern not to humiliate other members of the family was a major reason why people with HIV/Aids maintained silence. Mothers knew, for example, that any child from a family with a known infected member was likely to suffer cruel mockery from other children.[49] To shame the family was to risk alienating those on whose care one must rely. Nor was it thought necessary to inform caregivers; as close kin, their care was an obligation. Tact and courtesy, equally, dictated discretion:

> Who among her closest relatives in Addis Ababa is willing to risk offending her, hurting her feelings, shaming her, and causing her to lose face, in order to talk to her about the importance of getting tested for the disease? To this day, we are stuck at the crossroad where the Ethiopian heightened sense of shame and fatality meet and mingle like lovers.[50]

Even to suggest that a person might have an incurable disease was to display hostility. Such discretion often bred loneliness. 'Many people are just dying inside in silence,' a young woman with HIV warned.[51] It also assisted the expansion of the epidemic and increased its danger, as health workers pointed out. Yet the open discussion of sex, sickness, and death advocated by the WHO and its disciples was profoundly distasteful to honourable Africans. Only slowly and under circumstances of grave crisis did it win African adherents, converting sex for the first time from a physical activity into a subject of discourse in African cultures, as contraception and feminism had done in the West.[52]

Behind this silence, above all, lay the fear of stigma. The roots of Aids stigma – as with leprosy and syphilis – lay mainly in fear of contagion:

> Even when I feel like having a beer in the bar next door, the customers get up, quickly settle their bills, timidly say good bye to me and disappear. Others often buy me a beer and when I get up to shake their hands and thank them they refuse to shake my hand.... At home, when the meal is ready, no one wants to sit to eat with me. Everyone manages to eat before or after me; never at the same time. But my

portion of food is always kept for me and is always generous. My mechanic refuses to fix my moped because, according to him I may have cut myself and if my blood has touched the engine, he could contaminate himself.[53]

Such fears could expand to absurd lengths, as when parents forbade children to attend the funeral of a person suspected of Aids or a judge attempted to stop an infected person from giving evidence in court.

Moreover, because the disease was widely thought to be contracted by promiscuity or as a punishment for it, people with HIV/Aids were seen as morally contagious and worthy of contempt:

AIDS patients who are sent home after counselling at AIDS centres in Dodoma Region [in Tanzania], are rejected and segregated by their families, including being locked up in flat-roof houses and treated as people with leprosy.

Patients, who are mainly women, when they return home to be treated by their families, are refused food, are not given any services, are not even greeted and many times when people pass outside these flat-roof houses, they shout insults at them telling them they are adulterous and prostitutes fit for the graves.[54]

Fearing such maltreatment, some people with HIV/Aids reacted with intense sensitivity. A Ugandan likened them to wounded animals.[55] Others stigmatised themselves, felt ashamed, and either hid, suffering great loneliness, or believed that everyone they met despised them. 'You seem to think that everyone knows about it, that it is written on you,' a teenager said. 'If you climb into a taxi you'll find people laughing. You become uncomfortable. You feel like they are laughing at you.'[56] Often the fear of discrimination was worse than the reality.

The extent of stigmatisation in Africa varied greatly. Some careful observers of highly infected Ugandan provinces early in the epidemic denied the existence of stigma while others described it as 'very strong'.[57] The explanation may have been that individual attitudes and behaviours were diverse. Stigma tended to focus on the vulnerable – poor people, the young, women, and especially sex workers – while mature people with economic independence rarely suffered it.[58] Men were commonly more tolerant than women, while knowledge of HIV/Aids, education, urban residence, and higher economic status all increased tolerance.[59] Enquiries in Kagera early in the epidemic showed that rural communities with low HIV prevalence proposed more ruthless treatment of infected people than did urban residents where prevalence was high. Other evidence showed high levels of stigmatisation even in highly infected rural areas. In parts of KwaZulu, for example, it was reported in 2001 that 'people known to be AIDS sufferers have had their homes burnt to the ground. Some barely able to walk, have been chased by mobs into the bush.... Teachers and pupils act together to chase the children away because they are "unclean".'[60] Yet although growing experience of the disease did not necessarily reduce stigma, that was the general pattern. It was first observed in Uganda. 'In the beginning of the epidemic,' a villager there recalled in 1996–7, 'people thought it was contagious and were afraid of catching it. People who were ill were left with the door closed, but this doesn't happen any more.' Most accounts agreed that stigma had declined but had far from disappeared. Evidence from neighbouring Kagera suggested the same.[61] 'The disease is so common that it has lost much of its social stigma,' it was reported from Zambia in 2003, 'but people still do not talk about it publicly.' Stigma was often stronger where the disease was more recent or the prevalence lower.[62]

In these circumstances, it took great courage for people with HIV/Aids to disclose their status publicly. Some did so from a sense of duty. 'I want others not to be exposed as to what has happened to me,' an Ethiopian wrote in his diary. 'I want to share my experience with the youth. This is all I have.' Others, like Maria Ndlovu of Johannesburg, could not bear to live a lie: 'I made up my mind that this needs to be talked about because it is not right to feel as if you are dying when you are not. I wanted to normalise the situation.' Many found disclosure liberating and empowering: 'the minute you talk about it you are free'.[63] For some it was easier to declare themselves in public than to tell their families, who might resent the consequences. 'I was embarrassed. I was humiliated. I was not ready for this,' one wife protested.[64] Some who 'came out' in this way met sympathy and admiration, but it was probably more generally true, as a leader in Burkina put it, that 'you have to be prepared to face up to rejection, you have to be financially independent, and your family must be prepared to put up with the criticisms that will be made against you'.[65] Many met cynical suspicion that they were doing it for money. Others suffered more brutally. 'I remained isolated for two years,' the first Malian to disclose his condition recalled. 'Even my relatives abandoned me.' His counterpart in Sierra Leone 'had his house ransacked, his personal possessions set alight and was forced to seek refuge with his HIV-positive wife and live in a hospital cubicle'. Most tragically, Gugu Dlamini was stoned, kicked, and beaten to death in a Durban township by those who thought her disclosure had dishonoured the neighbourhood.[66]

People with HIV and their families sought desperately for a remedy amidst Africa's great variety of medical specialists. One Ugandan industrialist is said to have offered a building worth US$2 million to anyone who could provide a cure. A sociologist at the Aids clinic in Abidjan found that patients had not only tried every type of treatment – traditional, modern, and religious – but had often tried several varieties of each. 'If I heard that there was a healer in a particular part of Uganda,' recalled Noerine Kaleeba, a trained physiotherapist,

I would drive there and come back with a bottle or jerry can of preparation.... Relatives were bringing medicines by the jerry can too, and soon there were medicines for wrapping, medicines for sniffing, medicines for drinking, and so on.... Chris took all these remedies faithfully, alongside the [hospital] medicines he had been given.[67]

Some traditional healers professed to be able to cure the disease. One of the more serious was a Ghanaian shrine healer, Kofi Drobo II, who claimed in 1990 to have cured 60 Aids patients at his 750-patient medical centre, administering herbal remedies in capsule form and by injection. 'What matters,' he explained, 'is to make the foul buboes and sores disappear. In brief, to make an invalid preparing himself for burial into a human being, healthy in body and full of life.' Less convincingly, Yawanina Nanyonga, a Ugandan woman, dispensed therapeutic mud to thousands of pilgrims from as far away as Kenya and Rwanda, leaving a hole a metre wide and two metres deep when her practice was banned.[68] Nanyonga claimed direction by a vision of the Holy Spirit, one of the many spiritual healers and millennial prophets to emerge in Uganda at this time of catastrophe. Some were humble people dispensing prayer and holy water, but in Kampala the Apostle Deo Balabyekubo of the Prayer Palace Christian Centre attended healing sessions in a white Mercedes, while in Lagos the Prophet Temitope Balogun Joshua of the Synagogue Church of All Nations 'claims to heal hundreds of HIV/Aids patients every Wednesday.... Even before they return to the hospitals to confirm their negative status, the victims hail their healer, claiming he has cured them on the spot.'[69] Biomedicine, too, offered ambitious and often lucrative remedies: MM-1 in Egypt and the DR Congo, Mariandina in Uganda, Vanhivax in Cameroun, Kemron and Pearl Omega in Kenya, AKB in Tanzania, Herbiron-Tisaferon in Zambia, Virodene in South Africa, and the vaccine with which Dr Jeremiah Abalaka of Nigeria claimed to have cured over 900 HIV patients. 'It will only be justice,' a Congo-Brazzaville newspaper commented on MM-1, 'that a malady, of which Africa is suspected to be the genitor, should be conquered by Africans. Persons reputed rebels against science are today going to relieve the world's anguish.'[70]

Beneath the competing miracle cures the epidemic witnessed a dialogue between two views of the causation of disease. One was the biomedical view, propounded by the WHO and Africa's Western-trained doctors, which concentrated on explaining *how* the epidemic occurred, attributing it to the virus. The other was a moralistic view, expressed in different ways by traditionalists and religious leaders, which focused on *why* the epidemic occurred, attributing it to human immorality. Similar conflicts between medical and moral responses to epidemic had taken place in the nineteenth century in Western countries. In the United States, for example, the dominant response to the first cholera epidemic in 1832 was moralistic: it was the wicked who died. During the next thirty years, however, sanitary reform in expanding cities strengthened the champions of public health. When cholera returned in 1866, it was treated chiefly as a social rather than a moral problem, public health measures restricted mortality, and medical interpretations of epidemic became predominant because they worked.[71] In Africa this confrontation between medical and moral thinking had been played out since the nineteenth century in the lives of African medical assistants, nurses, and physicians. It reached a climax in the Aids epidemic, sometimes in personal controversies, as between Dr Malegapuru Makgoba and President Thabo Mbeki in South Africa, described later, or between the scientist-politician Pascal Lissouba and the moralist-politician Bernard Kolelas in Congo-Brazzaville.[72] The rationalism of French medical traditions made the contest especially bitter in francophone countries. Benin's Aids strategy of 2001, for example, listed among its chief obstacles 'The weight of tradition and culture, [the] magical representation of the disease', along with 'the ferocious and aggressive opposition of the Catholic

Church towards the promotion and use of condoms'.[73] Medical pragmatists also confronted both a racial nationalism that resented Western accounts of the epidemic and a deep popular suspicion of Western medical practices. The first large research programme in Rakai had to be suspended temporarily 'because people were running away from the teams of researchers' whom they suspected of draining their blood, a long-standing fear shared in Kagera. On World Aids Day in 1988 the District Medical Officer in Masaka had to announce publicly that doctors did not give Aids patients lethal injections. In 1994 an anthropologist watched Malawi's ancient *nyau* dance society satirise doctors equipped with camera and portable telephone reporting that they had found wasted villagers sick with Aids.[74] Ironically, the very sophistication of the scientific understanding of HIV – the fact that doctors knew almost everything about it except how to cure it – made their knowledge more difficult to convey. The notion of an invisible virus might be presented as a tiny insect. Ethiopians tried to explain a fatal but symptomless disease by the analogy of termites hollowing out a tree before it fell, yet many doctors found it impossible to convey the profoundly alien idea that people 'are understood as ill before they are ill'.[75] Some patients thought the doctors were lying. Even if their ability to test for HIV might give them credit, their inability to cure it, reinforced by their obligation to say so, gravely damaged their prestige. The conclusion of the Durban Declaration of 2000 – 'Science will one day triumph over AIDS, just as it did over smallpox' – sounded like bravado.[76]

It certainly sounded that way to traditional moralists, for whom the epidemic was primarily an evil consequence of Western innovations, of towns, prostitution, promiscuity, youthful disobedience, and the abandonment of inherited morality. Such moral explanations of disease were normal in pre-scientific societies, to which disease on a collective scale was a consequence of collective offence and a symptom of social disorder. The confrontation between this traditional moralism and medical rationalism was most acute in Botswana, the most vigorously modernising of African states, whose leaders, until late in the epidemic, made only timid attempts to integrate the indigenous healers whom President Mogae once described as 'a nuisance and a distraction'.[77] Botswana's medical authorities championed the WHO's safer sex message – Abstain, Be faithful, Condomise – against hostility to public discussion of sex and the perceived immorality of condoms as unnatural, distasteful, and likely to encourage promiscuity and spread disease. Against this programme many of Botswana's influential traditional healers set the belief that HIV/Aids was in fact an old 'Tswana' disease reactivated by neglect of Tswana culture and morality. This disease was *boswagadi*, hitherto caused chiefly by having sex with a widow or widower whose year of mourning had not been ended by ritual purification. The diagnosis offered an explanation of *why* an individual had been infected, gave a reassuring sense that the epidemic was potentially controllable, and, because the infected person might not have known the condition of his partner, reduced the implicit guilt and shame. Analogies between HIV/Aids and older diseases incurred through violations of sexual prohibitions were widespread throughout southern Africa, although the connections were generally disputed by other healers who insisted that Aids was entirely new. Similar dispute surrounded possible analogies with *mwanza* disease in Gabon and Congo-Brazzaville, *chira* among the Luo of Kenya, and *amenmin* in Ethiopia.[78] Identical or not, in all these cases Aids and the old diseases were explained in moral terms as almost automatic consequences of sexual irregularity. By contrast, the use of indigenous religious resources to protect communities against HIV has seldom been described outside the DR Congo,[79] perhaps because HIV had generally established itself silently before such protection could be mounted.

A second explanation of HIV/Aids in indigenous terms ascribed it to witchcraft. This was common early in the epidemic west of Lake Victoria, when little was known of the disease and the numbers affected were small enough to be blamed on personal malevolence, but once HIV spread widely it was seldom attributed to witchcraft there, although this remained a more common explanation in less developed areas.[80] Perhaps that was a general pattern. The areas where the association was strongest were the western equatorial region, where witchcraft was especially prominent in popular thought of all kinds, and remote rural districts, notably in Zambia. In the Chiawa area on the border with Zimbabwe, for example, villagers urged by Aids educators to take action against the disease did so in 1994–5 by simultaneously applying for a World Bank loan and calling in a witchfinder, 'Chaka Zulu', who caused sixteen deaths before the authorities suppressed him. Ten years later, in Kaoma on Zambia's western border, vigilantes called Karavinas (from 'carbine') killed numerous suspected witches alleged to be responsible for the symptoms of Aids. As a Kenyan pointed out, to blame Aids on witchcraft, rather than individual behaviour, reduced stigma and 'creates another dimension of hope', since counter-measures might be possible.[81]

As both HIV/Aids and elements of scientific explanation were incorporated into indigenous thought, hybrid and often contradictory understandings took shape, as was normal during epidemics elsewhere. People might believe simultaneously, for example, that tiny insects caused the disease but that witchcraft explained why it infected them.[82] This hybridity was equally clear in traditional medicine. Despised by colonial and modern African doctors, it had regained some prestige after independence as an expression of cultural nationalism, had enjoyed WHO backing, and had attracted patients neglected by the decaying modern medical systems of the 1980s, but HIV/Aids further swelled the numbers seeking treatment and gave indigenous healers the opportunity to demand a more equal relationship with Western medicine. Although some healers made extravagant claims to cure Aids, most – often following official warnings – professed only to treat opportunistic infections. HIV ideally fitted this strategy, with its brief spell of fever at the time of infection followed by a long, asymptomatic period. 'We can make the viruses sleep for some time but not kill them,' a Zambian healer explained in 1998. 'Provided the sick person comes to us early enough, he or she can have the virus sleep continually for up to ten years before he or she can die. You just give the person bitter herbs and then the virus sleeps again.'[83] Moreover, healers were very numerous: estimates in South Africa ranged up to

350,000.[84] They could offer the personal attention that patients sought fruitlessly in overcrowded modern institutions. As a patient explained:

> When I can, I come to stay with a traditional healer. He prays for me and warms and blesses water that he puts over my whole body. I had a big ulcer on my back and the healer applied herbs that took the sore away. The healer allows me to drink hospital medicine for my TB. He prays to God, not the ancestors, for the cure. He will be able to make me better but he will not be able to cure the virus.[85]

As this quotation shows, although healers were individualistic entrepreneurs, they were often keen to incorporate modern practices and gain official recognition. One successful specialist in Côte d'Ivoire maintained a 100-bed 'hospital', a hostel for visitors, a pharmacy, a plantation of medicinal herbs, and a factory to process them.[86] Western-trained doctors had long resisted merging of the two medical systems. Members of the Nigerian Medical Association declared that recognising traditional healers would be like licensing killers.[87] But some nationalist regimes, led by Zimbabwe in 1981, had given them legal recognition and many moved in this direction during the Aids epidemic, arguing, in Museveni's words, 'that since modern medicine has no answer to this problem, let us encourage our people to carry out their own research either by scientific methods or by empirical observation'. Even Nigeria admitted that traditional healers might be useful 'when armed with accurate information'.[88] Often the medical authorities intended 'cooperation' to mean little more than encouraging healers to distribute condoms, adopt hygienic practices, educate their patients, and refer Aids cases to modern medical institutions. South Africa's Traditional Health Practitioners Act of 2004 specifically banned unregistered healers from diagnosing or treating terminal diseases such as Aids.[89] But sometimes the collaboration went further, notably in Uganda, where in 1992 activists from TASO and Médecins sans Frontières created THETA (Traditional Healers and Therapies Against Aids) to foster 'active respectful collaboration between traditional healers and medical doctors combating AIDS in Uganda ... a forum where a dialogue between doctors and healers could be initiated at an equal level, given the absence of cure or vaccine for AIDS'. THETA subjected herbal medicines to formal testing, found remedies for *herpes zoster* and chronic diarrhoea allegedly more effective than Western drugs, packaged these for wider distribution, and by 2004 had trained 1,700 healers in Aids treatment and counselling. 'A client may come convinced of bewitchment,' one explained, 'but since the THETA training I know that the client may need to go for an HIV test. I provide treatment to cleanse the bewitchment and suggest that the client get a medical check.'[90]

The conflict between traditional and Western medicine was echoed in other responses to the epidemic. One subject of intense controversy in several areas was 'widow inheritance', by which a widow in a patrilineal society might be expected to enter the household of a male relative of her dead husband. The advantage was that she could continue to care for her children, who belonged to their father's lineage. The disadvantage in the time of Aids, in addition to the constraint on the woman's freedom, was that an infected widow might transmit disease to her new husband, possibly during the ritual 'cleansing' by sexual intercourse that customarily inaugurated the new relationship – a custom itself offensive to Christians and many widows. In southern Zambia, where the custom was widespread, the ritual intercourse was largely replaced during the 1990s by more symbolic acts, despite opposition. In the Nyanza province of Kenya the issue became the focus of deeper antagonism between born-again Christians and traditionalists, one blaming the custom and the other its neglect for the area's high HIV prevalence. Some suspected that moral opposition to the custom concealed anxiety to evade responsibility for supporting widows and orphans.[91]

Similar controversy often surrounded other potentially dangerous customs such as initiation rites and promiscuous sex at weddings or funerals. Ethiopia created a special National Committee on Traditional Practices to handle these issues. But there were also vigorous attempts to restore abandoned customs thought to have restrained promiscuity. Uganda attempted to revitalise the *senga*, the father's sister who had given sexual instruction to adolescent girls. Senior Zulu women, with royal approval, launched a campaign in 1993 to restore the testing of unmarried girls' virginity, a campaign denounced by South Africa's Gender Equality and Human Rights Commissions but quite widely accepted by girls as a source of solidarity and respect in a dangerous environment.[92]

Although Christians and traditionalists might quarrel over customs, they generally shared a strongly moralistic view of HIV/Aids. It was mainly from such religious perspectives that Africans viewed the epidemic, as they viewed other large issues of the time, especially where political leaders seldom took strong positions.[93] Many initial Christian responses to HIV were as hostile as secular reactions. Some Protestant churches in Kenya refused to admit people with HIV/Aids or to bury those who died from it. A Catholic priest there is also reported to have refused to conduct funeral services, saying that 'the church might be seen to be encouraging the spread of the disease'. These extreme reactions passed, but people with HIV/Aids continued to complain of discrimination in church and moral condemnation remained strong, especially perhaps where a harsh protestantism was superimposed over traditional moralism.[94] From that perspective, in the words of an independent church leader in Botswana, HIV/Aids was 'a punishment sent by God, as Sodom and Gomorrah. Today we have all kinds of unnatural things – homosexuality, Satanist cults who practice cannibalism, ritual murders, bestiality. Christ is the one who said that those who do such things are cursed already.' A study in South Africa found that sternly moralistic pentecostal churches were the most successful in disciplining their members' sexual behaviour.[95] The larger historic churches, by contrast, generally avoided a crude providentialism, as those in Zambia declared in 1988:

> We may admit that in many cases AIDS is the result of moral faults, without falling into an over-simple view that the epidemic is a direct intervention by God into human history to punish us for sins committed. We must rather recognise a revolt of nature against being abused and ask ourselves what God its Author is saying to us through this plague which in His providence he has allowed to afflict us.[96]

Other religions also struggled to respond to the epidemic. In Botswana the Sedimo healing cult was swamped by supplicants for protective amulets, which were refused to advanced cases.[97] The most striking use of indigenous religious ideas, although blended with Christianity, was the movement in Malawi in 1994–5 surrounding Billy Goodson Chisupe, an elderly adherent of the Providence Industrial Mission, who dreamed that ancestral spirits instructed him to use tree bark to make a cleansing medicine to cure HIV/Aids. Recipients called it *mchape*, a generic term for such medicines in this area. For success it required the recipient to abandon promiscuity. By May 1995 perhaps 300,000 people had made pilgrimage to Chisupe, including staff of the Aids Control Programme:

> As one ... middle-class professional mused, wouldn't it be wonderful if *mchape did* work! It would put Malawi on the world map; it would show Westerners that Malawi had something to offer, that Malawian traditional medicine wasn't so stupid. That *they* weren't so stupid, she also seemed to imply. Of course, she added, it was admittedly only a wild card, but afraid as she was she might be infected with HIV from her former husband, she radiated hope.[98]

Muslims, too, had to respond to the epidemic. In remote areas the reaction was probably often harsh. 'Encountering HIV/AIDS is a sign of punishment from Allah,' a leader in southern Ethiopia declared. 'A victim is believed to have contracted it because he/she broke Allah's guidelines.... Helping a patient could be justifying his/her acts.' Others were struck by the low HIV prevalence in many Muslim regions. Abbasi Madani, the Algerian fundamentalist leader, stressed that the skills of modern medicine were helpless against Aids, for which the only remedy was moral reform.[99] Yet Muslims were also active in public education. When Dr Babatunde Osotimehin was appointed to head Nigeria's National Aids Commission, his first action was to gain the support of the Sultan of Sokoto, the country's most influential religious leader. Cooperation between the Aids Control Programme and Muslim leaders in Senegal began in 1988. There and in Mali the disease and the behaviour it compelled were regular topics in Friday sermons. In Uganda the Chief Kadhi declared a *jihad* against Aids in 1989.[100] The most progressive leaders insisted that people with HIV/Aids must be embraced within Islam's powerful charitable traditions: 'Since very long ago, Islam has rejected stigmatisation, marginalisation. Islam has invited people to accept the sick. We are not the judges; only God is judge.'[101] Everywhere, however, teaching was within a moralistic framework.

This was true also of Christians as they moved from condemnation to active measures against the disease. The Ethiopian Orthodox Church began to train priests in Aids work in 1998. Its Patriarch instructed his clergy to include Aids education in their sermons and Sunday Schools. He took a leading part in the first National Religious Aids Week – declaring the church's policy to be 'virginity from birth to marriage and loyalty from marriage to death' – and he sat with other religious leaders on the National Council on HIV/AIDS, as was normal in most African countries.[102] Uganda's Aids Commission was chaired successively by Protestant and Catholic bishops. Clergy and doctors gradually realised that the epidemic required both medical and moral responses. Moreover, as will be seen later, the Christian churches had from the first provided care for those suffering from the disease. In 1998 Archbishop Bonifatius Haushiku launched Namibia's first national church-based programme of prevention and care after himself undergoing training as an Aids worker.[103]

Two issues especially divided religious moralists from medical pragmatists. One concerned the use of condoms, over which there was extreme diversity of opinion and practice. Roman Catholic leaders generally denounced them as contravening the divine purpose of procreation, encouraging promiscuity, and actually fostering HIV. They were legitimate only between married couples where one partner was infected. Protestant fundamentalists generally agreed, as did the Ethiopian Church and almost all Muslim leaders. In 1996 Cardinal Otunga and the Imam of Nairobi's central mosque jointly presided over a public bonfire of condoms.[104] This opposition led to numerous confrontations with medical and social workers. 'We go around teaching people about condoms and encouraging them to use them if they can't avoid sex. The [Catholic] church follows in our steps telling people how those who use condoms pave their way to eternal hell,' a District Medical Officer in Rakai complained.[105] Under this pressure, and because Museveni himself doubted the efficacy of condoms, Uganda was slow to popularise them and long banned their advertisement on television and radio. Similar controversy and hesitation ruled in Zambia, where the born-again President Chiluba prohibited television advertising but his successor restored it.[106] Generally, however, medical opinion prevailed and most African states mounted condom promotion programmes, although they preferred to let American social marketing organisations operate them. As the director of Senegal's Aids programme put it, 'We let the Imam talk about religion and fidelity, while we talk about condoms.'[107] Nor was religious opinion united. The powerful Anglican church in Nigeria supported use of condoms, as did some branches of the Lutheran church and the All-African Conference of Churches. One representative of the Ethiopian Church described its attitude in practice as 'not see, not hear'.[108] That was also true of some Catholic dioceses, apparently including Kinshasa and Kigali. Some casuists argued that in the circumstances of a generalised Aids epidemic, condoms might be a means of protecting life rather than destroying it.[109]

Similar conflict surrounded sex education – often called life skills education – in schools, where moralistic pressure was more effective because it generally had the support of parents, who viewed such instruction as encouraging promiscuity, and of many teachers, who found the subject embarrassing. Uganda was the pioneer here as part of its general policy of openness, but plans to follow suit in Kenya were vetoed by President Moi in response to religious opposition, while in Tanzania, Zambia, and Ethiopia controversy obstructed the incorporation of sex education into the syllabus well into the 2000s. Rwanda, Botswana, and Zimbabwe, by contrast, had extensive coverage, but in 2002 no Aids teachers were yet active in Senegalese schools. In equatorial Africa the Catholic church introduced its own programme of 'Education for life and love'. UNAIDS reckoned that in 2003 nearly 60 per cent of primary school pupils in sub-Saharan Africa received basic Aids education.[110]

The moralistic response to Aids drew strength, especially in eastern and southern Africa from a pervasive sense that the epidemic was only part of a wider crisis afflicting late twentieth-century Africa, a crisis combining destabilisation of indigenous cultures with failure of the modernisation expected at independence. Meja Mwangi's novel, *The Last Plague* (2000), captured this sense of crisis, and Gabriel Rugalema, perhaps the most perceptive analyst of the rural epidemic, observed it in Kagera:

> What is distinctive about the local views ... is the integration of the disease with wider socio-economic problems, as opposed to the prevailing scientific approach in which HIV is seen to cause AIDS and consequently adult mortality. Villagers are not reductionists. Their view is that AIDS and its effects cannot be separated from the wider social and economic environment.[111]

This was in a tradition of African thought, which had commonly attributed famine or epidemic to the breakdown of the social and political order. It was also in a tradition of religious thought, for some Christians saw the epidemic as a prelude to the end of the world. And even a medical pragmatist like Kapita Bila, perhaps the first man to witness the epidemic, diagnosed a crisis in the very modernity that his medical skill embodied. 'The Aids of the late twentieth century,' he wrote, 'judges our society, our morality, and the direction of our economic progress. Today's society seems to have attained the level of evolution required for its own destruction.'[112]

10
NGOs
& the Evolution of Care

Just as the nature of the immunodeficiency virus chiefly determined its pattern of expansion, so it also compelled societies to erect particular kinds of defences. Whereas easily transmitted and rapidly fatal diseases like the 'three-day flu' of 1918 had demanded brief, urgent, and predominantly medical responses, the years of incubation and months of terminal decline characteristic of HIV created an overwhelming need for long-term care. African governments, impoverished by economic depression and structural adjustment, could not provide this. Instead, late twentieth-century culture offered another model: the non-governmental organisations already active both in global relief work and in many smaller welfare functions in African countries. Along with government bodies, NGOs were largely responsible for preventive work and the support of HIV-positive people during the incubation stage. Initially they also attempted to care for those sick with Aids, but the numbers quickly overwhelmed them and instead this burden fell chiefly on the patients' families. It was a cruel burden, for in their final months of illness people with Aids needed much intimate and distressing care. Family responses varied, but predominantly they – and 'they' meant chiefly women – provided care with a selflessness that was one of the most heroic features of the epidemic. This was not unique to Africa: Aids epidemics everywhere evoked remarkable displays of compassion.[1] What was unique to Africa was the scale of the response in a continent where HIV/Aids was, in this as in other senses, a family disease. Had Africa's family systems been less resilient, the impact of the first Aids epidemic could have been terrible beyond imagining.

The scale and diversity of NGO action defy summary. In 1992 Uganda already had over 600 NGOs involved in Aids work; by 2003 there were about 2,000. Kisumu, the provincial capital of Kenya's heavily infected Nyanza province, had over 200 NGOs and community-based organisations combating Aids in 1999.[2] Senegal was also rich in organisations, over 700 receiving public subsidies during 2004, the same number as those affiliated to Nigeria's Aids programme. South Africa had a vigorous NGO tradition, inherited especially from the anti-Apartheid movement, and counted over 700 bodies engaged in Aids work as early as 1993. Ethiopia, by contrast, lacked such a tradition and had suffered between 1974 and 1991 a government with totalitarian aspirations; in 2002 it had only 103 NGOs concerned with Aids.[3] The number in the DR Congo is unknown, but none attracted wide attention.

NGOs everywhere were a jumble of established national welfare bodies (church organisations, Muslim charitable societies, medical-related associations like the Red Cross), international relief agencies, and locally constituted organisations of all kinds, operating at every level down to the individual town or neighbourhood. Most do not appear to have grown out of existing networks and organisations but to have been created ad hoc to meet immediate needs. Some held to a single function or target group. Others frequently began with such a function but branched out to meet a diversity of needs, tending to move from prevention towards care as the epidemic itself evolved. Others again were vast multi-purpose operations like World Vision, which in 2000 was engaged in 786 projects in 25 African countries.[4] The most common motive for involvement was religious, followed by simple compassion, personal experience of HIV in oneself or one's associates, desire for rewarding employment amidst a scarcity of opportunities for educated people, and doubtless the hope of access to donor funding. Perhaps only organisations concerned with the rights of women or people with HIV/Aids had substantial political aims. NGOs were both a consequence and a cause of the depoliticisation of the epidemic.

Africa's best-known NGO was The Aids Support Organisation (TASO) in Uganda, 'the first indigenous NGO in Africa to respond to the needs of people living with HIV'.[5] It was founded in 1987 by Noerine Kaleeba, a physiotherapist whose husband had died painfully of Aids, together with Elly Katabira, who needed trained counsellors for his newly opened Aids clinic, and a group of acquaintances, nearly all of whom soon died of the disease. They aimed to combat the prevailing stigmatisation and neglect of people with Aids by teaching them to 'live positively'. As Kaleeba put it, 'We emphasised *living* rather than *dying* with AIDS.'[6] Initial finance came largely from a British agency, Action Aid, and TASO remained heavily dependent on overseas donors, who provided 97 per cent of its income in 1999.[7] Its offices were generally at government medical institutions and some of its techniques were learned from similar bodies in Britain. Its methods became a model for many parts of the continent. Its counsellors generally met clients before and after testing for HIV. If the test was positive, the client was told its implications, encouraged to inform at least one trusted person, advised on how to protect health and practise safe sex, guided to plan purposively for the future, invited to participate in a supportive post-test group of infected people, given access to basic medical care, and provided if necessary with small quantities of food and other assistance. Many clients were trained as counsellors, which became the most important element of TASO's work without, as happened with some other NGOs, replacing its direct care for large numbers of clients. In 2003 TASO held 75,263 counselling sessions. By the end of that year it had supported over 100,000 people with HIV/Aids, about two-thirds of them women, and was the largest organisation of its kind in Africa, although it reached fewer than 10 per cent of infected Ugandans from its nine regional centres, having deliberately limited its expansion in order to maintain its effectiveness.[8] TASO made an interesting contrast with its closest Senegalese counterpart, the National HIV/Aids Alliance, formed in 1995 as the agent of an international support organisation, providing services similar to TASO's but operating through branch committees (*cellules*) dominated by state welfare employees rather than private activists and people with HIV/Aids, with whom there was often considerable tension.[9]

To provide counselling and train counsellors were among the first tasks taken up by NGOs in many countries. In Zambia, hospital staff in Lusaka established the Kara Counselling Trust in 1989 to complement testing facilities. In 1994 its director described the counsellors' difficulties in discussing sexual behaviour with their clients, explaining the operation of the virus, and handling their own fears of infection. Of the 101 counsellors she studied, only 24 had themselves taken a test and only 27 had ever used a condom.[10] To meet these difficulties, the Trust, like TASO and many similar organisations, increasingly concentrated on training people with HIV/Aids, who were generally thought to make particularly sympathetic and convincing counsellors.

In the field of preventive education, another early priority for NGOs, the pioneer organisation in Zambia was the Copperbelt Health Education Project (CHEP), created in 1988 by a doctor whose inability to cure HIV/Aids convinced him to concentrate on trying to prevent it. 'Our work,' he later wrote, 'was based on the assumption that ordinary people, once informed about the disease and how it is spread, would be able to make the necessary changes in their sexual behaviour. We have since realised that this assumption was somewhat simplistic, but it seemed reasonable at the time.'[11] They were especially concerned to combat the negative character of official Aids campaigns, adopting the slogan, 'We spread knowledge not fear.' With Norwegian financial aid, CHEP became known for the sophistication of its mass education techniques, ranging from literature of all kinds through radio and television programmes to extensive use of peer educators, mainly targeting youth and high-risk groups. Special concern for these was another NGO priority. In 1989 a Nigerian doctor and his sociologist wife founded Action Health Incorporated, initially at their own expense, to spread Aids information among young people from a youth centre in northern Lagos. With external funding, it created Health and Life Planning Clubs in local schools, trained hundreds of peer educators, and took the lead in producing guidelines for sex education in Nigeria.[12] Another target group were sex workers, addressed, for example, by Tasintha, a Zambian organisation, formed in 1992, that conducted community education in schools, helped sex workers to protect themselves by using condoms and seeking treatment for sexually transmitted diseases, and in particular sought to train them in vocational skills by which they could make alternative livelihoods. By 2000 it had trained 5,005 sex workers and could provide instruction in textile design, processing, and printing; knitting, crocheting, and embroidery; design, tailoring, and sewing; producing building materials; sisal weaving; baking; and book-keeping.[13]

Sex workers were naturally a special concern of the women who made up the bulk of NGO activists. Top leadership positions were often held by men, but this was not the case with the many organisations designed to care for and advance the general interests of women with HIV/Aids. Beatrice Were created the National Community of Women Living with Aids (NACWOLA) in Uganda for the women she cared for at Nsambya Hospital, after testing positive herself in 1991. By 1999 it claimed 46,000 members in 18 branches, provided mutual support groups and income-earning opportunities, and was active in advocating women's rights.[14] On a continental scale, the Society for Women and Aids in Africa (SWAA) was initiated in 1988 by professional women attending the Stockholm Aids Conference. Its most active leaders included Dr Eka Esu-Williams, who pioneered Nigerian interventions to aid sex workers, and Dr Nkandu Luo, later Zambia's Health Minister. While concentrating on advocacy on the continental scale, SWAA was unusually successful in creating a network of about thirty national branches frequently engaged in active Aids work. Tasintha in Zambia was one such outgrowth, while the Senegalese branch developed a micro-credit facility for women, Botswana's branch trained carers, Kano's was active in counselling, and Tanzania's was particularly engaged with Aids orphans.[15] Although HIV/Aids bore especially hard on women, it also provided them with opportunities to regain the active political role that they had often played in nationalist movements but had lost at independence. Their demands became increasingly effective as it became clear that improvement in the status of women was essential if the epidemic was to be controlled.

Like TASO, all but the smallest NGOs generally depended heavily on external funding, often to the extent of 95 per cent. The effect was seen dramatically after the establishment of majority rule in South Africa in 1994, when foreign money hitherto given direct to NGOs was channelled instead to the government, creating a crisis in the NGO sector. Poor people and those with HIV/Aids often viewed NGOs cynically as pork barrels for the elite. In 1995 Zimbabwe's Aids Counselling Trust, once a pioneer, was dissolved after auditors had found that in the previous year it had spent only 13,400 of its income of 1,400,000 Zimbabwean dollars on counselling, 670,000 on salaries and benefits for its 19 staff members, and 63,000 on the director's attendance at an International Aids Conference in Japan. Corruption and embezzlement by 'briefcase NGOs' became especially rife in the early 2000s when huge sums of money became available to provide antiretroviral drugs. In many countries a large proportion of NGOs were concentrated in the capital: 51 of the 66 registered in Cameroun in 2001, for example.[16] Their relations with governments were often uneasy. The impoverished Zambian government largely abandoned responsibility for HIV/Aids to NGOs, while seeking to prevent excessive foreign interference. In Uganda, too, governmental weakness before Museveni's take-over in 1986 led NGOs to establish direct ties with foreign donors, but one effect of the WHO's Global Programme was to strengthen the government's position, so that its subsequent relationship with NGOs, although sometimes fractious, was beneficial to both sides and to the country. Although the Ugandan government did not merely preside over an Aids campaign run by NGOs and international agencies, it did allow them considerable freedom of action. The situation in Senegal and Côte d'Ivoire was broadly similar, with the state concentrating on the medical sphere.[17] Other governments chafed at these constraints. The ANC regime in South Africa largely excluded NGOs – often white-controlled – from the policy formulation in which they had shared before 1994, leaving them to concentrate resentfully on grassroots work. Mali tried to confine each NGO to one *cercle*, which it would serve under government contract.[18] In 2004 UNAIDS rejected pressure from southern African ministers to channel all funds through governments rather than direct to NGOs, no doubt fearing that it would intensify corruption and political manipulation.

During the 1990s, as the number of infected people passing from the incubation period to the stage of Aids increased, NGOs focused increasingly on care. Initially, many tried to provide that care themselves, but the need soon overwhelmed them and most withdrew to a role of supporting the family members who did the actual caring – 90 per cent of all care in Africa, according to a UNAIDS estimate in 2004.[19] That primary caregivers were family members was true of Aids epidemics in other continents; the remarkable features in Africa were the sheer scale of the task and the difficulties under which it was carried out.

Everywhere in the continent, it appears, families had a unique and morally inescapable obligation to care for their own. 'I have no choice, she is my sister,' a man in southern Malawi explained, 'the world would laugh at me if I did not take care of her.' This was doubly true of Aids, for the task was so demanding: 'If it is not your relative you can't do it.... It needs courage.... A mere neighbour will not agree to care.' Such physical care was indeed often the definition of love: 'to love a relative means not to be disgusted with patients' dirty things'.[20] But this widespread feeling left two questions open. One was whether the wider community also had a caring role. That varied between different regions, according to different circumstances, and at different times, for increasingly, as the epidemic worsened, charitable people realised the primary carer's need for community support. The other question was what constituted the family in this context: whether it was those who lived together, those who provided reciprocally for one another, or those of the same blood.

The evidence from Ghana is particularly interesting. In 1992 Joseph Anarfi interviewed patients and caregivers in several parts of the country. A few patients had been abandoned in hospitals by their relatives. Eleven per cent were caring for themselves. Only 9 per cent were being cared for by their wives and none by their husbands. Almost all the rest were in the care of blood kinsmen, above all their mothers, who were generally most sympathetic towards them. Sisters and (less) brothers were also relatively sympathetic but were not expected to become primary caregivers. Care could be rudimentary:

In one example, a young woman aged 20 years had been abandoned by the whole family but her mother. She had her own drinking cup, plates, and a bucket for washing and other purposes. She did all her toiletries in her room partly because she was too sick to move and partly due to the fact that she was not welcome on the public toilet in the village. In another case, the patient had been locked up in her room and food was passed to her under the door post. The fear of the members of the community is that knowledge of the presence of an AIDS-infected person in the family may result in others shunning it and, thereby, refusing to let their relatives marry into the affected family.[21]

This was a society where individuals always remained members of their natal clans and where marriages were easily broken by circumstances much less disastrous than HIV/Aids. Moreover, as Anarfi wrote, 'AIDS tends to weaken relationships with non-relatives. The family turns in on itself as neighbours reduce contacts with its members because of the shame attached to the disease.'[22] Another anthropologist remarked, 'The social "safety net" once offered by the corporate clan to its members appeared to be undergoing changes; it does not seem to provide the individual with the protection and support it once gave.'[23] Yet 80 per cent of the patients expressed satisfaction with their care. Four years later an anthropologist working in the Asante area of Ghana described less satisfied patients but a broadly similar situation, stressing that people with Aids often received only reluctant care because their youth contradicted the intergenerational reciprocity on which care normally rested, although they could nevertheless rely upon the kindness of their mothers. More distant relatives contributed little. The anthropologist quoted an Asante proverb: 'The family is like a forest. Standing afar it looks together, but when you get closer you see that each tree is different.'[24]

Both the importance and the limits of reciprocity emerge from research in 1999 in the Otukpo area of Benue state in central Nigeria, the most severely infected part of the country, with 23 per cent antenatal prevalence in what was still the early stage of an epidemic. The researchers identified three broad attitudes towards those with Aids. The wider local community was strongly hostile, as we have seen, to those with 'the Abuja disease', supposedly contracted as sex workers or migrants in the capital before they 'come home almost dead', bringing nothing but their disease to endanger and batten upon the area. Closer neighbours were somewhat less hostile but still unwilling to provide care or even to visit: 'Once AIDS is confirmed normal interactions with the family are curtailed. Usual practices like asking for drinking water, fetching fire, or even passing through the compound stop.' The family resented this stigma, complained of the burden of caring, and did everything possible to conceal their sick member, but they did nevertheless provide care: 'If you look at people's behaviour, you will not accept them but when yours is sick, he or she cannot be thrown away like dogs.' Moreover, for the family the shame of not caring was worse than the shame of Aids. The care it gave, however, was sometimes less than an ordinary invalid might expect, for Aids patients might be isolated, left alone, and visited only to serve food or when they called for assistance. The patients spoke of themselves as the living dead.[25]

The reasons why care in these West African cases was grudging were perhaps that prevalence was still relatively restricted there, disease was widely attributed to promiscuity outside the community, and marriage was fragile, at least in matrilineal Ghana. By contrast, Angela Chimwaza's study in 2000 of another matrilineal area, in southern Malawi, suggested a higher level of acceptance, not least because the disease was longer established and more widespread. Chimwaza stressed that care was immensely burdensome, fell overwhelmingly on one female relative – usually mother or wife – but was nevertheless accepted resignedly in rural areas as a self-evident obligation of kinship: 'there is nothing I can do but look after her'.[26] Yet she showed also that caregivers did receive a degree of material and moral (but rarely physical) support from community members, especially because the community's core was a group of related women. 'We find that the social safety net is still functioning,' she reported. 'There was little evidence that either patients or caregivers were stigmatized.'[27] Other studies in Malawi broadly confirmed these findings, some showing a high level of support from friends and wider kin. 'We eat from the same plate,' one patient explained, 'they come to visit me whenever they see me sitting alone, they come to cheer me up.'[28]

A study in south-western Uganda, earlier in the epidemic, showed a broadly similar but perhaps less generous pattern. The thirty patients received care chiefly from their mothers, sisters, or wives. In thirteen cases the main caregiver received no assistance, while in fifteen there was help from close relatives, usually female. Neglect contributed to three of the seventeen deaths during the study period. The researchers described the extended family in this area as 'a safety net with holes', a description probably applicable very widely.[29] Across the Tanzanian border in Kagera, Gabriel Rugalema found, similarly, that 'Illness in Buhaya is perceived as a family affair and thus the rest of the village community has really no input in it besides visiting a household with a sick person to wish them well. Care provision was and continues to be shouldered by few female relatives.'[30]

Urban attitudes towards patients tended to be harsher, as they were reported to be also in later-infected rural areas, such as central Kenya, and especially in rural Ethiopia, where Aids cases were still quite rare in the early 2000s.[31] Studies in South Africa, similarly, revealed many cases of family rejection, but a survey of 728 Aids-affected households concluded in 2002 that 'Despite all the pressures, the safety net provided by the extended family was still holding, although often starting to fray.'[32] Everywhere there was great diversity of experience.

Although most Aids plans of the late 1980s did not make care a priority because few people had yet reached the stage of needing it, nevertheless patients already choked the beds at Mama Yemo, Mulago, and other hospitals in areas of early infection. Often they were discharged after only the most cursory treatment: 'A few days in bed, some aspirin, and then home to die,' as one observer put it. Uganda's plan of 1987, a model for others, specified that 'As soon as possible the AIDS patient should be referred to outpatient care, preferably in the extended family setting.' 'It is now essential,' a senior physician in Kinshasa insisted a year later, 'to prepare communities to accept and provide services for healthy HIV carriers and AIDS cases.'[33] Several strategies were attempted. One was the outpatient clinic pioneered by Katabira in 1987, drawing on TASO's counselling services. This model was implemented most extensively in francophone Africa, where the first was established at the University Hospital at Treichville in Abidjan in 1990 in association with a voluntary welfare organisation called Espoir. This was later imitated by outpatient treatment centres (*centres de traitement ambulatoire*) partnered by local welfare associations in ten other West and North African cities.[34] Yet this model could not serve the countryside or the bedridden who made up an increasing proportion of people with HIV/Aids in eastern and southern Africa. Many of these – as many as 94 per cent in Ethiopia in 2003, it was thought – never sought modern medical treatment at all.[35] Some method was needed to reach those dying in their homes with only the unskilled care of their families.

The first attempts to do this were made during 1987 by medical workers in Zambia and Uganda. Hospital-based home care, as it became known, had precedents in the treatment of tuberculosis and leprosy patients in the community and was extended to people with HIV/Aids in southern Zambia in 1987 by the Salvation Army Hospital at Chikankata, which found itself unable to provide beds for growing numbers of patients. By leaving patients in their homes to be visited by a mobile medical team from the hospital, it was argued, the system could treat larger numbers more cheaply, expand local knowledge, reduce stigma, foster family life, and allow patients to die in the home environment which they preferred to hospital. 'In 183 cases counselled in 1987,' it was reported, 'only four patients opted for hospital care rather than home-based care.' The cost was met largely by external donors. The Chikankata scheme was widely regarded at the time as a model of community-based activity.[36] By 1993 some 22 mission hospitals in Zambia were running home-based care programmes, although not all on the same pattern.[37] Meanwhile, such programmes were also launched during 1987 by two major Catholic hospitals in Uganda: Nsambya, which served mainly the poor of Kampala and its environs, and Kitovu, in Masaka district.[38] They were imitated by hospitals at Jinja in eastern Uganda and at Rubya in the Kagera region of Tanzania. The Catholic hospital at Agomanya in the highly infected Eastern Region of Ghana appears to have set up West Africa's first scheme of this kind in 1988. A group of hospitals in KwaZulu established a similar programme in 1991 on the model of Chikankata.[39]

Very soon, however, the number of patients and the cost of treatment made even hospital-based home care impracticable. In the countryside, especially, it was expensive in transport, which took up to three-quarters of the total cost, and in staff time, three-quarters of which was often spent travelling. The figures varied, but one home visit might cost as much as three to six days in hospital, even leaving aside the cost to the family caregivers. In the early 1990s both Chikankata and Nsambya were finding the expense insupportable, as very soon did the KwaZulu project.[40] Meanwhile the need became ever more urgent. 'When you visited houses,' a pioneer relief worker wrote of Rakai in 1989, '... there were dead bodies and hopeless relatives not knowing what to do, full of fear and hurt and shame.'[41]

The alternative developed in the early 1990s was to replace or supplement the travelling health staff by trained lay people based in the community to act as intermediaries between medical institutions and family caregivers. This reduced the cost by more than 90 per cent, according to a study in Zambia,[42] while greatly increasing the time that support workers could devote to each patient and family. Moreover, the new system could be implemented by NGOs not based in hospitals. It could even be implemented by community inter-mediaries themselves, perhaps by creating their own NGO. Either way, it released a force of largely female religious charity and community spirit that broke through Africa's widespread tradition that caring was almost entirely a family responsibility. It became also a community responsibility and the result came to be known as community-based home care, a term used very loosely to embrace both systems run by large NGOs and those launched by com-munity members. UNAIDS was later to describe it as 'one of the outstanding features of the epidemic'.[43]

The precise origins of community-based home care are hard to locate and probably diverse. TASO's lay activists, often themselves people with HIV, began to train and support family carers after the organisation's foundation in 1987.[44] The hospitals unable to sustain their initial schemes also helped to pioneer the new procedures. By 1993, for example, the more than 4,000 clients of Nsambya's home-care system were supported by volunteer com-munity caregivers backed by the original mobile health team:

> The community makes sure that patients are taken to the hospital, leads mobile medical teams to those who are too sick to travel, and even collects money every month to feed the poorer patients and help them wash and bathe. Their devotion has, it is reported, helped doctors at Nsambya reach 3–4 times as many AIDS patients as they could have without such a community support.[45]

This system illustrated the continuum of care from family to medical institution that became one of the principles of community-based home care. Chikankata moved in the same direction shortly afterwards, but the main pioneer in Zambia was the Catholic diocese of Ndola, which in 1991 initiated a programme that engaged 500 volunteer community workers in 25 town-ships at the end of the decade. Like many programmes it cared for all forms of chronic sickness in order to avoid stigmatising those with HIV/Aids.[46] Its counterpart in Zimbabwe was the Family Aids Caring Trust (FACT), founded in Mutare in 1987 on a strongly Christian base and active in all branches of welfare work connected with HIV, including a home-based care programme launched in 1989–90. By 1994 FACT employed 17 staff and 400 paid and unpaid volunteers.[47]

There were at least 67 home-care schemes in Zimbabwe in 1993, over 100 in Zambia in 1996, and over 85 in Malawi in 1998.[48] Most were run by charitable NGOs, with rather few organised by the carers themselves. Botswana, with a slightly later epidemic and a more effective government, adopted the system as national policy in 1992, to relieve its hospitals, but it was not until the late 1990s that communities responded with much enthusiasm, often preferring direct intervention by health workers. Gradually, however, energetic Tswana women broke through the prevailing silence:

> Tsholofelo Dibeela, Gakekgatlhege Lekgotla and Khumoetsile Sesiyane belong to a group of 21 volunteers who care for AIDS patients. With one exception, they're all women.

They visit in groups. So they can divide the tasks – feeding or bathing patients, counselling, collecting wood and water, or doing laundry – amongst themselves. Sometimes, families leave all the chores to them....

These three volunteers say they haven't taken a break from their work since they started. They don't fear possible infection during care, and they're confident about what they do. 'We have the necessary materials like heavy duty gloves, disposable gloves and gowns, but we do need masks,' says Sesiyane.

They love the work, they say. But they feel helpless and disheartened by the poverty their patients live in.[49]

Many activists hoped to be paid and it was often necessary to introduce incentives to sustain early enthusiasm. But there were other rewards. 'Since we began volunteering other people look at us differently,' a Mozambican community worker explained:

Often, when we pass someone on a walkway in the barrio, that person will give us a special gesture of dignity because of our work.... They say that we are people that can help others.... When someone is sick, the community leaders come to us for help. Before we were nobodies. So now we feel good; we feel honoured.[50]

In Uganda the first community-based home-care programmes established by TASO and Nsambya were supplemented in the early 1990s by a revival of *munno mukabbi* (friend in need) groups among women in heavily infected areas like Rakai. Trained by an Irish NGO, Concern, they offered both herbal medicine and basic care to needy families, especially those with Aids patients, each of the more than 400 caregivers being responsible for one zone of a village. 'The driving forces keeping these volunteers active are the underlying companionship of other group members, monthly meetings and ongoing support from the village coordinator,' it was reported.[51] Nearby, in Masaka, Kitovu Hospital trained community social workers who operated in pairs in their home areas, visiting and caring for Aids patients and orphans. They elected their own coordinator and, if still active after 18–24 months, received bicycles to increase their mobility.[52] The most important home-care organisation in Tanzania, WAMATA (from the Swahili for People Struggling Against Aids in Tanzania), was founded in 1989 in response to deaths among the elite in Dar es Salaam, but with training from TASO and Chikankata it focused increasingly on the poor and grew into an NGO of the hierarchical variety, with six major urban branches and fifty smaller ones by the late 1990s.[53]

Kenya was slower to develop home-care programmes of any kind, but the Medical Mission Sisters initiated a remarkable scheme in the Korogocho (Rubbish) shanty town of Nairobi, where they worked in 1998 through some 68 trained volunteer health workers from the township's Christian communities, who were supervised by professional nurses, served without material reward, helped to nurse the sick, and trained the children of Aids patients to care for their parents and eventually their siblings.[54] Ethiopia was also slow to move in this field. An Organisation for Social Services for Aids began to train home-care workers in 1992, but a year later 90 per cent of respondents in part of Addis Ababa stated that people with HIV should be cared for in hospital rather than at home, while a survey in 2000 found that reluctance to care for an infected relative at home was twice as high in the countryside as in towns. Little had by then been achieved outside the capital.[55]

In South Africa the activists who helped to draft the NACOSA plan of 1994 made home care their first priority. When they were then excluded from policy issues, their energies turned instead to organising care programmes, a field in which central government was slow to act. By 2003–4, South Africa had 892 recorded 'Home and community based care programmes ... with over 50,000 beneficiaries', implying that most were very small.[56] One of the largest was the Masoyi Home Based Care Project, which was modelled on FACT in Zimbabwe and was based in a remote area of the northern province of Mpumalanga but by 2002 had stimulated the formation of 28 similar projects scattered through Mpumalanga, Swaziland, Mozambique, and Zambia. Strongly Christian in ethos, it worked through uniformed volunteers who received between four and six months training and enjoyed a certain elite status in local eyes. More typical, in terms of scale, was Tateni Home Care Services, which was launched in Mamelodi, near Pretoria, by retired nurses who used a container as an office, taught their caring skills to family members, treated all manner of sickness in addition to HIV/Aids, and relied entirely on local and provincial funding.[57] Nearby, in Sebokeng, Grace Lengane, one of the founders of Vaal Aids Home-Based Care, recalled

> the bleak situation the programme had to grow from. When it first began in 1998, disclosure was synonymous to a death sentence. PLAs were not only ostracised by community members but also ran the risk of being rejected by their own families.... An additional stigma was attached to community members who were involved in HIV/Aids care and prevention. Ms Lengane remembers that several people in the community immediately thought that the whole staff of the fledgling Vaal Aids Home-based Care must all be infected. Otherwise, why would they care so much?[58]

The largest home-care organisation in southern Africa was in Namibia, where Catholic Aids Action, a countrywide organisation founded in 1998, had in 2002 some 39 staff and over 1,000 volunteers with 84 hours of training, organised into local groups with a formal status within the church. Hundreds more were waiting for training. Its model had been the Ndola Catholic Diocese programme.[59]

West Africa was remarkably slow to organise support for home carers, even taking into account that the epidemic spread more slowly there and prevalence was generally lower. Anglophone countries concerned themselves first, but to little lasting effect. By 1994 several Ghanaian institutions provided hospital-based home care, but the difficulty and cost of transport appear to have frustrated this, for Ghana's Aids plan for 2001–5 admitted that 'The provision of an effective and integrated continuum of care for PLWHA [people living with HIV/Aids] in health institutions and at home has not received adequate attention.' In Nigeria, too, initiatives to stimulate community-based home care during the 1990s achieved little. In Otukpo an energetic community programme launched with British funding in 1999 revealed the dangers of external intervention when a television documentary publicised the area as the epicentre of the national epidemic, leading local residents to complain that 'unworthy' people were being privileged, to ostracise those infected, and to close down the programme.[60] Of francophone countries, Côte d'Ivoire began to train a few home-care visitors during the mid 1990s and Burkina slightly later, but Aids plans prepared in 2001–2 showed little interest in the subject and it was only an international conference on community care of people with HIV/Aids in Dakar in December 2003 that alerted governments to their backwardness in this field. 'Community care is the weak link in Senegal's policy to counter Aids,' Professor Salif Sow observed at that time. 'Called continuum of care, this therapeutic approach has already proved itself in certain countries, above all in the anglophone world. Its results are considered positive.'[61]

Most patients and carers seem to have preferred home care during the last stages of disease, although a proportion of observers and caregivers disagreed, especially as the epidemic grew more burdensome.[62] At home the patient was protected from hospital infections and abuses, need not fear abandonment, could expect at least basic attention, and could die among kin rather than in the loneliness of a hospital ward. The caregiver, who would otherwise have to accompany the patient to hospital, avoided that cost, was spared the expense of transporting the patient's body home for burial, and could continue with domestic and agricultural work. This last advantage was especially important to the women who provided the vast majority of care, which was almost universally seen as a female duty within the customary sexual division of labour – in Lesotho women actively discouraged men from interfering – although as the epidemic proceded there were indications of greater involvement by men. Most patients were young adults and their most common caretaker was their mother, although wives and female relatives of all kinds might be involved. In the mid 1990s an estimated 21 per cent of all Zambian women were caring for someone with HIV/Aids.[63] Home care was indeed a euphemism for women's work. And it was terrible work:

> Looking after her son ... was ... difficult for Serina since he is a man. It was awkward caring for him physically and she had to listen to him cry and scream at night. He was heavy to carry and could not go to the toilet on his own. She had to tear up her bed sheets to clean him and to make nappies. Serina was upset by Tom's physical appearance during the illness. He had been a big man before he became ill and later she could 'see his bones'. However, she would not have wanted anyone other than family members to physically care for her ill children, i.e. to bathe them.[64]

Such tasks were especially difficult where running water, palliative drugs, and other facilities were lacking. Most caregivers had not been told their patient's diagnosis. Even if they suspected it – which observers thought was often the case – they could not protect themselves without revealing their suspicion to the patient.[65] To deny it was also necessary in order to avoid the stigma and isolation that caring for an Aids patient attracted. Moreover, few caregivers had equipment with which to protect themselves. There is some anecdotal evidence of carers contracting the disease and more of them fearing to do so. 'Last night I woke up screaming,' one said, 'I lit the lamp and jumped out of bed. I shook my clothes and rubbed my legs. I had been dreaming that my legs were covered with sores. After that I could not sleep. This dream has been occurring for the last two months every night, but some nights the sores are either in my mouth or on my face.'[66] Caregivers who were themselves already infected had the added distress of watching a fate that awaited them. In practical terms, too, Aids patients could be hypersensitive and difficult. A Ugandan woman who had nursed two dying daughters became partially paralysed whenever she heard a Land Rover that might be bringing home her only surviving child.[67] One study of caregivers found that about half spent up to three hours a day in patient care, a demand that grew as the disease progressed.[68]

For the patients the limitations of home care were even more painful. One group of people with HIV/Aids in Malawi described it as a dumping ground for those the hospitals wanted to be rid of. Others labelled it home neglect or managed death. A careful study of 33 home-care schemes in Zimbabwe in the mid 1990s found that almost half did not meet even half of the minimum criteria.[69] Not only did many caregivers have little idea how to care for their patients, but they were often too poor to provide the medicines, painkillers, and especially food that were needed. During a severe food scarcity in 2002, several patients in Zambia were reported to be refusing discharge from hospital for fear of dying from hunger at home.[70] The notion of a continuum of care from home to hospital seldom operated in practice because medical and welfare services lacked resources. One survey in Zimbabwe in the late 1990s found that only 2 per cent of the needed home visits were made. Even in Botswana, with a relatively well-funded welfare system, 58 per cent of home-cared patients studied in the mid 1990s were not visited by health workers. In South Africa, where the ANC government gave high priority to welfare grants, fewer than 16 per cent of Aids-affected households surveyed in the early 2000s received a grant, although all were entitled to one and over one-quarter benefited from an old age pension.[71]

Some observers believed that the most effective way to improve Aids care would be to subsidise the families who were still available and willing to provide it. For others, the major problem was that medical welfare or community support simply did not reach most households at all, not least because the numbers needing it were thought at the end of the century to be growing at least five times faster than the support networks. In Zimbabwe, FACT, one of the most effective organisations, reckoned in 1994 that support services reached fewer than 3 per cent of those needing them within its area of operation. A national survey of Zambia at the same period found that only 26 per cent of carers received support from any agency. The equivalent proportion in Botswana in 2002 was thought to be 57 per cent. In 2004, UNAIDS estimated that about 12 per cent of the people in sub-Saharan Africa needing assisted home care were receiving it.[72]

UNAIDS policy was that home care should be integrated with state health systems. Some feared that this might suffocate the community initiative on which the whole movement relied, but the most effective governments, as in Senegal and Botswana, began to move in this direction. Uganda sought to link home care to its decentralised local government structure. In South Africa the central government was slow to intervene in this field and the lead was taken by the provincial authorities in KwaZulu-Natal, who began to construct a network of paid carers linked to hospitals. Between 2001–2 and 2004–5, however, the central government's budget for home care rose from 25.5 million to 138 million rand, with the aim of eventually creating 2,400 home-care teams of paid volunteers.[73]

Perhaps the most glaring weakness of home care was its inability to relieve the acute pain that many terminal Aids patients suffered. In a study of terminal patients in home-care programmes around Kampala in 2000, 58 per cent declared pain and other symptoms to be their main concern.[74] Home carers lacked the necessary analgesics. So, frequently, did formal health institutions: in 1997 only two-fifths of university teaching hospitals surveyed had strong painkillers.[75] The main need was for morphine, rarely available in Africa but suitable for administration by trained caregivers. In many cases, however, proper terminal care required specialised institutions, since most ordinary hospitals refused to provide it. South Africa already had a number of hospices for the dying, generally founded for white cancer patients. During the 1990s most came instead to admit chiefly Aids patients. Many were so overwhelmed by the need that they also began to organise home-care systems. By 2002 some 57 institutions belonged to the Hospice Palliative Care Association of South Africa.[76] Several other institutions in southern Africa offered more rudimentary care or in some cases little more than places to die, mostly from charitable motives but occasionally as profit-making enterprises.[77] Hospices were rare in tropical Africa. One pioneer was Hospice Uganda, opened in 1993 as the nucleus of an outpatient scheme on condition that morphine should be made available to the terminally ill. In the early 2000s Uganda became the first African country to make palliative terminal care part of its national health plan, introduce specialist training in the field, and provide morphine free of charge, a step that other countries in eastern Africa began to follow.[78]

11
Death
& the Household

HIV/Aids was not one epidemic but four: first the virus, then disease, next death, and finally societal decomposition, each superimposed upon its predecessors. The timing of each epidemic varied with distance from the western equatorial epicentre and from the initial focus of infection in each region, but the sequence was the same everywhere. The process highlighted two distinctive features of heterosexual HIV/Aids as an epidemic disease. One was its slow incubation, which meant that individual deaths were spread across many years rather than concentrated in a brief period of mass mortality. During the influenza epidemic of 1918 in the South African town of Kimberley, so a missionary recalled, 'No coffins could be provided, as there was no one to make them; the dead were wrapped in blankets and piled one upon the others and taken in carts to the cemetery. Thirty at a time I have buried in a long grave, and we buried many three deep.'[1] During the Aids epidemic burials were equally common but for the most part individualised, with much of the ceremony that Africans had long devoted to them. This compounded another consequence of the virus's slow incubation: HIV/Aids was an impoverishing disease, disabling advanced cases from working while imposing heavy costs for months of medical care and the eventual funeral.

Here the second distinctive feature of the African epidemic was crucial. Heterosexual Aids was a family disease whose impact fell first and most heavily upon the household, with young adults as the chief victims. The result was a proliferation of orphaned children and elderly grandparents caring for them. The vulnerability of these new, misshapen households became clear during the famine that struck much of southern Africa in 2002, a 'new variant famine' that might herald a phase of societal decomposition. Yet here, too, the slow action of the virus shaped the epidemic, for by 2005 there was no evidence of the social disorder that had sometimes accompanied more explosive epidemics in the past. Nor was there necessarily reason to expect it.

Recognition that deaths were occurring on an unprecedented scale spread slowly behind the virus, between five and ten years after the epidemic struck each locality. A journalist reckoned that Kinshasa's people began to realise the scale of the crisis in 1986, at much the same time as Aids deaths became common in southern Uganda, Kagera, and Abidjan. An anthropologist working in Gaborone noticed few deaths among young adults in 1993, little discussion of the subject in 1995, and everyone talking about it in 1997. In Durban's cemeteries, burials of young people killed by disease rose rapidly from 1996, the year when deaths of young women first became markedly more frequent in South Africa as a whole.[2] In rural Masaka district in western Uganda, at the peak of the epidemic in 1990–2, the death rate among people aged 13–44 was 60 times higher for those with HIV than for those without. By 1999 Aids was sub-Saharan Africa's leading cause of death. Six years later, more than 13 million Africans had died of Aids and over 2 million were dying each year, or four each minute.[3]

Death became a central preoccupation. Because Africans generally rejected cremation, space for burials was a major concern for southern African city managers. By 2004 all but two of Durban's 53 cemeteries were full and the city needed to find between 14 and 22 hectares a year, public opinion having obliged the authorities to abandon the recycling of graves.[4] Almost every country town in South Africa had its stark field of freshly turned graves. Elsewhere, most Africans still buried the dead in their homesteads, a daily reminder of loss, although in parts of KwaZulu-Natal rural cemeteries were opened 'as kraals filled up too quickly'. 'They are burying them as if it is a competition,' a Zambian woman complained.[5] Catholic Aids Action in Namibia made and marketed *papier maché* coffins for the poor, but a respectable funeral might take four months of a worker's wages in southern Zambia and eleven months (for a child's funeral) in Kinshasa. A family plot in a South African private cemetery, complete with electrified security fence, could cost US$2,500.[6] The fence was to prevent grave robbing, a growing practice that mourners in Lusaka sought to prevent by immediately cementing over the grave.

'There are so many deaths these days, but most of them don't really make me feel much at all,' an anthropologist was told in Gaborone.[7] In southern Malawi or the Nyanza province of Kenya in the early 2000s it was normal for an adult to attend a funeral almost every weekend. Some southern African churches held collective weekly funerals.[8] Not to attend was to deny community and to risk being buried alone. Although funerals had always been major social events, they now pushed weddings and other ceremonies into the background, much as concern for death and grief might displace healing in the rituals of charismatic churches.[9] Yet an Aids death was not a normal death, hard as mourners tried to assert normal causes and enter them on the certificate. Whereas Africans had commonly buried the old amid celebrations of a life well lived, they had seen the death of young adults as unnatural and occasions for suspicion and grief. To these were now added the stigma of a shameful disease. In rural areas of the DR Congo several peoples devised rites to warn the ancestors that the addition to their ranks had offended lineage customs and to ensure that the deceased's spirit did not return to trouble the living. The corpse might be buried face down, with a large stone on the coffin, and the lineage elder might say: 'We do not know where your death has come from, but we ask you to take your fatal diarrhoea with you into the grave. Do not return to infect others. Go away! Never again return to the village.'[10] In Kenya, where some Protestant churches initially refused to bury people dying of Aids, Charles Nzioka reported that 'those who die of AIDS or related illnesses are assumed not to have the chance of life-after-death'. Their funerals, he claimed, were often ill-financed, ill-attended, and conducted at inconvenient midweek times far from their homes. In 1993, 26 per cent of Kenyans questioned believed that Aids could be contracted by touching an infected corpse. A visibly emaciated corpse was commonly concealed from all but the closest relatives and friends.[11]

The frequency of funerals compelled other innovations. Rites often became less elaborate and time-consuming. The range of those expected to attend might narrow. Instead of the initial burial being followed after a long interval by an elaborate 'second funeral', the ceremonies were frequently merged. The customary feasting became less elaborate and expensive for both relatives and guests. A goat rather than a bull might be slaughtered. Children might begin to attend what were now familiar occasions. The long mourning period, which had often required all members of the community to abandon agriculture for several days, was radically shortened or observed by only the closest relatives. Some communities formally enacted these innovations.[12] Occasionally, perhaps where the epidemic was still recent, the innovations applied only to Aids deaths, but generally they seem to have extended to other funerals.

Deaths could be occasions for conflict. At one funeral in Lusaka in 1991 the dead woman's father insisted that she had not died of Aids, but her brother, a staunch Adventist, announced that she had 'bewitched herself because she lived a shameful life. ' "What worries me most is that she has missed heaven," he said before his father stormed out of the house and shouted at him, "Go back to your parents!"'[13] By contrast, twelve years later a family of activists in Soweto 'told the world' the cause of their daughter's death: 'Dladla's mother said ... that far from being ashamed that her home would now become a landmark, she was glad that her daughter's last wish had been fulfilled.'[14]

In some this 'preoccupation with terminal illness and death' bred a deep pessimism. In others it bred defiance. Devotees of *sape*, the Congolese cult of elegant dress, invented a dance to celebrate the death of a true *sapeur*. Young people in Nyanza, so their elders complained, danced all the more wildly at the now so frequent funerals. Most, perhaps, concentrated on observing the proprieties, on ensuring especially that no one in their family joined the growing numbers subjected to the indignity of a pauper funeral. Terrible as it was, Aids was only one African preoccupation. Southern Africans commonly ranked it below unemployment and crime.[15]

Like the burden of care, the weight of death fell principally upon the household. In 1996 Gabriel Rugalema studied the process in a heavily infected Kagera village, stressing that the slow action of the Aids virus gradually fragmented households, through the illness and death of young adults, impoverishing them by depriving them of labour and forcing them to dispose of assets in order to meet the costs of health care and funerals. Rather than 'coping' with the crisis by a variety of expedients, as previous studies had claimed, Rugalema insisted that many households failed to cope and were either pauperised beyond recovery or completely destroyed. In their place emerged new kinds of households in which elderly people and orphaned children struggled to survive while imposing burdens on hitherto unaffected relatives. By 1996, 32 per cent of households in the village had lost a member and another 29 per cent had incurred a major obligation.[16] Elsewhere the impact was often less dramatic because infection rates were lower, many young people who died were not household heads, and lasting impoverishment affected chiefly households that were already poor.[17]

In Rugalema's village the average period from sickness to death was about eighteen months, some twelve of which were spent in bed. A sick man tried, successively, herbs and self-medication, the nearest clinic, the government hospital, and a mission hospital, often incurring heavy transport costs. Sick men continued to seek treatment until the last days of their lives. They decided whether to dispose of assets to cover the costs, selling cattle if available but seldom if ever land, although another study in the area found cases. The total cost of treatment might equal a year's household income. Meanwhile a wife caring for a husband would spend 45–60 per cent less time than normal on agriculture, allotting tasks where possible to children, especially girls who might be removed from school for the purpose. Less was spent on a sick wife, who seldom received hospital care.[18] Exact comparisons are difficult, but studies elsewhere suggested health expenditures as proportions of household income both higher (in Chad and Ethiopia) and lower than in Kagera, the latter especially in South Africa where some medical treatment was free and households caring for a member with Aids spent on average one-third of their income on health care in 2002.[19]

To the expense of medical care was added the cost of death. Rugalema thought that a funeral cost a Kagera household substantially less than medical treatment, partly because it received contributions from relatives and neighbours, thereby helping to impoverish the whole community. Another study in the area, however, recorded average funeral expenditure nearly 50 per cent higher than medical costs.[20] There was evidence elsewhere on both sides but agreement that the two expenditures together could cripple poor households and that most of the help they received came from community contributions to funeral expenses. In South Africa, Zimbabwe, and Botswana, a minority of households belonged to contributory burial societies. Under the financial pressure of the epidemic these seized any opportunity to reject a contributor's claims, but they nevertheless enabled many households to provide respectable funerals.[21] In Kagera and western Uganda women established informal mutual assistance groups for this purpose, while most Ethiopians belonged to traditional *iddir* burial societies – there were said to be about 2,500 in Addis Ababa alone – whose finances came under severe pressure during the epidemic.[22]

Households burdened with medical and funeral expenses might suffer further from the loss of labour and income resulting from the death of a young adult, but the impact varied with household circumstances. In Kagera, for example, per capita food consumption in the poorest 50 per cent of households fell by 15 per cent after such a death, whereas in the richest 50 per cent of households it rose by 10 per cent. The richer households also received far more assistance and credit, for no one wanted to lend to the poor, although they might obtain the ill-paid employment that often took the place of mutual aid.[23] Most affected households in Kagera recovered fairly quickly from an Aids death, but a proportion – probably the poorest – did not. In 20 of the 164 households in Rugalema's village the death of an adult member led one or more other members (young or elderly) to move to another household, while six households dispersed and disappeared completely, which probably happened more often than later researchers could discern.[24] Research elsewhere often showed less dramatic consequences of death, but it agreed that the impact was most severe on households whose male head had died. This reduced household income by more than 80 per cent in more than two-thirds of a group of affected households studied in Zambia. If the mother died, the household was more likely to disintegrate, as did 65 per cent of such households studied in Zimbabwe.[25]

As this evidence suggests, the impoverishing effects of Aids commonly fell especially heavily on widows and their children. Despite TASO's prompting, in 2001 only 6 per cent of its clients made wills.[26] Instead, the fate of property and survivors was generally left for the family to decide in accordance with current custom. The husband's kinsmen might blame the widow for his death and seek to appropriate his property and children. Noerine Kaleeba lost her marital home in that way, while a spokesman for people with HIV/Aids in Senegal complained in 2004 that children contracting the disease from their parents were usually barred from inheritance.[27] Alternatively, the husband's family might press the widow to remarry one of their number, but widows potentially infected with HIV were not always in great demand. Instead, a young widow might be left on the land, often in poverty, to manage it for her children to inherit. In Rugalema's village none of the 37 widows remarried. A Zambian study in the late 1990s found that 16 per cent of households were headed by widows and 2 per cent by widowers, who found it easier to remarry. In 2002 almost three-quarters of Aids-affected households in South Africa were female-headed.[28]

In 2004 sub-Saharan Africa had an estimated 12 million Aids orphans, defined by UNAIDS as children under 15 who had lost at least one parent to the disease. They were about 95 per cent of all the world's Aids orphans, because HIV prevalence was highest in Africa and late twentieth-century African families were exceptionally large.[29] The slow incubation of HIV was again crucial here, for it gave parents time to produce children before Aids intervened. The orphan problem first attracted attention in 1989 in Uganda, where a survey in Rakai district found that 25,364 children under eighteen – 13 per cent of all such children – had lost at least one parent, not necessarily to Aids. In the early 2000s Uganda still had the largest number of Aids orphans in the world, although HIV was no longer exceptionally prevalent there, because some twenty years separated the peak incidence of HIV from the maximum prevalence of orphanhood.[30]

A small number of children – about 3,000 a year in South Africa – were simply abandoned.[31] More of those from elementary families who lost both parents during the epidemic lived by themselves in child-headed households, with or without the assistance of adult relatives or neighbours, often in their parental home or in a house where a grandparent had cared for them until death. Some had themselves cared for dying parents or grandparents. 'When AIDS takes a parent,' it was said, 'it usually takes a childhood as well.'[32] Child-headed households were first noted in 1989 in Rakai, where one household had 'heard rumours that the government's solution to the AIDS problem requires extermination of all the victims' children'.[33] The numbers of these households were often exaggerated, but in 2000 Rakai district was said to have more than 2,000, a number roughly paralleled in the Luweero district, where 10 per cent of orphans were caring for themselves. Similar proportions were quoted in parts of the Nyanza province of Kenya. In Zimbabwe every village was said in the early 2000s to have at least one household headed by a child. Generally, however, fewer than 1 per cent of households were headed by someone under eighteen, although many must have disappeared.[34] Often these children were anxious to stay together in their home and avoid the control of an unwelcome relative. Such households coped best when headed by a girl who had already learned to cook, care, cultivate, and sell small quantities of produce. Some were enterprising and resilient. One early account of Rakai described five siblings aged between nine and fourteen who survived by growing food and making themselves useful at funerals, winning the neighbourhood's admiration.[35] Others lived in great misery:

> The children were blank, the 16 year old girl who headed the household in particular, was utterly passive. She sat in a heap averting her eyes, helpless, hapless and almost beyond reach. The others stood like objects, the most dejected and unresponsive children in the entire universe ... they lacked what an adult could give them; love, encouragement, socialization, hope and some measure of direction.[36]

Urban children who lost both parents faced special difficulties, for they might lack kinsfolk in the town and have no claim to urban accommodation. UNICEF estimated in 1996 that about 40 per cent of Zambia's street children had lost both parents, but this was a subject with few hard data and much exaggeration.[37]

Most people questioned in South Africa during the 1990s thought that the government should care for orphans,[38] but elsewhere it was generally regarded as a family responsibility and one that most families accepted with remarkable generosity. It was a traditional obligation – care workers observed that no Zambian language had a word for orphan that would include children living with adult relatives[39] – but the scale of the burden imposed by the epidemic was novel, as also was the identity of the relatives who bore it. The 1998 Malawi census showed that 95 per cent of maternal orphans, 97 per cent of paternal orphans, and 94 per cent of those who had lost both parents were living with relatives. A slightly later survey found that 25 per cent of Ugandan households contained an orphan, a proportion probably rivalled or exceeded in Zimbabwe and Zambia.[40] A study of orphans' caregivers in Nyanza found that 59 per cent had accepted the obligation as automatic next of kin and 29 per cent had volunteered themselves; for a family not to provide a caregiver was considered shameful everywhere.[41] A synthesis of 40 country surveys during 1997–2002 showed that three-quarters of paternal orphans were living with their mothers and slightly over half of maternal orphans were living with their fathers. When both parents died, however, the burden of caring for double orphans passed increasingly to grandparents who had not in the past generally undertaken this task.[42] Often the grandmother first cared for her sick and widowed daughter and her children, then took charge of the children when the daughter died.

As the epidemic grew, so did the proportion of orphan caregivers who were grandparents. In eastern Zimbabwe the proportion increased between 1992 and 1995 from 14 to 44 per cent. In Namibia in 1992, 44 per cent of orphans not living with a surviving parent were with grandparents; in 2000 the figure was 61 per cent. In 2002 a grandparent was the primary caregiver for 20 per cent of all South African children aged between two and fourteen. 'I do not see how I could not care for them since I am their grandmother,' a Zimbabwean woman explained.[43] The grandmother's burden, as Aids has been called, could be overwhelming:

> Life is very difficult because I have a pension of 500 Rand per month. With that I have to support my two daughters Nomhlahla and Samkeliswe who are ill, my other two children who are unemployed and seven grandchildren who I take care of.... At my age of 59 it is hard to be a mother once again to all these children, but I try to give them all the love that I have.[44]

In most countries for which data exist, a majority of the households sheltering orphans were headed by women, with the highest proportion (approximately 72 per cent) in South Africa, where it was sometimes thought mistakenly that the extended family had been unusually weakened, whereas in reality it had often become female-linked. It was striking, too, that the households most willing to accept orphans were commonly those already with numerous dependents and those that had themselves suffered an Aids death. In several tropical countries the more prosperous households accepted orphans most readily, but in South Africa the opposite was the case.[45]

Caregivers often found orphans difficult to manage. Some were anxious, depressed, moody, and occasionally suicidal. 'It's my fault because I don't have parents,' one said. 'I was not supposed to be born,' said another. Some were angry, the main feeling expressed in a book that TASO kept for children's thoughts.[46] The anger might be directed at parents who had ruined their lives:

> Thabang faced a lot of complications after my disclosure. After his father died, I told his teacher I was HIV positive. All the teachers at the school said, 'Don't touch this child, his mother has AIDS.' After that, Thabang said to me, 'Don't touch me, mommy, you're going to give me HIV.' ... Thabang never wanted to go to school again so he actually stayed back a year.[47]

Most painful of all was probably the merciless teasing from other children, who widely assumed that children orphaned by Aids must automatically be infected, a view often shared by caregivers. Many orphans felt unwanted. 'I was taken to the relatives, and I used to be mistreated,' a child complained. 'Whenever I made a mistake I was beaten, told all sorts of insults and always told I am an orphan. They used to remind me about my parents and I just cried.'[48] Resentment could also fester where caregivers had their own children of similar age competing for attention. 'I stay with my aunt,' one girl explained. 'Sometimes I used to fight with my aunt's child.... I feel like I could go somewhere to people who will love me.'[49] That orphans were liable to maltreatment was proverbial; in Botswana a maltreated child might be said to be 'living the life of an orphan'. 'You can tell orphans by their appearance – their clothes are worn out, they are dirty and their hair is not combed,' a Zimbabwean headmaster said, echoing a view widely held by teachers and social workers. Yet there was also evidence on the other side. Surveys found few physical signs of discrimination against orphans; rather, the condition of children depended chiefly on the household's wealth.[50] Orphans, especially double orphans, were more likely than other children to be working for pay and somewhat less likely to receive schooling. A study in eastern Zimbabwe found that paternal orphans had a better chance of education than those who had lost their mothers. More remarkable was the widespread concern to ensure that orphans did go to school, a concern shared by governments, NGOs, caregivers, and orphans themselves. In Kagera, for example, 'orphans unanimously cited lack of school fees and school uniforms as the most important problem they had to face – more important problems than clothing and housing'.[51]

Although there was little evidence that extended families rejected orphans on any scale, the growing numbers bred increasing reluctance to accept them[52] and difficulty in caring for them, moving NGOs of all kinds to provide support. Uganda was a pioneer in this field. One of the first organisations involved was UWESO (Uganda Women's Effort to Save Orphans), originally founded in 1986 by Museveni's wife to care for war orphans but gradually refocused on the Aids epidemic. Working through some 35 branches manned by women activists, it concentrated on supporting extended families in rural areas, first by short-term relief, then by subsidising school fees, and in the late 1990s through a rotating credit scheme. In 2000 it claimed to have helped over 40,000 orphans.[53] Other pioneers were the home-care programmes based on Nsambya and Kitovu hospitals. Nsambya supported families with orphans, paid school fees, and established orphan houses with housemothers. Kitovu entered this work in 1988 and dealt with 5,000 orphans in 1994. TASO concentrated on paying school fees. World Vision launched the largest operation in Rakai in 1990, expecting it to be only a three-year programme. Working through communities, it targeted vulnerable children of all kinds, later extending the programme with World Bank support to Masaka and Gulu. In 1992 it assisted 18,000 orphans to attend school, in addition to support for foster parents, income-generating projects, house building, and training schemes. By 2000 it had helped some 125,000 children. All these support bodies shared the general African rejection of institutional care as impossibly expensive, depriving children of family life, and making them vulnerable to abuse. In 1990 Uganda's 70 children's homes contained only some 2,500 children, only 15 per cent of whom were thought to need such care.[54] In South

Africa, which had a number of small orphanages caring for particularly needy children, only one orphan in 400 was thought to be in an institution in 2000. Rwanda and Zimbabwe initially relied more heavily on orphanages but found the expense unsustainable.[55]

As an activist pointed out, African communities were quicker to organise care for Aids orphans than for Aids patients, although the orphan care was heterogeneous and unsystematised. Malawi, with UNICEF support, was quick to establish a network of community groups and childcare centres. FACT in eastern Zimbabwe organised a similar system of church-based women's groups. Also in Zimbabwe, the Farm Orphan Support Trust worked among the million children estimated to live on commercial farms.[56] Kenya was especially slow to arrange orphan care, but several urban institutions cared for the most needy, usually under religious auspices. In the DR Congo, where care institutions of all kinds were sparse, Avenir Meilleur pour les Orphelins (Better Future for Orphans) was a local NGO with French financial backing paying school fees for nearly 2,000 orphans in the mid 1990s. Yet most Aids orphans – perhaps 90 per cent in Zambia and 95 per cent in Uganda in 2000 – enjoyed only family support.[57] International bodies other than UNICEF largely ignored the orphan problem during the 1990s, prefering to stress Aids prevention. National governments also neglected what they saw as quintessentially a field for community and charitable action. Zambia's social services reached only an estimated 2 per cent of the needy in 2000. South Africa's system of old age, fostering, and child support grants was immensely important to the poor but was often difficult to access and ignored a large proportion of needy children.[58] Botswana launched its National Orphan Programme only in 1999, Uganda in 2003, Ethiopia in 2004, and Namibia in 2005, when Kenya was still planning one. West Africa, with fewer orphans, was far behind the east and south. Although women's organisations in Senegal and elsewhere involved themselves at earlier dates, discussion of national strategies began for the most part only in 2004.[59] By then it was widely recognised that the worst of Africa's orphan problem was still to come. Long-term projections were of little value, but USAID estimated that by 2010 Africa would have about 35 million Aids orphans; in Swaziland orphaned children would then make up more than 10 per cent of the entire population. Many would lack grand-parents as well as parents.[60]

Disease and death within the household impacted on agricultural systems already stressed by rapid population growth on limited good land, unfavour-able rainfall, falling commodity prices, mistaken agricultural strategies, and the economic crisis that began in the late 1970s. Perhaps the best of many uncertain estimates is that between 1960 and the mid 1980s food production per head in sub-Saharan Africa fell by about 1 per cent per year. Between 1963 and 1990 the proportion of Ugandans holding less than one hectare of land tripled.[61] Kagera, Nyanza, and southern Malawi were only the most obvious areas where population growth, land scarcity, and agricultural decay preceded high HIV prevalence. The epidemic's impact on agricultural systems was chiefly to intensify existing adverse trends. Its first effect, in areas of high HIV prevalence, was to reduce household labour, either through caring duties or death. At the same time hired labour became more expensive – in Kagera costs tripled during the 1980s[62] – as disease interrupted supplies. The result was smaller cultivated areas and lower output. In Swaziland, for example, an Aids death in the early 2000s roughly halved the average area cultivated. Labour scarcity also obliged some poorer households to sacrifice higher value cash crops like cotton and coffee in favour of domestic food crops like maize and cassava, a 'tuberisation' of agriculture that damaged nutrition. Disposal of stock to raise cash or supply funerals exacerbated this trend. Many young men with uncertain life expectancy abandoned the drudgery and long-term goals of farming in pursuit of short-term earnings in towns or other commercial enterprises. Disease interrupted the transmission of rural skills. Not all households suffered. The more prosperous could generally survive a single death and a successful minority might accumulate land and cattle at low prices from poorer neighbours.[63] But new categories of impoverished households – the 'Aids-poor' – came into being, notably widows or elderly grandparents caring for numbers of orphans. Not all regions were affected. There was rather little evidence of change in the Ethiopian countryside, where HIV prevalence was low, or in South African farming, where peasant production was relatively unimportant. Labour-exporting areas like Burkina could be badly affected as illness and death among migrant workers reduced remittances and made it impossible to maintain the two households that migration demanded. The most vulnerable areas were the savanna grain-farming regions with a single wet season into which labour was concentrated, whether in West Africa – although HIV was less prevalent there – or especially in the drier parts of eastern and southern Africa where prevalence was so high. By contrast, areas such as Kagera and western Uganda, enjoying year-round rainfall and permanent crops like bananas, might be less affected agriculturally than their high disease prevalence suggested.[64]

This did not mean that the high-prevalence regions west of Lake Victoria were spared. 'Drive through Rakai and Masaka, the worst-hit districts along Lake Victoria,' it was reported in 1998, 'and the effects of the pandemic are obvious: abandoned banana groves, overgrown fields, empty, closed houses, fresh graves next to homes, coffin-making shops and funeral processions.' There were reports of starvation in western Uganda in 1990 and famine relief was needed in the drier parts of Masaka and Rakai during 1999.[65] But the major famine related to the Aids epidemic took place in the dry-grain lands of central and southern Africa during 2001–3, centring in Malawi, Zambia, and Zimbabwe but extending also into Mozambique, Lesotho, Swaziland, and vulnerable parts of South Africa. Excessive rains early in 2001 reduced Malawi's maize harvest by 32 per cent. By the end of the year NGOs reported growing distress, but it was not until some hundreds of southern Malawians died early in 2002 that the authorities took action. Throughout 2002 the scarcity spread more widely, exacerbated by another poor harvest, until over 15 million people needed aid. Between 1,000 and 3,000 Malawians may have died, with unknown but much smaller numbers elsewhere, before the worst of the crisis passed during 2003, although aid was still needed in Zimbabwe and scattered areas elsewhere as late as 2005.[66]

The deeper roots of the famine lay in the growing pressure on resources and the impoverishment of many rural areas over several decades. Between 1980 and 1999 average calorie intake in Zambia fell by 15 per cent. In 1998, a 'normal' year, 68 per cent of Malawians were short of food. To this was added the climatic instability that usually triggered famine in Africa, but it was mild compared with earlier experiences. Malawi's inadequate harvest of 2001 was more than twice that of 1991–2, yet the earlier scarcity had not caused famine deaths. One reason for the disaster in 2001–2 was that governments and donors ignored the early signs of approaching famine. Another was that during the intervening decade, under pressure to liberalise, Malawi had dismantled its public anti-famine measures without first ensuring that private enterprise could replace them, a policy compounded during 2001 by selling (apparently corruptly) the entire national grain reserve rather than some two-thirds of it, as donors had recommended. At the same time the normal defence against famine in the region, Zimbabwe's surplus maize production, was removed by its government's seizure of commercial farms. Finally, the Malawi government's intervention was less effective than in earlier scarcities.[67]

Yet a closer analysis of the famine of 2001–3 shows that its novel and distinctive character was due to the Aids epidemic. In the phrase of Alex de Waal and Alan Whiteside, this was the first 'new variant famine' shaped by young adult deaths and the 'Aids-poor' households they had left behind.[68] The most careful study, in Zambia, showed that per capita consumption during the famine fell by 25 per cent in households without an adult aged 15–59 and by 28 per cent in households whose head was sick. Not all these disabilities were due to Aids – there was no medical testing – but most clearly were. Disadvantaged households were especially likely to grow non-nutritious root crops and to rely partly on wild foods. Other evidence suggests that one reason why the 2001–3 famine was worse than that of 1991–2 was that households no longer had assets to sell, partly owing to impoverishment by disease and death from Aids. Mutual aid also seems to have been abnormally slender in 2001–3, while relief was especially difficult to distribute to those bedridden or immobilised by caring duties. In other ways, too, Aids gave a new character to the famine. It happened in democracies, which current theory had thought impossible. It was exceptionally difficult to end, because Aids-poor households had little recuperative power. In 2002–3 poor Zambian households with a sick head planted 69 per cent less than in 2001–2 and doubtless often became permanently dependent.[69] 'The ... most alarming factor that makes this crisis unique is its prophetic character,' a United Nations team reported. 'Rather than anticipate the conclusion of this crisis, the affected populations, governments, and the international community are concluding that this crisis marks the start of an unwelcome trend: health, education and other sectors are equally vulnerable to collapse under assault by HIV/Aids.'[70]

For several years economists had been trying to estimate the impact of the epidemic on African development, without reaching any consensus. Most estimates were quite low. The World Bank suggested in 1997 that a general-ised epidemic (as in eastern and southern Africa) reduced the growth of per capita GDP by about 0.5 per cent per year, which it thought manageable for all but the weakest economies. Roughly similar figures were often quoted for South Africa. In 2002 UNAIDS reckoned that the epidemic had reduced sub-Saharan Africa's economic growth by 2–4 per cent.[71] Some economists and national governments took gloomier views. Botswana, for example, reckoned in 2000 that HIV/Aids was reducing its growth rate by 1.5 per cent per year and would make its economy 31 per cent smaller in 2025 than it would otherwise have been.[72] The main fears were the cost of health services, the death of skilled workers, the potential deterrent to foreign investment, and failure to transmit knowledge and socialisation to new generations.

Attention also focused on the impact on companies, which was still relatively small. Of a thousand companies surveyed in South Africa in 2003, only 9 per cent had yet felt a serious impact. A conference on the subject arranged in Port Elizabeth in 2004 was cancelled for lack of interest. Some 77 per cent of East African businesses questioned at the same period did not know what the impact had been, while most Nigerian manufacturing firms did not regard HIV as a management concern.[73] Among unskilled workers the chief cost resulted from absenteeism, either from sickness or to attend funerals. More damaging and expensive was the loss of skilled and managerial staff that multiplied training costs, pension payments, and other benefits. Consequently, HIV impacted most heavily on firms with high levels of skill. One study of six enterprises in southern Africa, published in 2004, found that the increase to wage and salary bills ranged from 0.4 to 5.9 per cent and was greatest for those providing the most extensive benefits to workers. Firms producing consumer goods foresaw shrinking markets. Large companies feared that HIV might threaten their global competitiveness.[74] South African mining companies, with 20–30 per cent of their huge labour forces infected during the early 2000s, reckoned that HIV added between $4 and $6 an ounce to the production costs of gold then selling on world markets at nearly $300 an ounce. 'The impact is not as huge as one would gain the first impression from reading a lot of the literature,' a spokesman for the Anglo American Corporation said in 2000. Many companies transferred costs to their workers by reducing medical scheme benefits and excluding new employees from them, shifting pension schemes to provident funds, outsourcing non-core activities, investing in more capital-intensive technology, and imposing retrenchments and early retirements.[75]

Insurance companies were especially vulnerable. Malawi banned them from testing applicants, as a result of which the industry virtually disappeared, as also in Uganda. Kenyan companies refused to cover HIV-positive patients. Zimbabwe's firms quadrupled their premiums in two years.[76] South Africa's sophisticated and powerful companies were exceptionally quick to assess the new risks, insist on HIV testing, impose exclusions, and devise new and restricted policies open only to those in the early stages of the disease, but by 2000 some firms were suffering losses consequent on the epidemic.[77] Pension funds faced similar difficulties. So did medical schemes; several in Kenya collapsed, South Africa's were legally obliged to cover HIV/Aids costs (except antiretroviral drugs) at the price of ever-higher contributions, and the Namibian government had to inject taxpayers' money in order to keep its own scheme afloat.[78]

The epidemic had an especially early and severe impact on professional groups. During the 1990s Barclays Bank of Zambia lost more than one-quarter of its senior managers to Aids.[79] The alleged deaths among teachers are sometimes difficult to credit – the Central African Republic is said to have lost over half its teachers during the 1990s and to have closed 107 of its 173 schools – but more teachers died than were trained in several countries with high HIV prevalence. A survey in 2000 found that 20 per cent of South African health workers aged 18–35 were infected.[80]

Doomsday predictions of the demographic consequences flourished early in the epidemic. By simply projecting current growth rates of prevalence into the future, a Johannesburg physician predicted in 1991 that by 2010 South Africa's population would be reduced by 75 per cent.[81] Some sophisticated early projections were also deeply pessimistic. The most influential, by Roy Anderson and others, predicted that the epidemic might convert sub-Saharan Africa's high population growth rates of 3 per cent per year into population decline 'over timescales of a few to many decades'.[82] During the early 1990s, by contrast, most demographers came to believe that continued high fertility would cushion Africa against the epidemic, but two developments undermined this confidence. One was that prevalence rates mounted to unexpected levels in many countries. The other was that birthrates in several of the more developed African countries fell dramatically for reasons unconnected with the epidemic and due more to the availability of artificial contraception, lack of economic opportunity, and desire to give children the best possible education. Whereas Uganda's total fertility rate at the end of the century remained at a high 6.9 births per woman, Zimbabwe's had fallen to 4.4, Botswana's to 4.1, and South Africa's to 2.9.[83] Since these countries also had amongst the highest levels of HIV, by the late 1990s demographic opinion was swinging back towards the pessimistic view propounded by the United States Bureau of the Census, which predicted that the populations of all three countries would decline during the early years of the new century. In 2005 a United Nations report added Lesotho and Swaziland to the list, while removing South Africa.[84] In the meantime, pressure for family planning, which had peaked in 1984 when African governments collectively accepted its necessity, faded before 'the painful "family planning" by Aids'.[85]

The pessimistic view of Africa's demographic future current at the beginning of the new millennium was matched by pessimistic predictions of the epidemic's social and political consequences. 'What kind of shrivelled wasteland will my nation become?' a young doctor asked from Zimbabwe. 'Young orphans and the old ekeing out a crabbed, hand to mouth existence in dusty forgotten rural homes, while in the towns, industry falls silent, businesses and stores lie closed and derelict while the wind blows rubbish and old leaves down deserted, dead streets.' An extravagant prophet warned that by 2010 'South African society could be living out the values of a movie gangland dystopia such as Mad Max.'[86] The prophets pointed out that because Aids chiefly killed people aged between 25 and 45, countries with adult HIV prevalence of 25 per cent or more would become polarised between the old and the young, with more people over 60 than in their 40s and 50s, and with perhaps a quarter of South Africa's entire population aged between 15 and 24.[87] Many of these young people would have grown up as orphans, unsocialised, alienated, and potentially 'sliding into lawlessness and anarchy' – although there was no evidence for this. With few years of adult life ahead of them, the young might neglect education in favour of opportunistic behaviour and instant gratification. They might breed hurriedly, reducing the status of women. Skills would not be transmitted. The state might well lose control of violence, not least because half its soldiers and (in South Africa) perhaps 35 per cent of its policemen might themselves be infected. Institutions would be weakened, property rights disrupted, and democracy threatened. Wide social divisions might open between high-risk people dying young and low-risk people surviving to normal ages, between the skilled and protected and the unskilled and dispensable, between Africans and the rest of the world. Medical and welfare services for the old and weak might atrophy. Many, it was suggested, might flock to millenarian promises or retreat to millenarian dreams.[88] Africa was threatened by 'social involution of a scale probably unprecedented in human history'.[89]

These predictions, like long-term demographic projections, took no account of the positive developments taking place within the epidemic during the 1990s and early 2000s: the demonstration, especially in Uganda, that ordinary people could change their behaviour to minimise the risk of HIV; the discovery of antiretroviral drugs that could suppress viral infection; a greater international willingness to fund measures against the epidemic; and the emergence of people with HIV/Aids as political actors more apt to re-engage society with the state than to retreat into anomie. These positive developments will dominate the remainder of this book.

12
The Epidemic Matures

During the 1990s the epidemic's character changed in most African regions that it had first infected. HIV prevalence grew more slowly, stabilised, or began to decline, either because deaths overtook the incidence of new infections or, more controversially, because incidence also declined. Preventive measures claimed their first successes, provoking debate on which measures were effective and how they might be replicated elsewhere. Instead of spreading rapidly among people with high-risk behaviour, the virus increasingly attacked vulnerable members of the general population, especially poor women. In short, the epidemic matured. It remained widespread and fatal, but without the explosive quality of its youth, although with the equally alarming prospect of permanence. This, however, was true only in areas of early infection. Even in the mid 2000s there were still parts of the continent, hitherto isolated by distance, disorder, or some other obstacle, where HIV was spreading with epidemic vigour. At the end of 2004, an estimated 25.4 million people in sub-Saharan Africa had HIV, one million more than two years earlier.[1]

The first half of the 1990s was the worst period in the epidemic's early history. Expansion in southern Africa was at its peak. Preventive measures seemed to make no impact on behaviour. There was no progress with vaccines or curative drugs. Many national programmes were corrupt or ineffective. International interest was low and aid was declining. The WHO's Global Programme, attacked from within and without, was wound up at the end of 1995, leaving many national programmes bereft of funds.

News from Uganda restored hope. In retrospect, epidemiologists came to believe that the incidence of new infections in southern Uganda had peaked in the later 1980s and then fallen rapidly.[2] The first indication that HIV prevalence there was declining came from the antenatal clinic at Mulago Hospital in Kampala, where infection among pregnant women fell between 1989 and 1993 from 28.1 to 16.2 per cent. Other urban hospital clinics in southern Uganda showed similar reductions from 1991–3, as did rural Rakai district. The Aids Control Programme checked its testing procedures before giving the news maximum publicity during 1995.[3] Thereafter prevalence rates

126

in southern towns dropped steeply and continuously, from 29 per cent in Kampala in 1992 to 8 per cent in 2002.[4] Decline was slower in the southern countryside and was temporarily reversed during the later 1990s in war-ridden Gulu district in the north, while expansion continued into the 2000s in some outlying areas. Overall, however, UNAIDS reckoned that Uganda's adult HIV prevalence fell from 13 per cent in the early 1990s to 4.1 per cent at the end of 2003.[5] Across the border in the Kagera region of Tanzania, too, urban prevalence nearly halved and rural prevalence fell by roughly one-third between 1987 and 1996.[6]

The first reports of decline met scepticism. Some suggested that the antenatal figures were unreliable: that less rigorous testing was allowing positive cases to go unnoticed, that more rigorous testing was excluding those falsely tested positive in the past, or that the epidemic was increasing the number of HIV-positive women whose low fertility artificially reduced antenatal prevalence figures. Later sample surveys of entire populations suggested that antenatal statistics often somewhat exaggerated overall HIV prevalence, so that many official estimates were reduced in 2003, making long-term comparisons difficult, but as Uganda's antenatal returns showed ever lower prevalence during the 1990s it became clear that more than statistical distortion was involved. Some observers suggested political distortion, whether by the Aids Control authorities, for whom evidence of declining prevalence became an argument for desperately needed funding, or by the natural tendency to exaggerate good news. 'They don't believe that any country in Africa can do anything positive,' Uganda's Minister of Health complained.[7] More serious doubts suggested that declining prevalence might not indicate success against the virus but arise from its own dynamics. As the epidemic matured, it was suggested, high-risk sections of the population might be saturated, infection less quickly transferred, individuals become less infectious, and perhaps the virus itself lose some of its initial virulence.[8] Most important, declining prevalence might simply mean that more people were dying of Aids, rather than any reduction in the incidence of new infections. This was argued especially by Ugandan and American researchers in Rakai who had since 1988 conducted one of the three long-term projects in the region, the others being a joint British and Ugandan programme in Masaka and a Tanzanian and Swedish project in Kagera. The Rakai team pointed out that although prevalence had declined there during the early 1990s, the incidence of new infections had not. Instead, 'excess mortality among HIV-positive persons could almost entirely explain the decline in HIV prevalence'.[9]

The objection to this pessimistic conclusion was that the most dramatic reductions in HIV prevalence had taken place among people aged 15–19 who rarely died of Aids. At Nsambya Hospital's antenatal clinic in Kampala, for example, prevalence among women of that age fell between 1991 and 1996 from 28 to 10 per cent. Other institutions recorded similar figures.[10] They suggested a decline in the incidence of new infections, which would imply that the epidemic itself was waning. That, however, could be measured directly only by surveying the same large population repeatedly over several years. Such data from the Masaka project began to emerge during the 1990s and were published fully in 2002, covering a ten-year period that the researchers considered necessary in order to reveal change. They showed that the incidence of new infections among adults aged over 13 fell between 1990–4 and 1995–9 by 37 per cent. The fall occurred in all age groups, although the total number of new infections concerned was only 190. 'The most likely explanation for the falling incidence and prevalence,' the project's director wrote, 'is risk-lowering sexual behaviour change in response to the severe HIV epidemic itself or to health education messages from government and non-government sources and in the media.'[11]

As encouraging evidence from antenatal clinics and the Masaka project accumulated, argument about its explanation sharpened. The Ugandan authorities naturally claimed the credit. The decline of infection especially among the young and educated implied a particular role for the HIV instruction compulsory in schools since 1987. Several studies supported this, one finding that each additional year of schooling reduced the risk of HIV infection by 6.7 per cent.[12] Museveni and other leaders had spoken relentlessly about HIV/Aids on all occasions, the press had been remarkably frank, while the decentralised local government system and the mass of NGOs and religious bodies had contributed to high levels of communication, often backed by threats and coercion.[13] Uganda's success became a matter of national pride and attracted delegations from many parts of the world. 'In Uganda,' a journalist from equally proud Senegal wrote in 2004, 'the retort to Aids concerns everyone. It has become a matter of patriotism that demands a general commitment and mobilisation.'[14]

How this general awareness had translated into behavioural change was more contentious. Some analysts pointed to a reduction in casual sex, especially but not only among the young, for whom there was something of a return to earlier and more restrained sexual behaviour. According to personal accounts given to behavioural surveys, the average age of sexual debut in Uganda rose between 1989 and 2001 from 14 to 16. The proportion of those aged 15–19 with sexual experience fell between 1989 and 1995 from 69 to 44 per cent among men and from 74 to 54 per cent among women. In rural Masaka the age of marriage for women rose by about a year during the first half of the 1990s while the number of unmarried teenage pregnancies more than halved.[15] Teenage girls, it was reported from Rakai in 1995, 'are truly frightened of contracting AIDS. Many of them believe that one can only be safe through sexual abstinence.'[16] This behavioural change had begun very early, during the late 1980s, almost as soon as the epidemic was widely visible, demonstrating once more how destructive the yet earlier, silent epidemic had been. But change was cumulative. In 2000–1, 72 per cent of unmarried women and 65 per cent of unmarried men (including 78 per cent of both aged 15–19) said that they had not had sex during the previous twelve months. Among the sexually active, fidelity to one partner – locally known as zero grazing – also increased markedly and became perhaps the most important form of behavioural change. Between 1989 and 1995 the proportion of men and women admitting casual partners fell by over 60 per cent, while the number of men admitting three or more casual partners during the last year fell by 80 per cent.[17] The trend continued, for in 2000–1 some 88 per cent of married men and 97 per cent of married women said they had had only their regular partner during the previous twelve months. Only 1.6 per cent of men reported commercial sex during that period. Similar changes took place in Kagera.[18] Perhaps the most striking aspects of behavioural change were that those who knew themselves not to have HIV were most likely to change behaviour, that the initiative was often taken by young women who had often been thought unable to control their own sexual lives, and that behavioural change commonly took the form of moral self-control supported either by religious belief or notions of return to a purer, traditional morality. Ironically, the apparent role of behavioural change in reducing HIV prevalence in Uganda was the strongest refutation of those who denied the importance of sexual behaviour in the growth of the epidemic.

Three other aspects of Uganda's experience were also distinctive. One was that its early and widespread epidemic ensured that an exceptionally large proportion of people had personal experience of the disease. In 1995, 89 per cent of Ugandans said they knew someone with HIV/Aids or dead of it; the equivalent figure in Zimbabwe in 1994 was only 50 per cent. In Uganda, more-over, young people were as likely as their elders to have this experience. Its impact was described as 'scary, shocking, painful, terrible, and demoralising'.[19]

A second special feature of Uganda's experience was the openness with which HIV/Aids was discussed and the fact that the main channel by which Ugandans learned of the disease shifted from official or media sources to personal contacts with friends or relatives that perhaps had a greater impact on behaviour. Such community involvement, it has been argued, has been essential in all successful campaigns to check the spread of Aids, as in Thai-land and among American homosexuals. As the visiting Senegalese journalist put it, Ugandans had internalised the threat of HIV.[20]

The third and most controversial aspect of Uganda's distinctiveness was the role of condoms. Until the mid 1990s Museveni wavered between his personal distaste for them, supported by strong traditionalist and Catholic feeling, and the view of doctors and NGOs that condoms were an essential part of HIV/Aids control. In 1995 only 16 per cent of Ugandan men and 6 per cent of Ugandan women said that they had ever used one.[21] This implied that the initial reduction of HIV prevalence among young people, if a consequence of behavioural change, must have been due mainly to the other forms previously described. At precisely this moment during the mid 1990s, however, the apparent failure of prevention programmes and a softening of overt religious opposition led to a new policy of 'quiet promotion'. The result was a sub-stantial increase in their use in casual and especially commercial sex, although seldom in regular partnerships. In 2000–1, only 4 per cent of men reported using a condom with their last cohabiting partner, but 59 per cent with their last non-cohabiting partner. Among nineteen African countries with known condom usage by men aged 15–24 with their last casual partner at that time, Uganda came third only to Botswana and Zimbabwe.[22]

Some observers drew from this the conclusion that increased condom use since the mid 1990s had reinforced the declining prevalence initiated by other behavioural changes.[23] A more radical interpretation emerged in 2005 when the Rakai project reported the results of its research between 1994 and 2003. Although prevalence there had fallen by 35 per cent, it had not fallen significantly among those aged less than nineteen, while incidence had not declined, as in Masaka, but had slightly increased. Moreover, Rakai had experienced exactly the opposite of the behavioural changes reported elsewhere: the age of sexual debut had fallen, the percentage of young adults sexually active had risen, the proportion of men reporting two or more partners during the previous twelve months had increased from 22 to 27 per cent, and the proportion of HIV-positive men reporting this had grown from 48 to 69 per cent. On the other hand, these trends had been balanced by greater condom use, which had doubled in intercourse between men aged 15–19 and their casual partners. Over 80 per cent of the reduction in prevalence, however, was due not to behavioural change but to increased deaths.[24]

These depressing findings fed directly into controversy surrounding Uganda's remarkable decline in HIV prevalence. Optimists argued that the positive evidence of behavioural change demonstrated that Africans were capable of solving their own HIV problem by their own methods of morally guided, community-based reform. Religious zealots used the Ugandan case to insist that the epidemic could not be defeated by condoms but by 'a return to moral values'. Fundamentalist elements in the United States Administration took a similar view. So did Museveni, who shocked the Bangkok Aids Conference of 2004 by claiming, inaccurately,

> that Uganda had managed to cut down the prevalence rate of the pandemic even though it has the lowest per capita use of condoms in sub-Saharan Africa.
>
> 'In our prevention campaigns we emphasised on abstinence and on being faithful rather than condom use. Ultimately we cannot become a condomised nation.... [C]ondoms is just a stop gap, improvised measure.'[25]

Museveni's speech aroused much opposition in Uganda. The Rakai report flatly contradicted it, giving his critics the opportunity to reassert the ABC programme – Abstain, Be faithful, Condomise – that sought to combine moral and medical approaches and had become the international orthodoxy. As Uganda's Minister of Health explained in his response to the Rakai report, 'Our position is still the same: that it is the ABC strategy that has been effective in checking HIV/Aids in Uganda. We would not want to go into a struggle with anybody over which is better than the other.'[26] That struggle, however, was already taking place, especially over the messages to incorporate into sex education in schools.[27]

As news of Uganda's declining HIV prevalence spread, other African countries scrutinised their antenatal statistics for similar signs. The first to find them was Zambia. As in Uganda, change appears to have begun among young urban women. Between 1993 and 1998 antenatal prevalence among women aged 15–19 in Lusaka fell from 28 to 15 per cent, with a somewhat smaller decline in Ndola. The change was concentrated among women with post-primary education, who had hitherto been highly infected, whereas young women with little schooling showed increasing prevalence levels. The decline among the more educated young women was also apparent, although less conspicuous, in the countryside. It slowed markedly in the late 1990s. A later recalculation of Zambia's statistics reckoned that national HIV prevalence among adults had peaked in 1994–5 at about 17 per cent and then declined very slowly to 16 per cent in 2003. There were no longitudinal studies from which to calculate incidence, but comparison with Uganda suggests that it is unlikely to have fallen. Overall, analysts concluded, 'these prevalence changes have been small, restricted geographically, and transient relative to those in Uganda'.[28]

Kenya's statistics were more difficult to interpret, but prevalence appears at least to have stabilised and possibly to have declined in the early 2000s. Again the first indication came from teenage women in the capital, whose infection rate fell between 1992–3 and 1996–7 from 18.1 to 12.5 per cent.[29] During the 1990s, however, the rural epidemic was spreading rapidly in Nyanza and elsewhere, outweighing urban changes. National prevalence may have levelled out around 2000, but the level is difficult to determine because subsequent studies showed that antenatal clinics recorded inflated figures and male prevalence was little more than half that among women. In 2003 adult prevalence was recalculated at 6.7 per cent, probably indicating a real rather than merely statistical decline. Nyanza, with 14 per cent adult prevalence, then outstripped even Nairobi, with 9 per cent.[30] Whether change was due to reduced incidence and behavioural change as well as increased mortality was not known.

The pattern of urban decline balanced by continued rural growth appears to have existed in several other countries. In Ethiopia, for example, the first evidence of falling prevalence rates came in the mid 1990s from young women in the inner city of Addis Ababa, where the national epidemic had begun. Initially it was not paralleled even in the remainder of the city, but between 1995 and 2003 antenatal prevalence in Addis Ababa as a whole declined from 24 to 11 per cent. In other towns, however, infection increased until the early 2000s, while the slow growth of the rural epidemic outweighed any urban change. Whereas urban incidence had fallen during the 1990s and then stabilised, rural incidence remained steady at a low level. During 2003 Ethiopia experienced more than twice as many new infections as Aids deaths, so that total prevalence continued to increase.[31]

A comparable shift of balance between urban and rural took place more brutally in Rwanda. In 1991, three years before the genocide, antenatal prevalence there was 27 per cent in towns and 3 per cent in the countryside. Eight years later it was 14 per cent in towns and 6 per cent in the countryside. The urban decline may have owed something to greater sexual restraint by the young, but the major reason for the change of balance was probably the genocide itself. Although rape spread disease to some degree, the major impact came from the mixing of urban and rural people during the crisis, both in refugee camps outside the country and especially among those internally displaced. In the early 2000s UNAIDS estimated Rwanda's adult prevalence at a stable 5.1 per cent, although it was a stability masking significant change.[32] By contrast, no such reordering of urban–rural relationships appears to have taken place in Burundi, at least by the late 1990s. Tanzania had yet another experience, with declining prevalence in rural regions of early infection like Kagera and Mbeya roughly balanced by continuing expansion into more isolated areas.[33]

Elsewhere in the continent, despite the absence of declining prevalence on the Ugandan scale, there were indications that the epidemic was stabilising and maturing. Senegal was the most obvious case, with adult prevalence held down in the early 2000s to 0.8 per cent. Burkina had a higher level, at 4.2 per cent, but this too appeared to have stabilised, with evidence of decline among young urban women.[34] Prevalence in Ghana fluctuated in the early 2000s within narrow limits and at somewhat lower rates.[35] A UNAIDS report in December 2004 also detected stabilisation in Malawi and Zimbabwe, although at much higher levels implying numerous new infections to balance deaths.[36] In Malawi's capital, Lilongwe, antenatal prevalence among women aged 15–24 fell from 22 to 13 per cent between 1997 and 2001, with a somewhat smaller decline in general antenatal prevalence. Blantyre experienced a slightly smaller reduction in the general prevalence, but among older rather than young women and most probably owing to deaths. This limited urban decline, however, was balanced by increased rural infection.[37] In Zimbabwe, Harare may have seen reduced prevalence among young women during the later 1990s, but otherwise little is known about the dynamics of its epidemic and the most likely reason for stabilisation of prevalence was that its very high death rate had caught up with the incidence of new cases.[38] The Botswana government also believed that prevalence was stable or falling and pointed to reduced infection in young urban women, although UNAIDS was unconvinced.[39] It was equally unconvinced by Namibia, but that was before its antenatal survey for 2004 first showed a modest decline in infection from the 21.3 per cent estimated by UNAIDS in 2003 to 19.8 per cent. At least the Minister of Health could claim that 'we are really not working in vain'.[40]

Like everything concerning HIV/Aids, this issue was most contentious in South Africa. Antenatal prevalence rates there rose rapidly until the late 1990s, including those among women aged 15–19, but thereafter the latter declined while the overall rate rose irregularly from 22.8 per cent in 1998 to 27.9 per cent in 2003. The government claimed that this demonstrated that the epidemic was 'slowly stabilising' and insisted that the true prevalence among women of childbearing age was only 20.7 per cent, as found by a population survey whose completeness the government's critics doubted.[41] All agreed that the growth of the epidemic had slowed, mostly because of increasing deaths but also because the incidence of new infections had fallen from a peak around 1997. Olive Shisana, chief author of the population survey, attributed this decline to 'major interventions like condom distribution and unbelievable behaviour change'.[42]

Pressed to specify the change, Shisana first pointed out that between surveys in 1999 and 2002 the proportion of youths aged 11–19 who said they had not had sex during the previous twelve months had risen from 60 to 70 per cent. A later enquiry questioned this, but all studies of the period showed levels of teenage sex lower than the stereotypes of the 1990s had suggested, although somewhat higher than those in Uganda after behavioural change. The median age of sexual debut in the early 2000s was between 16.5 and 17 years, slightly later than in Uganda and without clear evidence of change. Frequency of sex among unmarried young people was relatively low. In one survey, 17 per cent of those sexually experienced had not had intercourse during the previous twelve months.[43]

The most common behavioural change to avoid HIV reported by young South Africans was to use condoms, in roughly half of their last sexual encounters, a far higher proportion than had been reported for the general population earlier in the 1990s and little less than their use in Uganda. The increase in distributed condoms from 150 million in 1998 to 310 million in 2003 was the clearest evidence of behavioural change.[44] Young people greatly underrated their risk of contracting HIV, especially from apparently steady partners, and 10.2 per cent of those aged 15–24 were infected in 2003. Of these, 77 per cent were women, who were alert to their danger and for the most part, as in Uganda, were confident that they could refuse sex, although 10 per cent in one survey and 19 per cent in another said they had been forced to have it. Some 65–70 per cent of people aged 15–19 knew someone either with HIV or dead from it.[45] Schooling was their main source of information – bearing out its importance in Uganda – along with radio and television. Kevin Kelly's research found that in areas of high media penetration and strong community mobilisation, 'There are signs ... of development of cultures of risk prevention which are self-perpetuating,' especially among 'those who are less at risk and those whose life circumstances are most promising'. Another study noted how optimistic such young people were, in contrast to the disillusionment and fatalism of the earlier 1990s. Most now thought it wrong to force sex, have many partners, or have transactional sex.[46] 'There are no longer *amasoka*,' one declared in 2001, 'people are scared to die of AIDS.' Mark Hunter commented:

> Day by day, funeral by funeral, AIDS bears harder down on the *isoka* masculinity. The symptoms, recognised by even very young children in the township, couldn't be more emasculating – and de-masculinising: some of the most virile, popular, and independent bodies are steadily transformed into diseased and dependent skeletons, shunned by friends and neighbours.... Indeed, it is at the many funerals, as mourners walk in a slow circle around the coffin, taking a shocked glance at the deceased's diminutive body, where the contradictions of *isoka* are most tragically played out.[47]

Yet life circumstances were not promising for all young South Africans. *Isoka* behaviour survived among feckless men and the poor or ambitious young women obliged to use their sexuality to gain access to male wealth. *Isoka* behaviour was strong in neglected rural areas of the Eastern Cape, where 92 per cent of young people claimed sexual experience in 1999, 35 per cent of them by age thirteen. It was strong in informal housing areas around great cities, where both sexual experience and HIV prevalence among young people were highest.[48] Siphelo Mapolisa's study in 2000 of young men at an STD clinic in the Guguletu township of Cape Town – the most highly infected area in the Western Cape – described a virtually unchanged youth culture:

I found that their perceptions relating to HIV/AIDS are greatly influenced by peer pressure. Although there is a high level of knowledge amongst members of these groups on how HIV/AIDS and STDs are contracted and transmitted, little or no effort is made to put this knowledge into practice. Generally, the individuals in my study engage in unprotected sex, and in the process risk their lives because of their desires to experiment, achieve social, emotional, financial support and most of all gain acceptance by their peers.[49]

Resistance to behavioural change was strong, too, among migrant mining communities and the networks of commercial sex and informal enterprise surrounding them. The major attempt to transform such a community, the Carletonville Project, met such apathy and opposition that STD prevalence increased and mineworkers' knowledge of HIV appeared to diminish.[50]

The unevenness of behavioural change in South Africa paralleled its failure to experience the dramatic decline of HIV prevalence seen in Uganda, although causal relationships were uncertain while the reasons for Uganda's experience were disputed. The other countries where prevalence stabilised or perhaps somewhat declined at that time also showed uneven changes in behaviour. The age of sexual debut rose slightly in most African countries during the 1990s, but seldom to the extent seen in Uganda.[51] In Lusaka, where HIV prevalence declined, the proportion of never-married people reporting no sexual experience rose between 1990 and 1998 from 38 to 53 per cent for men and from 50 to 60 per cent for women, while the proportion of married men and women admitting extra-marital partners fell during the same period from 31 to 19 per cent and from 8 to 2 per cent respectively. These changes were reported chiefly by the young, especially the more educated young who were most susceptible to propaganda, but they were not paralleled in the countryside.[52] Similarly, reductions in sex with extra-marital partners among students in Ethiopia and factory workers in Tanzania seem to have been isolated examples.[53] Consequently, whereas in Uganda in 2000–1 only some 12 per cent of married men admitted a non-marital partner during the previous twelve months, the equivalent proportions were 16 per cent in Kenya in 1998, 18 per cent in Malawi in 2000, and 29 per cent in Tanzania in 1999. There was evidence, however, that men were increasingly careful in their choice of partners.[54]

Change was similarly uneven in the use of condoms. At the beginning of the epidemic this was very low throughout sub-Saharan Africa, partly for lack of access to them and partly from a widespread distaste. As Meja Mwangi put it, 'The men were too manly to use them and the women were too womanly to insist.' Supply expanded substantially during the 1990s, reaching some 724 million from official sources in 1999, although that was only about four per adult male per year.[55] As in Uganda and South Africa, they were used almost exclusively in casual or commercial sex and often served in effect to define it: 'the prostitute's identity card', as a Malian put it. Often the sex workers insisted on condoms: 'I don't want to die for three thousand francs.' One estimate in 2003 was that they were also used in 19 per cent of sexual encounters with non-cohabiting partners. As in South Africa, use was strongly associated with education, youth, urban life, and modernity in general – an association exploited in advertising campaigns. The highest rates of use were consequently in self-consciously modernising countries such as Botswana, Zimbabwe, Ghana, and Côte d'Ivoire.[56] Elsewhere, as in Uganda, it was only in the late 1990s that condoms were accepted by more than small minorities. Although careful studies showed that consistent use gave much protection against HIV, use was seldom consistent and it is difficult to identify any connection between condom use and HIV prevalence or its reduction. Botswana and Zimbabwe, with perhaps the highest rates of use in sub-Saharan Africa, also had two of the highest rates of infection.[57]

Perhaps the most striking differences between Uganda and the countries where prevalence only stabilised or declined slightly concerned the public visibility of the epidemic. Whereas in Uganda in 1995 some 89 per cent of people said they knew someone with HIV or dead from it, equivalent proportions were 70 per cent in Malawi, 68 per cent in Zambia, and 50 per cent in Tanzania in 1996, 50 per cent in Zimbabwe in 1994, and 41 per cent in Kenya in 1993. Most studies found that such personal experience encouraged behavioural change, which frequently took place first in those areas, like the inner city of Addis Ababa, where the epidemic also had begun.[58] Even more marked was the difference between the openness with which HIV/Aids was discussed in Uganda and the secrecy that long surrounded it in Kenya, Botswana, or South Africa. In 2001 only 3 per cent of South Africans questioned said they believed a friend or family member was HIV-positive, against 87 per cent of Ugandans.[59] Among nineteen countries surveyed during the 1990s, only in Uganda had people learned of the disease more from friends and relatives than from the electronic media. The nearest approximation in this respect was Zambia, which was also the next to show evidence of declining prevalence. 'Evidence suggests,' UNAIDS reported, 'that messages and activities developed at the grassroots level are much more effective than those developed by remote "professionals".'[60]

Alongside the stabilisation or decline of prevalence, a further indication that the epidemic was maturing was the changing social profile of infection. Many early epidemics had first affected relatively small numbers of sex workers and their more numerous male clients. Over time, as the infected men transmitted the disease to their other partners and the epidemic became generalised, perhaps half of new infections took place within regular partnerships. By the mid 1990s prevalence in Zimbabwe was higher among married than unmarried people, while a study in Lusaka in 2000–1 found that 52 per cent of post-partum women stating that they had no or little risk of infection were in fact already infected. 'Today it is not a question of promiscuity, it's just a question of sex,' Noerine Kaleeba had written in 1991. 'The level of infection in Uganda is such that every time you have unprotected sexual intercourse you are exposing yourself. Certainly most clients I have talked to have said nothing to make me suspect that they even know what promiscuity means.'[61] In this situation the gender balance among those infected shifted towards women, because they were generally younger than their partners, were especially susceptible when young, and survived longer with the disease.

A study in 1997–8 found that approximately 19 per cent of women in Kisumu and 23 per cent in Ndola contracted HIV within one year of sexual debut. In Senegal the number of women with HIV quadrupled between 1989 and 2004 while that of men only doubled. By 2004, some 57 per cent of Africans with HIV were women. In the extreme case of Kenya, they outnumbered men by nearly two to one.[62] Around 2000 the life expectancy of men overtook that of women in South Africa, shortly followed by Zimbabwe, Zambia, Malawi, and Kenya. As the proportion of infected women increased, so did the number of maternal Aids orphans – who outnumbered paternal orphans in sub-Saharan Africa by 2004 – and of infected babies. Africa had 90 per cent of the world's HIV-positive children.[63]

As HIV increasingly concentrated among women, so also it concentrated among the poor. This had not been true earlier in the epidemic, when those most likely to contract HIV had often been mobile people, as in Karonga, and frequently the more educated. In Lusaka in 1994, a pregnant woman with ten or more years of education had a 161 per cent higher likelihood of HIV infection than a woman with four years or less of education. By 1998, however, the educated woman in Lusaka was only 33 per cent more likely to be infected. The change was probably due to the educated woman's greater exposure to propaganda and her better opportunities to protect herself. At Uganda's main testing centre in the late 1990s, the higher a client's education, the less the likelihood of infection.[64] More broadly, the expansion of disease in the countryside, as in Rwanda and Ethiopia, was also an expansion among the poor. HIV came to justify its description as a 'misery-seeking missile'.[65]

Stabilisation of HIV prevalence might often mean only that deaths had risen to equal new infections, but it marked a difference from those countries where the epidemic was still visibly expanding. In many of these, especially in western Africa, the expansion was barely perceptible. In others it was more disturbing. Nigeria, with its huge population, caused much concern. Official antenatal prevalence figures showed an increase between 1993 and 2001 from 3.8 to 5.8 per cent, followed perhaps by a slight decline, but much doubt surrounded these findings, individual states within the federation recorded prevalence up to 12 per cent, and even the official figure implied that over three million Nigerians were infected, the largest number in the continent outside South Africa. 'The epidemic in Nigeria ... is now common in the general population,' a policy document warned in 2003; '... the nation is now threatened by an exponential and explosive growth.'[66] Cameroun also caused alarm when reported antenatal prevalence in Yaounde rose between 1996 and 2000 from 2 to 11 per cent and the latter figure was also reported for the country as a whole. Following further research, UNAIDS reduced the estimated national adult prevalence in 2003 to 6.9 per cent and the Ministry of Health to 5.5 per cent, but even these figures suggested a significant and unexplained increase in a country whose epidemic had been regarded as low-key.[67] The most disturbing of the established epidemics, however, was that in Swaziland, where adult prevalence was estimated at 38.8 per cent in 2003, the highest in the world, and it was not yet certain that the peak had been reached.[68]

The other cause for particular concern was the long-term impact of war. Violence itself might inhibit the spread of disease, probably by obstructing civilian mobility, but the aftermath of war was exceptionally dangerous when mobility resumed, refugees returned, and often highly infected combatants were reintegrated into the general population. This had occurred during the 1990s in Mozambique, where general adult prevalence rose to 12.2 per cent in 2003 and was thought still to be increasing.[69] Sierra Leone's prevalence at that time was still low, but was watched with trepidation. Liberia's had risen rapidly to 5.9 per cent and was potentially very dangerous.[70] In Sudan, where adult infection in the south was estimated in 2004 at 2.6 per cent, with higher proportions among refugees, it was feared that the prospect of peace at that time might open the possibility of an explosive epidemic.[71]

The two most uncertain situations were in the DR Congo and Côte d'Ivoire. Studies of Congolese provincial cities in 2002, after nearly 40 years of violence and insecurity, surprisingly found levels of antenatal prevalence between 3 and 6 per cent, much the same as at the time of Projet Sida, but unconfirmed reports suggested much higher prevalence in parts of the war-ridden eastern region bordering Rwanda and Uganda.[72] Similar uncertainty surrounded the impact of civil war in Côte d'Ivoire. Its epidemic was declining rapidly during the late 1990s in Abidjan, where antenatal prevalence fell between 1997 and 2002 from 14 to 6 per cent, and was probably approaching stability in the country as a whole at the latter date. In the north, however, near-secession during 2002 led medical workers to flee, closed most schools, and forced many young people into risky survival activities. Reports of the rapid spread of disease there awaited confirmation by a population survey during 2005.[73]

By 2005 the number of HIV-positive Africans was still increasing slowly. The chief reason why it was not increasing more quickly was that growing numbers of infected people were dying. Whether the incidence of new infections was declining anywhere, even in Uganda, remained uncertain. Pockets of rapid epidemic growth still existed and more gradual expansion into the countryside was widespread, but for the most part the HIV epidemic was stabilising and maturing, although it remained a fatal and terrible disease. In epidemiological theory, one major determinant of the duration of an epidemic was the length of time between infection and recovery or death.[74] With HIV/Aids that averaged about ten years. It would be a long epidemic.

13
Containment

During the late 1990s and early 2000s response to HIV/Aids was revitalised at both the global and the African levels. Leadership passed from the WHO to the Joint United Nations Programme on Aids (UNAIDS) in 1996, but the main dynamic came from the discovery of antiretroviral drugs (ARVs) that could suppress, but not cure, the disease. ARVs brought hope, the crucial quality needed to activate health workers and people with HIV/Aids. As with previous African diseases, it needed such a magic bullet – penicillin for syphilis, dapsone for leprosy – to stimulate a mass treatment campaign. Yet to make ARVs available to millions of infected Africans required radical changes of attitude among international donors, shifts of power in the pharmaceutical industry, and infusions of energy into African regimes – infusions that might in turn require pressure by those in desperate need of drugs. Here the source of HIV's power – its slow action and long incubation – became its weakness, for unlike many other epidemic diseases it gave infected people time to organise a counter-attack. By 2005 only a small minority of Africans needing ARVs were receiving them and it was increasingly obvious that the drugs, while immensely valuable to individuals, could not reverse the epidemic. The search for a vaccine, which in principle could achieve that goal, was still desperately slow. Nevertheless, between 1996 and 2005 the scene was transformed. Hitherto the virus had held the initiative. Now the victims were taking it.

UNAIDS took responsibility for coordinating international action against the epidemic in January 1996. It grew out of the impatience with WHO displayed by richer, more interventionist international agencies from the early 1990s as they developed separate and often competing Aids programmes. Only the United Nations, it was realised, could bring these agencies together, and even then there was doubt until 1994 whether the World Bank would join the coalition. Based alongside the WHO at Geneva, UNAIDS did not take over its medical functions or those of other agencies, nor was it a funding body. Rather, it sought to coordinate, define, and publicise policies, acting through 'theme groups' in each country bringing together the local representatives of the various international agencies. Its first Director-General was Peter Piot, a veteran of the first investigation at Mama Yemo in 1983.

Piot was quick to stress the continuity between UNAIDS and the WHO's Global Programme. Its principles, he declared, were 'a clear concern for human rights, a desire to meet the needs of young people, a commitment to ensuring a strong gender dimension in policy and programmes, and the need to ensure that people living with HIV and AIDS are properly involved at all stages'. But UNAIDS was more than a medical institution and it insisted that HIV/Aids must be seen as a multi-sectoral development problem, that 'people's vulnerability has social and economic roots, often including marginalisation, poverty and women's subordinate status'. To tackle this development challenge, each country must shift its HIV/Aids programme from its Health Ministry to the Office of the President or Prime Minister, who would preside over a council representing government departments and non-governmental interests, with an Aids component in each departmental programme. Multi-sectoralism, mainstreaming, and political commitment became catchwords of the new approach. 'I had two major objectives when I got into this job,' Piot later recalled. 'The first one was to bring AIDS onto the political agenda in the affected countries and the second one was in the north making sure that this remains a global issue.'[1]

Despite Piot's dynamism, UNAIDS made rather little practical impact during the later 1990s. The end of WHO funding created severe financial difficulties for several national programmes. Although UNAIDS was not intended to prepare national Aids plans in the manner of the Global Programme, in reality the new principles demanded a new generation of plans, targeted at potential donors. By 2002, 40 African countries had produced them, often with a large input from the local theme group. If not exactly 'hatched like chickens', many had a distinct family likeness, not least because UNAIDS organised a workshop on how to draft them. Large sections of the plans for Benin and Togo were identical.[2] Many lacked distinctive national character and showed signs of weariness. 'Despite advocacy efforts by the National Aids Control Programme,' Tanzania confessed, 'the National Response to the epidemic is yet to pick up a sufficient momentum. To a large extent things are still "business as usual".'[3] Some plans blamed what the DR Congo described as 'the feeble involvement of the highest political level of the state',[4] although several national leaders did show a new concern with the epidemic during the late 1990s, notably in Malawi, Botswana, and Ethiopia. All plans enthusiastically adopted the UNAIDS catchwords: multi-dimensionality, multi-disciplinarity, multi-sectoriality, decentralisation, and communitarianism. 'Lesotho has jumped on the global bandwagon that embraced the multi-sectoral approaches,' it proclaimed, proposing to undertake everything simultaneously, a feature of many plans that were in reality shopping lists for donors. As Tanzania put it, 'The National Multi-sectoral Strategic Framework does not attempt to prioritise among those objectives or strategies. It insists on the comprehensiveness of the Response.'[5] In reality, most national programmes remained under Health Ministry control.

The problem was that, beneath the rhetoric, the later 1990s produced few new ideas for dealing with generalised HIV epidemics in poor countries. This was clear from the two most important policy documents of the time, both produced by the World Bank, the most assertive institution. *Confronting AIDS* (1997) was strongly influenced by experience in Thailand and argued that the most effective preventive measure was to target high-risk groups like commercial sex workers, especially at an early stage but even in mature epidemics.[6] *Intensifying action against HIV/AIDS in Africa* (1999), by contrast, proposed a more diffuse approach, stressing the need to regard HIV/Aids as a development issue, to expand the resources available and the knowledge base, and to concentrate on 'specific interventions using voluntary counselling and testing ... condom social marketing, peer education, and treatment of sexually transmitted infections'. One critic described this as reinventing the wheel.[7] Of the two main interventions advocated, the targeting of commercial sex workers was questioned by a study of Cotonou, Yaounde, Kisumu, and Ndola, organised by UNAIDS, which found that the two West African cities with low HIV prevalence had levels of commercial sex as high as the two East African cities with high HIV prevalence; more important was that the latter had lower levels of male circumcision and higher prevalence of HSV-2. The other intervention especially pressed by the World Bank and the European Union, the treatment of sexually transmitted diseases, had spectacular initial success against an early epidemic near Mwanza in Tanzania, reducing the incidence of new HIV infections by 42 per cent, but had no impact at all when tried against mature epidemics in Rakai and Masaka where STDs were no longer a major risk factor for transmission.[8] The poverty of current thinking about the African epidemic emerged vividly in 2000 when a committee of the British House of Commons discovered that the country's official assistance to Aids programmes in Africa had declined, giving the impression that the department concerned did not know what to do about a generalised epidemic, whereas assistance to Asia had increased because there, as an official put it, 'we do have a window of opportunity'.[9]

One point on which these programmes of the late 1990s agreed was that antiretroviral drugs were no answer to the African epidemic. *Confronting AIDS* dismissed them as 'currently unaffordable and too demanding of clinical services to offer realistic hope in the near term for the millions of poor people infected in developing countries'. The British committee, likewise, concluded that the provision of antiretrovirals to 'people with HIV in the poorest developing world is clearly not a practical or sustainable development'.[10] The first antiretroviral, azidothymidine (AZT), had been synthesised in 1964 in the hope that it would stop cancer cells replicating. It failed and had such severe side-effects that it sat on a shelf at Burroughs-Wellcome's laboratory for twenty years until it was tested again in 1985 to see whether it would stop the process by which HIV converted its RNA into the DNA of the host cell.[11] Although initially spectacularly successful, its cost – about US$3,000 per patient per year in 1991 – was an absolute barrier, and during the early 1990s it was found to delay the deaths of people with HIV/Aids by only six to twelve months. In 1994, however, research showed that AZT was effective in another field: it could prevent transmission of HIV from mother to child.[12]

Perinatal transmission was, after sexual intercourse, the most important means by which HIV was passed on, especially in Africa, where 90 per cent of all such transmissions took place and about 10 per cent of all babies might be infected at birth in areas of high HIV prevalence.[13] Africans, indeed, often believed that all children of HIV-positive mothers inherited the disease, although in fact between one-quarter and one-half did so, roughly twice the proportion in Europe. The risk varied with the severity of the mother's infection and the extent and duration of breast-feeding, for it was reckoned that on average about 6 per cent of babies were infected in the womb, 14 per cent during birth, and another 14 per cent during breast-feeding, a proportion that could rise if breast-feeding extended beyond six months, as in Africa it often did. Between one-quarter and one-third of infected babies died during their first year and at least three-quarters by age five.[14] Surveys suggested that most women in highly infected areas knew of perinatal transmission in the early 1990s and that information spread to other regions during the decade. Knowledge that breast-feeding could transmit the disease spread more slowly; in the early 2000s only 46 per cent of women in Uganda and 53 per cent in South Africa knew this.[15] Transmission by breast-feeding had been demonstrated in 1985 but was initially declared unimportant and was deliberately played down for fear of discouraging an otherwise beneficial practice. In 1996 UNAIDS advised that HIV-positive mothers should be given the best information available and left to choose whether to breast-feed.[16]

Perinatal transmission caused African women terrible anxieties. If a pregnant woman knew she had HIV and might infect her child or not live to raise it, she had to decide whether to terminate the pregnancy, which few did. Probably more often, the mother did not know her HIV status and learned it only when her child sickened and died. In one series of cases at Bangui,

> The mother's reaction to the announcement of their child's serology was marked by resignation (87 cases), evasion (14 cases) and rejection of the results (2 cases).... Parents informed of the serological status of their children practically never return to medical care, save sometimes to report the news of the child's death.[17]

'At first I could not even walk on the street,' a young mother in Durban recalled. 'I felt that everybody was just looking at me and blaming me for making my baby sick. For them it was me who was killing my baby.' Breast-feeding was immensely important to African women, both culturally and because its abandonment might reveal their infected condition and expose them to violence for failing to care for their child. Yet HIV corrupted even this: 'All the time I thought I was breastfeeding my baby, but I was giving him poison.'[18]

The discovery in 1994 that AZT could reduce mother-to-child transmission by 68 per cent transformed the situation in developed countries. After 1998 fewer than 3 per cent of the babies born to HIV-positive mothers there were infected. But AZT administered during pregnancy, at delivery, and during the neonatal period cost about US$1,000 per case.[19] In 1998 trials in Thailand showed that AZT administered only in the last month of pregnancy and at delivery reduced transmission in a non-breastfeeding population by 51 per cent, at substantially lower cost. The WHO recommended this for poor countries, but in the meantime another reverse transcriptase inhibitor, nevirapine, entered trials in Uganda and was shown in 1999 to reduced transmission by 48 per cent at a cost of only US$4 per case for the drug, excluding the costs of administration. The WHO immediately approved it.[20] Nevirapine could have side-effects, did not combine well with standard tuberculosis medication, and rapidly provoked resistant mutations in the virus, which was not immediately important where only a single dose was given but could hamper later antiretroviral treatment. These difficulties and the drug's rapid testing and approval made it a subject of later controversy, but it came to be widely used in poor countries. Some argued, also, that the expense of administering it made it less cost-effective than it appeared, an argument against which Piot stressed the 'hope factor' that it offered.

Another problem surrounding prevention of mother-to-child transmission was that the drugs might protect the babies but not their mothers, thus swelling Africa's orphan population. As Ugandan women observed, 'Women are not incubators for babies. We deserve treatment in our own right.'[21] Moreover, antiretroviral drugs like AZT and nevirapine gave no protection against infection by breast-feeding. The only agreement on this point was that mothers should either breast-feed exclusively during the early months or should use only formula foods; to use both, as was common, was to expose the baby to the dangers of both.[22] Exclusive use of formula foods was generally acceptable, however, only to better-off mothers and in the more modern settings such as Botswana, Côte d'Ivoire, and South African towns where water supplies were good and women who did not breast-feed were less likely to be stigmatised. These were also the areas where women were most willing to be tested for HIV, which was essential if they were to be selected for antiretroviral treatment. By contrast, acceptance of testing and antiretroviral treatment elsewhere was often low, both from fear of stigmatisation and possible violence and because no treatment was offered to the women themselves.[23]

Botswana was the first African country, in 1999, to launch an extensive programme to prevent mother-to-child transmission. By late 2002 some 34 per cent of pregnant women with HIV were receiving AZT, transmission was estimated to have fallen by 22 per cent, and the main hospital at Gaborone was the largest antiretroviral treatment site in the world.[24] Uganda, with more infected women and less money, also began in 1999 but had fewer than 5 per cent of eligible women under treatment in 2002 and perhaps 15 per cent in 2004, when every district hospital offered the service.[25] UNAIDS estimated that in 2003 only 10 per cent of pregnant women with HIV in sub-Saharan Africa were offered antiretroviral medication. 'My concern as a parent who has lost a child to AIDS,' a Swazi woman declared, 'is the lack of drugs that prevent the transmission of the disease to babies. Those drugs are the only way we know that has been effective in the fight against this disease.'[26]

This issue became especially acute in South Africa. Once the African National Congress had taken power there in 1994, its alliance with Aids activists began to break down. The government could not afford NACOSA's unrealistic Aids plan and gave higher priority to unifying the country's health systems, reducing expenditure on high-quality hospital treatment, giving free treatment to infants and pregnant women, expanding primary health care for the poor, and decentralising its provision to the provinces. Although real public health expenditure per capita fell during the later 1990s, the percentage allocated to 'basic health services' rose between 1992–3 and 1997–8 from 11 to 21 per cent. By 1998 the new government had built some 560 rural clinics.[27] Yet this drastic reversal of policy threw medical structures and staffing into disorder for a decade, not least because it was carried through with the jealous authoritarianism of an inexperienced and insecure regime. Demoralised nurses struck over pay and conditions while doctors withdrew to private practice or left the country. In the poorest provinces like the Eastern Cape, health systems were gravely weakened. As a result, the HIV/Aids epidemic was neglected at the moment of its most rapid expansion, apart from measures like condom distribution and the treatment of STDs and tuberculosis that could be given through the primary health care system. For much of the later 1990s a large proportion of the national Aids budget was not spent. In contrast to Uganda, the regime refused to work in partnership with NGOs except as its agents, cutting their state support in 1998 from 19 million to 2 million rand.[28] Instead the government marginalised the (largely white) activists and the Aids Treatment, Information, and Counselling Centres whose experience of the epidemic was thought to be outweighed by their location in high-risk urban areas and their inability to fit into the primary health care system.

Conflict between Aids activists and the regime escalated during 1996–7 when scandals in the Department of Health also embroiled the ANC executive and the Deputy President, Thabo Mbeki, who was appointed during 1998 to head an inter-ministerial committee controlling Aids policy. Meanwhile the capacity of AZT to prevent mother-to-child transmission had aroused excitement, especially at the Vancouver Aids Conference of 1996, which also focused world attention on inducing the patent holders to make AZT available more cheaply to poor countries. Doctors at major South African hospitals began to experiment with AZT, showing in 1998, as in Thailand, that a shorter and cheaper course of the drug was effective. At the same time Glaxo-Wellcome sought to divert pressure by reducing the price of AZT for pregnant women in poor countries by 75 per cent. Although doctors argued that AZT was cheaper than treating pediatric Aids, South Africa's Department of Health decided in October 1998 that it could not afford the drug and ordered pilot tests to stop. 'If you have limited resources,' the Minister explained, 'you may decide to put your resources into preventing mothers getting infected in the first place. These are difficult issues we have to face.' Many suspected that other reasons included the overburdened health system's difficulty in implementing an AZT programme, the fear that it would encourage pressure to supply AZT to adults with HIV/Aids, and the government's desire to oblige pharmaceutical companies to reduce their general price levels.[29]

This was a vital decision in the history of the African Aids epidemic because it provoked the first major political action by HIV-positive Africans, the intervention by patients into their own treatment that was a distinctive feature of the global epidemic and was, once more, a consequence of the long incubation period that enabled patients to organise themselves in substantial numbers. Organisations of people with HIV/Aids had existed for some time in tropical Africa, although little is known about them. The first may have been Zambia's Positive and Living Squad (PALS), founded in or before 1991 by a small group of HIV-positive people led by Winston Zulu, the first Zambian to make his condition public. It provided both care and advocacy.[30] By contrast, another body formed in 1991, in Senegal, was inspired by a Dakar hospital as the first of many associations stimulated from above by NGOs or governments, often to provide national representatives at international gatherings or to popularise official programmes.[31] An international umbrella organisation, the Network of African People Living with HIV/Aids, was also formed in Dakar in 1993 and was estimated in 2005 to have affiliated organisations with some two million members.[32] Another early organisation was Lumière Action, created in 1994 by HIV-positive people in Abidjan; its founder-president, Dominique Esmail, died in 1996 after refusing antiretroviral treatment until it became generally available.[33] Normally, however, these African associations lacked the radicalism that made people with HIV/Aids such a powerful force in epidemics in the United States, Australia, and Brazil. In those countries homosexuality provided a community basis and often a tradition of activism on which to found powerful pressure groups, advantages not available to heterosexual Africans with HIV/Aids, who were also slow to declare themselves publicly for fear of a stigma to which homosexuals were already accustomed. Instead of homosexuals, therefore, many activists in Africa, as in Thailand, were women, sometimes in separate organisations like NACWOLA in Uganda, so that the epidemic had the effect of empowering numerous women.[34] It has been suggested, also, that Africa's clientelist politics fostered private manipulation rather than public agitation, but, if so, it was a recent pattern due to the depoliticisation of the continent by its one-party states once the activism of the nationalist period was quelled, and it was a passivity broken again by the democratisation movements of the 1990s to which concern with Aids contributed.

South Africa was an exception to the otherwise remarkable lack of political turbulence created by the African epidemic during its first two decades, for in South Africa the nationalist experience had been more traumatic, more recent, and had left many internal activists marginalised once the returning ANC leadership took control. South Africa's first small organisations of HIV-positive people were established by white homosexuals, notably Body Positive, founded in Johannesburg in 1987. In 1994 the various groups came together, with backing from NACOSA and the Department of Health, to form the National Association of People with Aids (NAPWA), an organisation of the officially sponsored kind designed 'to be the assertive, legitimate, and respected voice of all people living with HIV/AIDS'. With paid officers and provincial branches financed by the state, it was active in education and training but did not create a grassroots movement.[35] Late in 1998 its refusal to contest the government's Aids policy led radicals to form a ginger group within NAPWA known as the Treatment Action Campaign (TAC), apparently named after a section of ACT UP, the American organisation dedicated to direct action on behalf of people with HIV/Aids. When NAPWA's leaders refused in March 1999 to organise demonstrations demanding provision of AZT at affordable prices to prevent mother-to-child transmission, TAC broke away as an entirely independent body.[36] Its most prominent leader, Zackie Achmat, an HIV-positive homosexual, had been an underground youth organiser for the ANC and insisted on TAC's loyalty to the party.[37] He drew into the movement legal and medical expertise to strengthen its insistence, as another activist put it, 'that, as a person living with HIV, you have to take prime responsibility, you have to know as much as the doctor; you have to follow the politics'. Achmat was later to claim that 'the most important thing that we've done is to challenge the paternalism of public health'. Equally important was to revive the protest tactics of the anti-Apartheid struggle and attract the support of the young, poor, and female who were primarily affected by HIV and provided most of the tens of thousands of members in TAC's 110 branches (in 2004). Achmat himself became a hero by refusing, like Dominique Esmail, to take antiretrovirals until they were generally available.[38]

The TAC had not expected the government to resist the provision of antiretrovirals for pregnant women once it was clearly feasible. That the government did resist had many reasons, but probably the central one was political: an insecure regime's anxiety to maintain control over a situation perceived as threatening. The threat was that pressure from a coalition of HIV-positive people, Aids activists, political opponents within and outside the ANC, pharmaceutical companies, and international opinion might oblige the government to undertake an antiretroviral programme that it could neither administer nor afford at current drug prices, at the expense of its authority, its health priorities, and its wider development programme. Thabo Mbeki, once he became president in 1999, felt especially threatened, for he lived in the shadow of a still-active Nelson Mandela and aspired to challenge entrenched white power structures on a national and global scale. His many and varied pronouncements about HIV/Aids expressed his racial bitterness, his intellectual vanity, and a politician's search for an understanding of the epidemic capable of rallying support and countering the weight of scientific opinion deployed by the coalition against him.

The first major political threat to the regime's Aids policy was a decision in January 1999 by the provincial government of the Western Cape, which was hostile to the ANC, to defy the ban on providing AZT to pregnant women. At Khayelitsha, outside Cape Town, it allowed Médecins sans Frontières to establish a pilot scheme designed to prove that treatment was feasible in a poor area and to use HIV/Aids to spearhead demands for cheaper drugs and larger global aid.[39] The programme halved transmission. Soon after his election as president in June 1999, however, Mbeki publicised claims that AZT was toxic. A month later the Minister of Health doubted the drug's effectiveness.[40] Mbeki was to return to these claims frequently. In the meantime he invited dissident scientists, mainly from the United States, to meet with leading African Aids specialists to devise a response to the distinctive crisis of Africa's mass, heterosexual epidemic. The meetings were predictably inconclusive, but these contacts provided Mbeki with the argument, which he set out when opening the International Aids Conference at Durban in July 2000, that the real health problem was poverty.[41] As he later insisted, he did not doubt that HIV was *one* cause of Aids, 'But you have got to take into account the fact that extreme poverty destroys the immune system of people as well. So we cannot, this government, narrow our response to Aids to merely an anti-[retro]viral response. It's got to be more comprehensive.'[42]

Mbeki may have hoped that his stress on poverty would find resonance among ANC supporters, for evidence suggested that many South Africans saw Aids as only one among many consequences of poverty.[43] Yet his stance also provoked resentment:

> The president seems to be playing games with foreigners while our children and young people are drying up and dying like beautiful cut flowers in a vase.... Thabo Mbeki is too proud to admit he was wrong about this HIV thing. Pride is a sign of a weak leader.... Mbeki, if you want to be a world leader, go to the UN. Let us find a president who cares about his own people.[44]

During 2001 South Africa's liberal newspapers, themselves recently accused by ANC leaders of racism, replied by attacking Mbeki savagely as a scientifically illiterate denialist arrogantly disputing medical orthodoxy: 'President Thabo Mbeki and his entire government must either get their act together in combating the HIV/Aids catastrophe – now – or get out of government.'[45] The country's leading black scientist, Malegapuru Makgoba, protested that 'To conflate causation with cofactors through a mixture of pseudoscientific statements is scientifically and politically dangerous in societies where denial, chauvinism, fear, and ignorance are rampant.'[46] More dangerously, opposition surfaced within the ANC when its national health committee called on Mbeki and his Health Minister to acknowledge that HIV caused Aids in accordance with 'the predominant scientific view'. And in the local government elections of 2000 the ANC lost votes to parties that promised free antiretrovirals to pregnant women.[47]

In October 2000 Mbeki told his national executive that he was withdrawing from 'the public debate' on the science of HIV. Although this proved untrue, it created a space during which developments on other fronts changed the situation. Between mid 2000 and April 2001 the price of antiretroviral drugs to poor countries fell by 90 per cent owing to competition from generic producers in India and elsewhere and attempts by multinational companies to head off the challenge by reducing their own prices. In April 2001 the Pharmaceutical Manufacturers Association of South Africa abandoned a long-standing legal attempt to prevent the government from importing generics, largely because TAC intervention had led the court to require the companies to produce details of their pricing procedures.[48] Although the TAC hoped that this would lead to rapid provision of antiretrovirals for adults with HIV/Aids, in fact the government's intentions went no further than the prevention of mother-to-child transmission. In April 2001 Nevirapine was at last approved for this purpose. The first of 18 planned pilot sites began to make it available, but the Health Minister insisted that this was designed to test the drug's toxicity and the feasibility of administering it. Exasperated at delay in providing a treatment widely available elsewhere in the world, the TAC filed a legal case in August 2001 demanding that the government institute a general programme to satisfy citizens' constitutional right to life.[49]

This challenge to executive authority brought Mbeki back into the dispute. In October 2001, at the black university at Fort Hare, he expressed most fiercely the racial bitterness provoked by Apartheid and early Western theories of the origin of Aids. 'Convinced that we are but natural-born, promiscuous carriers of germs, unique in the world,' he declared, 'they proclaim that our continent is doomed to an inevitable mortal end because of our unconquerable devotion to the sin of lust.'[50] Three years later he told the National Assembly:

> I for my part will not keep quiet while others whose minds have been corrupted by the disease of racism, accuse us, the black people of South Africa, Africa, and the world, as being by virtue of our Africanness and skin colour – lazy, liars, foul-smelling, diseased, corrupt, violent, amoral, sexually depraved, animalistic, savage, and racist.

A critic described these views as 'the ultimate victory of the apartheid mindset'.[51]

In December 2001 the Pretoria High Court ruled that 'a countrywide mother-to-child-transmission programme is an ineluctable obligation of the state' wherever the capacity to provide it existed.[52] Government appealed to the Constitutional Court on the grounds that this was an interference in the functions of the executive, but without success. The Health Department tried to insist that experience at its eighteen trial sites must be analysed before wider treatment was attempted, but in February 2002 the provincial governments in Gauteng and KwaZulu announced that they would make it generally available. This split within the ANC leadership produced the most ferocious crisis in the entire sequence, for Mandela backed the demand to expand the programme and Mbeki's loyalists in the national executive accused the former president of undermining his successor and flouting party loyalty.[53] In doing so they distributed an extraordinary document, apparently authored by Peter Mokaba, soon to die of suspected Aids, which denounced antiretrovirals as poisons and the orthodox interpretation of HIV/Aids as propagated by vested interests including pharmaceutical companies, 'governments and official health institutions, inter-governmental organisations, official medical licensing and registration institutions, scientists and academics, media organisations, NGOs and individuals'.[54] This paranoia was too much for the senior African civil servants in the Health Department, who threatened resignation, for several powerful figures around Mbeki, and eventually for the Cabinet, which in April 2002 appointed a Task Team to arrange the general provision of nevirapine to HIV-positive pregnant women and agreed to multiply the Aids budget five times between 2001–2 and 2004–5, while declaring that it would seek to reduce the price of antiretrovirals further before they could be made generally available to people with Aids.[55] Three months later the Constitutional Court ordered the government to make nevirapine available to pregnant women in all sectors of the public health system. By March 2003 most provinces were complying, but this revealed the incapacity of many health systems to supply more than a fraction of those in need.[56]

The struggle over perinatal provision in South Africa was a key point in making antiretrovirals available to Africans, for it not only stimulated political activism among people with HIV/Aids and campaigning organisations like Médecins sans Frontières but introduced the generic drugs that were to make antiretroviral treatment more generally accessible. Highly active antiretroviral therapy (HAART) became widely available in rich countries during 1996 through the discovery of drugs known as protease inhibitors that prevented the virally corrupted DNA in cells from maturing into an infectious virus. When combined with reverse transcriptase inhibitors like AZT or nevirapine, usually as a three-drug combination, HAART avoided much of the drug resistance provoked by monotherapy and proved remarkably effective in repressing, but not eradicating, HIV, so that the treatment had to be taken for life. 'Nobody can call Aids an inevitably fatal, incurable disease any more,' Piot told the Vancouver Aids Conference of 1996. Between 1997 and 2001 the death rate from Aids in Europe and North America fell by 84 per cent. It was perhaps the greatest achievement of the chemotherapeutic research that had come to dominate twentieth-century medicine, but it was initially complicated to administer and monitor, and it was very expensive, costing $10,000–15,000 per person per year in 1996.[57] This was why the World Bank and the British Department for International Development held in the late 1990s that HAART could not be a basis for Aids policy in poor countries. HIV/Aids, as a fatal complaint, was becoming another Third World disease.

HAART reached Africa through several routes. One was private purchase by wealthy South Africans. The first protease inhibitors were registered there in 1996, facilities for monitoring viral load were set up in the same year, and an HIV Clinicians Society was launched in 1998. Four years later most of the 20,000 South Africans receiving antiretrovirals obtained them in the private sector. Most were financed by medical schemes, which had discovered that antiretrovirals were cheaper than hospital treatment.[58] Others gained access through their companies. Early in 2001, as the price of antiretrovirals fell, Anglo American decided to provide them for its 200,000 employees in South Africa, as did the Debswana diamond-mining company in Botswana. Other major companies in southern Africa adopted the same policy, followed by some of the most progressive employers in the east and west.[59] There, during the late 1990s, a few wealthy individuals also bought antiretrovirals from pharmacies or received them from relatives abroad, often taking only one or two drugs intermittently rather than the recommended daily triple therapy. In 2000 a study described private drug use in Harare as 'therapeutic anarchy', threatening to breed permanent drug resistance.[60] Three years earlier, however, UNAIDS had launched two Drug Access Initiatives in the capitals of Uganda and Côte d'Ivoire to examine more orderly methods of provision. In Uganda nearly a thousand patients were recruited into the scheme, many in very advanced stages of disease. There were remarkable recoveries, but patients had to pay for the drugs, at up to US$700 a month for triple and US$200 for dual therapy, so that some dropped out, others struggled to comply, and many outside the programme complained that it was only for the rich. The main achievement was perhaps to train nearly 200 medical workers to administer antiretrovirals.[61] In Côte d'Ivoire the scheme also treated about a thousand patients but operated on different lines, beginning with the cheaper dual therapy, subsidising the price for most patients, admitting them at earlier stages of disease, and selecting them chiefly by ability to pay or by their active participation in associations for people with HIV/Aids. When dual therapy stimulated resistance, so that many patients abandoned a scheme that seemed to do them no good, it was dropped in favour of triple therapy and higher subsidies, although the expense still led many to fall away. Further expansion was frustrated by the country's growing political disorder. Meanwhile, Senegal launched a successful antiretroviral programme of its own in 1998, but for only 58 patients.[62]

The chief obstacle to these initiatives in the late 1990s, the cost of drugs, was broken in February 2001 when Cipla, an Indian manufacturer of generics with no research and development costs, offered to sell triple therapy drugs for $350 per person per year. The effective minimum price remained at or slightly below this level for the next four years. Producers also simplified medication by combining the drugs into a single tablet. Activists within and outside UNAIDS realised that this breakthrough created an opportunity to revitalise HIV/Aids programmes and raise new levels of international funding that, for the first time, might have a dramatic effect on the epidemic. The World Bank had already taken the initiative in September 2000 by making a billion dollars available in grants or concessional loans. In June 2001 a special session of the United Nations General Assembly agreed to establish a Global Fund for Aids, Tuberculosis, and Malaria with an ambitious target of providing US$10 billion a year for low- and middle-income countries, whereas total HIV/Aids expenditure there in 2001 was only US$2.1 billion. In reality, by January 2005 the Fund had approved some US$1.7 billion in grants for HIV/Aids projects, mostly in Africa. In addition, the United States government announced in January 2003 a Presidential Emergency Programme for Aids Relief (PEPFAR) to make available US$15 billion over five years to fifteen countries with high HIV prevalence, twelve of them in Africa. Some US$2.4 billion of this money was allocated during 2004.[63] Other funds were made available at the same period, whether by philanthropic bodies like the Gates Foundation (especially in Botswana), debt relief (as in Cameroun), bilateral donors, or other sources. Between 2001 and 2004 global funding for HIV/Aids in low- and middle-income countries trebled to US$6.1 billion per year. UNAIDS reckoned at that time that such aid provided 50 per cent of all HIV/Aids spending in sub-Saharan Africa, national governments provided 6–10 per cent and the remainder came from development banks or from families and individuals.[64]

Not all of this money was spent on antiretrovirals. By 2004 some US$550 million per year were devoted to vaccine research and there was talk of multiplying this by factors of two or ten.[65] This was a new enthusiasm. In principle a vaccine was the only known way to end a viral epidemic. In the early days of HIV/Aids optimism was high. A leading American specialist estimated in 1984 that it might take two years to produce a vaccine. In 1991

Montagnier stretched that to five. Before long, however, it was realised that this 'will be one of the most formidable challenges ever assigned to health sciences'.[66] Three fundamental difficulties faced the scientists: whether a vaccine could stimulate an effective immune response if the virus itself did not do so; whether a vaccine could overcome the defensive effect of HIV's extraordinary speed of mutation; and whether any single vaccine could be effective against the many HIV subtypes.[67] In practical terms, moreover, there was no animal model on which potential vaccines could be tested and no researcher dared produce an attenuated live vaccine of the kind generally most effective, lest it should prove only too live. In addition, there was no great public pressure in developed countries for a vaccine, since HIV was relatively easy to avoid there, and little incentive for pharmaceutical firms to invest in it, since any profits likely to come from poor countries after a long research programme would be far outweighed by the costs of lawsuits if the vaccine failed. By 1997 only about 1 per cent of international HIV/Aids research spending had been devoted to vaccines,[68] but it had become clear that publicly funded research was essential. It began substantially in the late 1990s in the United States and through the International Aids Vaccine Initiative.

Several African countries were involved in the new vaccine experiments. In 1999, after much controversy, Uganda undertook Africa's first small-scale trial, which 'demonstrated the feasibility of conducting scientifically valid vaccine research' there.[69] Five years later a more ambitious trial in Kenya was successfully conducted, but demonstrated the ineffectiveness of the vaccine. An important South African research programme began in 1999 and put its first vaccine into initial trials in 2003.[70] By 2004 none of the 30 vaccines subjected to trials had shown any serious promise, but 22 were still being tested. The responsible WHO official warned at that time that no vaccine could be ready for administration before 2015 at the earliest. Sceptics feared that none might ever be possible. There was more optimism about the possibility of developing a microbicide that women could use to prevent HIV entering their bodies during intercourse. Long neglected, this was hoped to yield a marketable product by 2010 or soon afterwards.[71]

Before the finance mobilised by the Global Fund and other institutions could be used for antiretroviral programmes, it was essential to expand HIV testing facilities to identify who needed the drugs. Voluntary counselling and testing (VCT) had been pioneered by TASO in 1990 at the Uganda Aids Information Centre, which by 2002 had expanded to 70 sites, had tested over 700,000 people, and had probably contributed significantly to Uganda's declining prevalence rates. VCT sites were opened in several other capital cities during the 1990s, but in 2000 UNAIDS estimated that only 5 per cent of HIV-positive people in the developing world knew their status.[72] Although there was evidence that such knowledge encouraged behavioural change, there was nevertheless much resistance to seeking the information so long as it might incur stigma without offering effective treatment. In one trial in Zambia, fewer than 4 per cent of those invited agreed to be tested and fewer than half of those returned for the result.[73] Once antiretrovirals became available in the early 2000s, however, medical authorities and donors undertook a massive expansion of the programme. By the end of 2004 Zambia had 172 VCT sites, Kenya over 400, and South Africa over 3,000 (at the great majority of primary health care facilities).[74]

The combination of VCT and antiretroviral drugs had important implications for the human rights principles that had governed international Aids policies since the time of Jonathan Mann. Health administrators in southern Africa had often chafed against these principles and demanded that HIV/Aids should become a notifiable disease that patients and doctors must declare and possibly accept treatment for. Extremists like Brigadier David Chiweza in Zimbabwe and his Citizens AIDS Survival Trust urged mandatory annual testing, the introduction of HIV status certificates, and the criminalisation of HIV transmission.[75] The appearance of antiretrovirals stimulated new demands for notification and led some to propose mandatory treatment. A less drastic alternative of routine testing was advocated by a veteran Aids researcher, Dr Kevin De Cock, and the Centers for Disease Control in the United States. Given the scale of Africa's generalised epidemic,

> We think that Africa would now benefit most from an approach to HIV/AIDS based on a public health model that includes voluntary counselling, testing, and partner notification; routine HIV testing in prevention services such as prevention of mother-to-child transmission, and treatment for sexually transmitted infections; routine diagnostic HIV testing for patients seeking medical treatment (e.g., for tuberculosis); and enhanced access to HIV/AIDS care.[76]

Routine testing meant that the patient could refuse. Although human rights advocates warned that it might put patients, especially women, at risk of violence, routine 'opt-out' testing was adopted as a counterpart to antiretroviral treatment in Botswana, where one in seven patients were reported to refuse the test. Zambia's Health Ministry sought to adopt a similar policy. So too, with slightly different emphasis, did UNAIDS and the WHO, which, while continuing to express their commitment to human rights, recommended in 2004 'that, particularly in key health care settings such as antenatal clinics and tuberculosis treatment facilities, counselling and testing be offered routinely'.[77] Specialists realised that antiretrovirals had 'the potential to change community perceptions of people living with AIDS'.[78] The evolution of the disease and its treatment was outdating early approaches, although it was fortunate that those had prevented formal discriminatory structures that might have been difficult to remove.

When the Global Fund was established early in 2002, there was still great scepticism in the West about the wisdom of investing so much in antiretroviral programmes. It was widely believed that Africa's impoverished and decrepit health systems could neither use large sums of money effectively nor administer complex medication. The result, it was feared, would be drug resistance, corruption, neglect of preventive measures and essential structural change, greater promiscuity, and perhaps even increased infection as was alleged to have happened in Thailand when antiretrovirals became widely available. The old rivalry between HIV and primary health care surfaced again. 'If all the drugs were free most people would not get them,' Britain's Overseas

Development Minister warned in January 2003. 'What we really need to do is to look at basic health care systems that reach everybody.... The whole Western, European obsession with antiretroviral drugs is not where Africa is, except in the cities.'[79] The activists of Médecins sans Frontières, the WHO, and UNAIDS disagreed. 'Antiretroviral therapy is not only an ethical imperative,' UNAIDS insisted, 'it will also strengthen prevention efforts, increase uptake of VCT, reduce the incidence of opportunistic infections, and reduce the burden of HIV/AIDS – including the number of orphans – on families, communities and economies'.[80] Vice-President Justin Malewesi, who headed Malawi's HIV/Aids programme, expressed a widespread African view:

> I think there is too much fear about antiretrovirals (ARVs) being introduced in a poor developing country and I think the fear is that we will not be able to manage these complex drugs and therefore will lead to resistance strains being developed in Africa, which will somehow find their way to the west. And therefore the best way to protect the west is not to allow these ARVs programmes in poor developing countries. But that is of course false. We have run in this country the best TB programme in the world. We have received awards for it. We have proved that you can have a directly observed therapy programme implemented in a poorly resourced country like Malawi. Now, what is so complex about ARVs? You take one tablet in the morning when the sun comes up. You take another tablet in the evening when the sun goes down. You don't even need a wristwatch.[81]

Africa's first national antiretroviral project was Botswana's *Masa* (New Dawn) programme, launched in January 2002 and financed equally by the Gates Foundation, the Merck pharmaceutical firm, and the Botswana government. It was driven by the political commitment of President Mogae, who warned his people that, with the second highest HIV prevalence in the world, 'We are threatened with extinction', and by the most efficient and wealthy government in tropical Africa. Yet it faced the intense stigma still attached to the disease. As a programme manager recalled, 'We assumed once we started giving out the drugs, people would flock to get tests. No way. Everyone still thinks: "AIDS isn't me. It's the other guy."'[82] After nine months only 1,600 people were being treated; after 22 months, nearly 10,000. For the first two years the patients were mainly the most advanced cases, with CD4 cell counts averaging only 50–60 cells per cubic millimetre, whereas the maximum entry point to the programme was 200 cells per cubic millimetre. However, even these disappointing numbers almost overwhelmed the medical staff, who learned – as later programmes learned – that the admission and initial treatment of patients, especially advanced cases, was extremely demanding on the time of trained physicians. Patients were expected to attend fortnightly for the first month, monthly for the next three months, and every three months thereafter. Each had a family member or friend to supervise regular drug taking. The programme managers learned that antiretrovirals were eminently filchable – they had to be locked away like narcotics – and that tracking mobile patients, ensuring adherence to the drug regimen, and monitoring progress required elaborate technical and administrative procedures. And they learned that they could not operate such a programme by themselves but must involve the private sector, NGOs, the community, and above all the patients, who 'must be empowered and equipped to participate maximally in their own care'.[83] Despite all these difficulties, however, by September 2004 the programme was treating between 36,000 and 39,000 people, or perhaps half those needing treatment, the major obstacle to further expansion being the scarcity of health workers, as throughout the region. 'Many of those who have taken the cocktail of ARVs talk of a "rebirth",' a newspaper reported.[84] It was certainly the most successful programme in southern Africa, rivalled in Namibia (7,500–11,000 treated, or 28 per cent of those eligible), Swaziland (5,000–6,500, or 16 per cent), and Zambia (18,000–22,000, or 13 per cent). The least successful was in Zimbabwe, obstructed by its acute financial crisis and the refusal of the Global Fund for three years to channel funds to a government whose probity it distrusted.[85]

In eastern Africa in September 2004 the most effective programme was Uganda's, which was treating between 40,000 and 50,000 patients, or some 40 per cent of those needing it. This programme had begun more slowly, because Uganda was a poorer country than Botswana and depended on international donors if it was to supply free drugs, which it did not begin until 2004. Before then, it was reported:

> Patients desperate to receive these drugs often go to extreme lengths to mobilise funds such as selling cattle or land, their most precious assets. Children may be denied their education because school fees are used to purchase drugs.... Often patients raise the money for a few months supply of antiretrovirals, but soon they can no longer afford drugs and treatment has to stop. Patients and their families are left destitute, having sold their land and cattle and yet are still in poor health.[86]

Once free drugs became available, however, Uganda had the experience and trained staff to expand the programme relatively quickly, delegating all but the most skilled duties to nurses and paramedics. It also opened in 2004 an Infectious Diseases Institute designed to train medical practitioners from across the continent in antiretroviral therapy.[87] Other countries in eastern Africa relied on international funding but lacked Uganda's preparatory experience. In 2004 Kenya launched a piecemeal programme estimated in April 2005 to embrace some 37,680 recipients. Ethiopia initiated a more coordinated campaign in January 2005, but Tanzania's plans were frustrated by repeated delays and a gravely depleted health service, so that in December 2004 only about 1 per cent of Tanzanians needing antiretrovirals were receiving them.[88]

Owing to civil conflict, Côte d'Ivoire, the pioneer of antiretroviral treatment in western Africa, was unable to build upon its early experience; in September 2004 only 5 per cent of its people needing the drugs were receiving them, although plans and funding for rapid expansion existed. Senegal gradually expanded its free drug supply from Dakar into the provinces.[89] The most active programmes were in Gabon, a relatively wealthy country with probably the best medical system in tropical Africa, where 29 per cent of those needing antiretrovirals received them in June 2004 and the first manufacturing plant in the region opened early in 2005, using Brazilian technology; Cameroun, where Médecins sans Frontières pioneered triple therapy in 2001; and Benin, which subsidised drug prices.[90] The main problem area in West Africa was Nigeria, with its large population and exceptionally weak public health service. In 2001 President Obasanjo ostentatiously bought enough Indian generic drugs to supply 10,000 adults and 5,000 children at heavily subsidised prices, at a time when over 500,000 Nigerians needed them. After some initial hesitation, uptake was enthusiastic, but capacity to administer the drugs was slender. By February 2005 some 20,000 patients were receiving anti-retrovirals. The international target for Nigeria was 400,000 at the end of 2005. It was one of the two African countries giving greatest cause for concern.[91]

The other was South Africa, where the conflict surrounding the prevention of mother-to-child transmission had been replayed over the provision of antiretrovirals to people with HIV/Aids, with the government again struggling grimly to retain control of the process and its timing. Once drug prices had fallen dramatically early in 2001, the crucial obstacle to a programme was the feasibility of implementation by a health system already acutely overburdened. As a rural doctor commented at that time, 'If they gave us ART free of charge tomorrow, all we could hope to do is to put it in a bucket with instructions on the outside and say help yourselves – and don't come back to us if you get sick!'[92] In order to demonstrate that antiretroviral treatment was feasible in poor communities, Médecins sans Frontières extended their programme at Khayelitsha to adult cases in May 2001, in alliance with the TAC and using free generic drugs. It gave priority to the poorest and most acute cases, recording 86 per cent survival after 24 months at a cost reckoned similar to that of caring for the same patients without antiretrovirals. 'Many people in the government say that poor people are too stupid to understand how to take the antiretrovirals,' one recipient commented. 'We love these drugs. We never forget to take them. This is the most important thing to us. Like air.'[93]

Yet the authorities remained cautious and in President Mbeki's case clearly hostile. In October 2002 the Cabinet announced that it was costing the possibility of providing universal access to antiretrovirals. The budget of February 2003 increased HIV/Aids funding by 75 per cent for 'medically acceptable' treatment, but the Minister refused to commit herself to an anti-retroviral programme until sure of its cost and feasibility. Exasperated, the TAC accused her of murdering 600 people a day and launched a programme of civil disobedience. Five months of friction followed until a Cabinet revolt in August 2003 – possibly stimulated by an approaching general election – accepted the outline costing, approved a national programme in principle, and instructed the Department to develop a detailed operational plan 'as matter of urgency'. Three months later the Cabinet approved a plan that still put its first emphasis on prevention and primary health care but proposed to provide at least one antiretroviral site in each of the country's 53 health districts within 12 months, treat 53,000 patients by March 2004, and cover all 1.5 million people needing antiretrovirals within five years.[94]

It was a wildly ambitious plan where little preparation had been made, the initial stages of a programme demanded so much professional time, 31 per cent of professional health posts were vacant, 16 per cent of health workers were themselves HIV-positive, and nearly half were 'exhausted and stressed'. Three months after the plan was approved, not a single person had started treatment except in the Western Cape. Only the TAC's threat of legal action started active drug procurement, although it took another year to award tenders, mainly to local and generic producers.[95] In April 2004 Mbeki announced that the target of 53,000 new patients would be transferred from March 2004 to March 2005. In fact the public system was probably treating about 30,000 patients in February 2005. In the public and private sectors combined, about 8 per cent of those needing antiretrovirals were receiving them. Waiting lists in most areas were said to be short, because the initial demand was disappointing and the criteria for treatment were interpreted stringently. For those who received the drugs, however, they often came as salvation: 'I can now once more dream and hope to live long enough to implement my dreams.'[96]

The TAC was especially important in hastening implementation and educating those receiving the drugs. Its style of activism bred resentment among government loyalists and conservatives, leading late in 2004 to a march against it by traditional healers demanding a larger role in countering the epidemic.[97] Nevertheless, 'globalisation from below' was spreading the TAC style to countries where people with HIV/Aids had hitherto been passive. As an Ethiopian newspaper reported, 'It was a heart-rending experience to watch on CNN the demonstration by a group of HIV-positive South African youth asking their government to speedily and effectively make antiretroviral drugs available.' Addis Ababa had seen its own first protest of this kind in 2001, when its main organisation of people with HIV/Aids, Dawn of Hope, held a demonstration, said to be 30,000 strong, to demand cheap antiretrovirals.[98] Most such organisations confined themselves to providing care, working through official channels, and increasingly acting as intermediaries for the distribution of drugs, an opportunity that attracted many new associations. ACT-UP Abidjan was thought to have been domesticated in this way by receiving free antiretrovirals.[99] But in Nigeria, Namibia, Kenya, and perhaps elsewhere, associations of HIV-positive people exerted significant pressure to accelerate drug distribution. In Malawi's general election of 2004, 'Candidates from the president down reached out to a constituency once shunned as untouchable by admitting that they had lost relatives to Aids and promising to provide free treatment.'[100]

At the Barcelona Conference on HIV/Aids in July 2002 the WHO gave an overall target for the antiretroviral campaign to supply 3 million people in low- and middle-income countries by the end of 2005. The strategy was to begin immediately and use the programme to strengthen the massive weaknesses in health systems. The programme began slowly but accelerated. During the second half of 2004, the number receiving antiretrovirals increased from 440,000 to 700,000, including an increase from 150,000 to 310,000 in sub-Saharan Africa, the last figure being about 8 per cent of those needing them.[101] The task for 2005 was daunting, especially in view of the fact that another 5 million people in the world were likely to be infected during the year. But Piot was optimistic: 'I believe 3 by 5 is already changing the dynamics of how we deal with AIDS.'[102] Some long-held fears were proving well-founded. Major allegations of corruption emerged in Kenya, where the head of the National Aids Control Council was gaoled and the Council was accused, early in 2005, of misappropriating vast sums of donor funds. A tribe of MONGOs (My Own NGOs) came into being. Bogus antiretrovirals were on sale in several African countries. Early in 2005 a syndicate was reported to have smuggled over 43,500 packets of cheap drugs from Africa to Europe.[103] Other fears, however, had not been fulfilled. As in Khayelitsha, adherence to drug regimens was generally higher than in Western countries, partly because the composite drugs used in Africa – one tablet twice a day – were easier to take. Study in Cameroun showed that this generic regimen was equally effective in reducing viral load. Drug resistance was no higher than in the West. Of the first patients treated in Senegal in 1998, 81 per cent were still alive after three years, a remarkably high proportion in view of the advanced condition at which treatment began.[104] How long patients on antiretrovirals might expect to live was unknown, although an estimate at Khayelitsha was an average of slightly over eight years. The fear that people taking antiretroviral drugs might practise risky sex was controverted by the only study made, in Côte d'Ivoire.[105]

Yet even if antiretroviral drugs were made available to all advanced cases, they would have little direct impact on the epidemic, because 80–90 per cent of infectious and sexually active people were still in HIV's long incubation stage.[106] The main impact of antiretrovirals could only be indirect, by inducing people to learn their HIV status and behave accordingly, by lessening stigma, and by reducing the number of orphans. In the short term, antiretroviral treatment was likely to withdraw resources – especially human resources – from other forms of medical work, although the campaign for cheaper drugs was likely to benefit health systems as a whole. Competition for access to antiretrovirals might breed dangerous conflict, although there was little indication of this by 2005. In the longer term, antiretroviral treatment was more likely to strengthen health services and enable them to penetrate deeper into African societies, as had been true of the great epidemics of the past such as the smallpox, syphilis, and sleeping sickness outbreaks that had first drawn colonial doctors into mass treatment of African diseases. As drugs converted HIV/Aids into a chronic disease, stigma was likely to decline and care to become less burdensome and more willingly undertaken. By demonstrating that women's disabilities endangered the entire society, the epidemic had already advanced female status and empowered many women activists. The mobilisation of people with HIV/Aids had not only introduced patient power into medical systems but was a major step towards the repoliticisation of Africa after the long stagnation of one-party rule, a repoliticisation to which NGOs had also contributed largely. In the long term that was likely to strengthen Africa's weak states, as might their control of access to free antiretrovirals, provided they could maintain that control and prevent it collapsing in a welter of piracy and corruption. HIV/Aids might, as pessimists predicted, reduce the continent to 'a Mad Max scenario', but responses to the epidemic might equally strengthen the state, as innovations had often done in the past. That, however, depended heavily on continued international funding, whose scale and duration were in 2005 still subjects for speculation. It depended also on the continued supply of generic drugs, either by middle-income producers – whose long-term interests did not coincide with those of African consumers – or by African manufacturers. In the last resort, however, the only effective counter to the virus was a vaccine. If these conditions could be met, the HIV/ Aids epidemic, so often seen as a metaphor for Africa's failure to achieve modernity, might instead be the vehicle by which medical modernity became predominant within the continent.

14
Conclusion

This book began by suggesting that a history of the African HIV/Aids epidemic to 2005 could offer four valuable perspectives. One was an answer to President Mbeki's question why Africa had suffered the most terrible epidemic. The book has argued that the presence of the natural ancestor of HIV and the full range of viral subtypes in the western equatorial region of Africa is compelling reason to believe that the epidemic began there. The virus existed in the Kinshasa region by 1959 and began to take epidemic form there by the mid 1970s, perhaps as a result of the wide sexual networks and decayed socio-economic conditions of the city. For nearly ten years, and perhaps more, it remained a silent and unrecognised epidemic. During that period, subgroups of the virus were carried away from the epicentre to infect eastern, southern, and western Africa. Their impact on each region was shaped by its patterns of communications and mobility, its gender relationships and sexual networks, its disease environment and socio-economic arrangements. But in this first HIV/Aids epidemic, the virus initially established itself silently within the general heterosexual population before any steps were or could have been taken to check it. Africa had the worst epidemic because it had the first epidemic.

Second, this silent expansion was one way in which the unique character of the virus – mildly infectious, slow-acting, incurable, fatal – decisively shaped the epidemic and human responses to it. Those responses were slow, for HIV's long, asymptomatic incubation period and the eventual appearance of diverse opportunistic infections defied prompt action and fostered uncertainty and denial. Instead, people with Aids faced a slow and painful death while their families undertook a heavy burden of care and mourning. Care and death impoverished households and multiplied the orphans to whom young adults gave birth before they died. Yet slow incubation also gave people with HIV/Aids time to organise themselves for mutual aid and political action.

The third perspective has been to set the epidemic in the longer context of African history. When compared with earlier epidemics, HIV/Aids stands out chiefly by its uniqueness: more enduring than influenza, less environmentally dependent than sleeping sickness, more fatal than tuberculosis. Yet it emerged both from Africa's long history of human colonisation, from its twentieth-century history of demographic, social, commercial, and intellectual change, and from its most recent history of economic and political crisis. Already, moreover, the epidemic is reshaping patterns of change, compelling women and young people to assert themselves for their own protection, obliging those with HIV/Aids to organise themselves to secure treatment, requiring governments to expand their medical and social care, and alerting the outside world as never before to the realities of disease and poverty.

Finally, a historical perspective reveals the changing character of the epidemic. In 2005 the reasons for Uganda's declining HIV prevalence were uncertain, but the fact itself was not, and it contrasted with continued expansion in parts of southern Africa and in regions affected by the aftermath of war. As the epidemic had matured, so the balance of infection had shifted between men and women, richer and poorer. Antiretroviral drugs, promising to convert an epidemic disease into a chronic complaint, had raised new questions about human rights, new dilemmas for medical administrators, new partnerships between donors and recipients, new dangers of corruption and political competition, new relationships between doctors and patients. Yet in 2005 the epidemic had reached only 'the end of the beginning'. Although over 25 million Africans had HIV/Aids, 12 million children had lost a parent, and over 13 million Africans were dead,[1] experts warned that the worst was still to come, both for Africa and the world. In 2003, Richard Feachem, Director of the Global Fund, speculated that the pandemic would not peak before 2050 or 2060.[2] Yet that was not inevitable. Although the means to eradicate HIV/Aids did not yet exist, the means to contain it were already at hand. The virus no longer held the initiative that had explained its success.

Notes

1 *Intentions* (pages 1–2)

1 President Mbeki's letter to world leaders, 3 April 2000, http://www.virusmyth.net/aids/news/lettermbeki.htm (accessed 7 March 2005).
2 J.C. Caldwell, P. Caldwell, and P. Quiggin, 'The social context of AIDS in sub-Saharan Africa,' *Population and Development Review*, 15 (1989), 185–234.
3 P. Piot, M. Bartos, and others,'The global impact of HIV/AIDS,' *Nature*, 410 (2001), 973.

2 *Origins* (pages 3--9)

1 A.G. Motulsky, J. Vandepitte, and G.R. Fraser, 'Population genetic studies in the Congo, I,' *American Journal of Human Genetics*, 18 (1966), 514–16; A.J. Nahmias, A. Motulsky, and others, 'Evidence for human infection with an HTLV III/LAV-like virus in central Africa, 1959,' *Lancet*, 1986/i, 1279–80; E. Hooper, *The river: a journey back to the source of HIV and AIDS* (reprinted, London, 2000), pp. 129–30.
2 For detailed accounts of these early cases, see Hooper, *River*, chs 8, 9, 19, 23, and the references therein.
3 L. Montagnier, *Virus* (trans. S. Sartarelli, New York, 2000), p. 122.
4 E. Bailes, Feng Gao, and others, 'Hybrid origin of SIV in chimpanzees,' *Science*, 300 (2003), 1713.
5 K.F. Kiple (ed.), *The Cambridge world history of human disease* (Cambridge, 1993), pp. 552, 612, 628, 807, 819, 1100.
6 N.D. Wolfe, M. Switzer, and others, 'Naturally acquired simian retrovirus infections in central African hunters,' *Lancet*, 363 (2004), 932–6.
7 F. Damond, M. Worobey, and others, 'Identification of a highly divergent HIV type 2 and proposal for a change in HIV type 2 classification,' *ARHR*, 20 (2004), 666–72.
8 B.H. Hahn, G.M. Shaw, and others, 'AIDS as a zoonosis: scientific and public health implications,' *Science*, 287 (2000), 607–14; J. Yamaguchi, A.S. Vallari, and others, 'Evaluation of HIV type 1 group O isolates: identification of five phylogenetic clusters,' *ARHR*, 18 (2002), 269–82; P. Bodelle, A. Vallari, and others, 'Identification and genomic sequence of an HIV type 1 group N isolate from Cameroon,' *ARHR*, 20 (2004), 907.
9 D. Candotti, C. Tareau, and others, 'Genetic subtyping and V3 serotyping of HIV type 1 isolates in Congo,' *ARHR*, 15 (1999), 309–14; N. Vidal, M. Peeters, and others, 'Unprecedented degree of human immunodeficiency virus type 1 (HIV-1) group M genetic diversity in the Democratic Republic of Congo suggests that the HIV-1 pandemic originated in central Africa,' *Journal of Virology*, 74 (2000), 10498–501.
10 This account is taken chiefly from J.M. Coffin, 'Molecular biology of HIV,' in K.A. Crandall (ed.), *The evolution of HIV* (Baltimore, 1999), ch. 1; J.F. Hutchinson, 'The biology and evolution of HIV,' *Annual Review of Anthropology*, 30 (2001), 85–108.
11 Crandall, *Evolution*, p. xii.

12 M. Peeters, C. Toure-Kane, and J.N. Nkengasong, 'Genetic diversity of HIV in Africa: impact on diagnosis, treatment, vaccine development and trials,' *AIDS*, 17 (2003), 2547–60.

13 Vidal and others, 'Unprecedented degree,' pp. 10500–1; A. Rambaut, D.L. Robertson, and others, 'Phylogeny and the origin of HIV-1,' *Nature*, 410 (2001), 1047; P. Roques, D.L. Robertson, and others, 'Phylogenetic analysis of 49 newly derived HIV-1 group O strains: high viral diversity but no group M-like subtype structure,' *Virology*, 302 (2002), 267.

14 F.E. McCutchan, 'Understanding the genetic diversity of HIV-1,' *AIDS*, 14 (2000), supplement 3, s32.

15 B. Korber, A. Muldoon, and others, 'Timing the ancestor of the HIV-1 pandemic strains,' *Science*, 288 (2000), 1789–96; K. Yusim. M. Peeters, and others, 'Using human immunodeficiency virus type 1 sequences to infer historical features of the acquired immune deficiency syndrome epidemic and human immunodeficiency virus evolution,' *Phil. Trans. R. Soc. Lond. B*, 356 (2001), 857.

16 M. Salemi, K. Strimmer, and others, 'Dating the common ancestor of SIVcpz and HIV-1 group M and the origin of HIV-1 subtypes using a new method to uncover clock-like molecular evolution,' *FASEB Journal*, 15 (2001), 276–8.

17 Bailes and others, 'Hybrid origin,' p. 1713.

18 B. Korber, J. Theiler, and S. Wolinsky, 'Limitations of a molecular clock applied to considerations of the origin of HIV-1,' *Science*, 280 (1998), 1868.

19 M. Gómez-Carillo, J.F. Quarleri, and others, 'Drug resistance testing provides evidence of the globalization of HIV type 1: a new circulating recombinant form,' *ARHR*, 20 (2004), 885; McCutchan, 'Understanding,' p. s33.

20 M.H. Schierup and J. Hein, 'Consequences of recombination on traditional phylogenetic analysis,' *Genetics*, 156 (2000), 888.

21 Hooper, *River*; J. Cohen, 'Disputed AIDS theory dies its final death,' *Science*, 292 (2001), 615, and references therein.

22 A. Chitnis, D. Rawls, and T. Moore, 'Origin of HIV type 1 in colonial French Equatorial Africa,' *ARHR*, 16 (2000), 5–8.

23 P.A. Marx, P.G. Alcabes, and E. Drucker, 'Serial human passage of simian immunodeficiency virus in Africa,' *Phil. Trans. R. Soc. Lond. B*, 356 (2001), 911–20.

24 P. Piot and M. Bartos,'The epidemiology of HIV and AIDS,' in M. Essex, S. Mboup, and others (eds), *AIDS in Africa* (2nd edn, New York, 2002), p. 202; R.H. Gray, M.J. Wawer, and others, 'Probability of HIV transmission per coital act in monogamous, heterosexual, HIV-1-discordant couples in Rakai, Uganda,' *Lancet*, 357 (2001), 1149–53.

25 C.D. Pilcher, Hsiao Chuan Tien, and others, 'Brief but efficient: acute HIV infection and the sexual transmission of HIV,' *Journal of Infectious Diseases*, 189 (2004), 1785; B.L. Rapatski, F. Suppe, and J.A. Yorke, 'HIV epidemics driven by late disease stage transmission,' *Journal of AIDS*, 38 (2005), 241.

26 D. Morgan, C. Mahe, and others, 'HIV-1 infection in rural Africa: is there a difference in median time to AIDS and survival compared with that in industrialized countries?' *AIDS*, 16 (2002), 600.

27 R.M. Anderson and R.M. May, *Infectious diseases of humans: dynamics and control* (Oxford, 1991), p. 31; S. Scott and C.J. Duncan, *Biology of plagues: evidence from historical populations* (Cambridge, 2001), pp. 22, 128.

28 A.Y. Sawadogo, *Le sida autour de moi* (Paris, 2003), p. 13.

3 *Epidemic in Western Equatorial Africa* (pages 10–18)

1 Nzila Nzilambi, K.M. De Cock, and others, 'The prevalence of infection with human immunodeficiency virus over a 10-year period in rural Zaire,' *NEJM*, 318 (1988), 276; J.B. McCormick and S. Fisher-Hoch, *Level 4: virus hunters of the CDC* (New York, 1999), p. 185.

2 G. Remy, 'Image géographique de l'infection à VIH 1 en Afrique centrale,' *Annales de la Société Belge de Médecine Tropicale*, 72 (1993), 136; G. Giraldo, E. Beth, and S.K. Kyalwazi, 'Role of cytomegalovirus in Kaposi's sarcoma,' in A.O. Williams, G.T. O'Conor, and others (eds), *Virus-associated cancers in Africa* (Lyon, 1984), p. 595.

3 F.H.N. Spracklen, R.G. Whittaker, and others, 'The acquired immune deficiency syndrome and related complex,' *SAMJ*, 68 (1985), 141.

4 L. Garrett, *The coming plague: newly emerging diseases in a world out of balance* (New York, 1995), p. 367; Kapita M. Bila, *Sida en Afrique: maladie et phénomène social* (Kinshasa, 1988),

p. 12; P. Piot, T.C. Quinn, and others, 'Acquired immunodeficiency syndrome in a heterosexual population in Zaire,' *Lancet*, 1984/ii, 68; McCormick and Fisher-Hoch, *Level 4*, p. 175; D. Fassin, 'Le domaine privé de la santé publique: pouvoir, politique et sida au Congo,' *Annales ESC*, 49 (1994), 749.

5 P. Aubry, G. Kemanfu, and others, 'La tuberculose à l'heure du SIDA en Afrique subsaharienne: expérience d'un pays d'Afrique centrale: le Burundi,' *Médecine Tropicale*, 54 (1994), 68.

6 J.J.M. Tamfum, O.M. Kibadi, and others, 'Cryptococcose à *cryptococcus neoformans var. gattii*,' *Médecine Tropicale*, 52 (1992), 435–6; J.-F. Molez, 'The historical question of acquired immunodeficiency syndrome in the 1960s in the Congo River Basin area in relation to cryptococcal meningitis,' *American Journal of Tropical Medicine and Hygiene*, 58 (1998), 273–6.

7 T.C. Quinn, J.M. Mann, and others, 'AIDS in Africa: an epidemiologic paradigm,' *Science*, 234 (1986), 957.

8 J. Sonnet, J.-L. Michaux, and others, 'Early AIDS cases originating from Zaire and Burundi (1962–1976),' *Scandinavian Journal of Infectious Diseases*, 19 (1987), 511–17; J.P. Coulaud, A.G. Saimot, and G. Charmot, 'Le syndrome d'immuno-depression acquise de l'adulte,' *Médecine Tropicale*, 44 (1984), 10.

9 *Global AIDS News*, 1993 no. 1. See also J. Cohen, 'The rise and fall of Projet SIDA,' *Science*, 278 (1997), 1565–6.

10 McCormick and Fisher-Hoch, *Level 4*, p. 193.

11 Piot and others, 'Acquired immunodeficiency syndrome,' pp. 65–9; *Salongo* (Kinshasa), 5 and 8 November 1983.

12 P. Boggio, 'L'épidémie de SIDA à Kinshasa,' *Le Monde*, 24 December 1986.

13 Garrett, *Coming plague*, pp. 347–50; WHO, 'Acquired immune deficiency syndrome emergencies: report of a WHO meeting, Geneva, 22–25 November 1983' (WHO/STD/84.1), pp. 6–11; McCormick and Fisher-Hoch, *Level 4*, pp. 175–6.

14 Bosenge N'Galy, and R.W. Ryder, 'Epidemiology of HIV infection in Africa,' *Journal of AIDS*, 1 (1988), 554; J.M. Mann, 'The epidemiology of LAV/HTLV-III in Africa,' *Annales de l'Institut Pasteur/Virologie*, 138 (1987), 114; J.M. Mann, D.J.M. Tarantola, and T.W. Netter (eds), *AIDS in the world* (Cambridge, Mass., 1992), p. 34.

15 J.M. Mann, T.C. Quinn, and others, 'Prevalence of HTLV-III/LAV in household contacts of patients with confirmed AIDS and controls in Kinshasa, Zaire,' *JAMA*, 256 (1986), 721–4.

16 J.M. Mann, H. Francis, and others,'Surveillance for AIDS in a central African city,' *JAMA*, 255 (1986), 3257; Ngandu Kabeya Dibandala and J. Courtejoie, *Le sida est la! Que faire?* (Kangu-Mayombe [1987?]), p. 13.

17 Kapita M. Bila, *Sida en Afrique*, pp. 50–1; Bosenge N'Galy, 'Epidemiology of HIV infection in Zaire,' in G. Giraldo, E. Beth–Giraldo, and others (eds), *AIDS and associated cancers in Africa* (Basel, 1988), p. 37; Mann, 'Epidemiology,' p. 114.

18 R.W. Ryder, Wato Nsa, and others, 'Perinatal transmission of the human immunodeficiency virus type 1 to infants of seropositive women in Zaire,' *NEJM*, 320 (1989), 1638, 1642.

19 Mann, 'Epidemiology', p. 116; Mann and others, 'Surveillance,' p. 3257; J.M. Mann, Nzila Nzilambi, and others, 'HIV infection and associated risk factors in female prostitutes in Kinshasa, Zaire,' *AIDS*, 2 (1988), 249.

20 Kapita M. Bila, *Sida en Afrique*, p. 28; *Salongo*, 26 November 1982; J.M. Mann, H. Francis, and others, 'Human immunodeficiency virus seroprevalence in pediatric patients 2 to 14 years of age at Mama Yemo Hospital, Kinshasa, Zaire,' *Pediatrics*, 78 (1986), 674.

21 Mann, 'Epidemiology,' p. 115; J. Mann, 'Global AIDS: epidemiology, impact, projections, global strategy,' in WHO, *AIDS prevention and control* (Oxford, 1988), p. 6.

22 Garrett, *Coming plague*, pp. 370–1; B. Auvert, 'Epidémiologie du sida en Afrique,' in J. Vallin (ed.), *Populations africaines et sida* (Paris, 1994), p. 82.

23 K. Magazini, G. Laleman, and others, 'Low and stable HIV seroprevalence in pregnant women in Shaba Province, Zaire,' *Journal of AIDS*, 6 (1993), 420.

24 Fassin, 'Le domaine privé,' p. 749; D.A. Eaton Jr, 'Men's lives and the politics of AIDS in the Republic of Congo,' PhD thesis, University of California, Berkeley, 2001, pp. 5–6; Remy, 'Image géographique,' p. 130; M.Y. Nzoukoudi-Nkoundou, L. Penchenier, and others, 'Séroprévalence des infections à VIH-1 à Djoumouna, Congo,' *Bulletin de l'OCEAC*, 26, 1 (March 1993), 10.

25 E. Delaporte, W. Janssens, and others, 'Epidemiological and molecular characteristics of HIV infection in Gabon, 1986–1994,' *AIDS*, 10 (1996), 903, 909.

26 J.P. Durand, S. Musi, and others, 'Prévalence des porteurs d'anticorps contre les virus de l'immunodéficience humaine (VIH 1 et VIH 2) dans le sud-Cameroun,' *Médecine Tropicale*, 48 (1988), 391; UNAIDS, *Accelerating action against AIDS in Africa* (Geneva, 2003), p. 10; J.M. Garcia-Calleja, S. Abbeny, and others, 'Review of HIV prevalence studies in Cameroon: what next?' *Bulletin de l'OCEAC*, 26, 4 (December 1993), 165; H. Kamngo, 'Rôle, statut de la femme et SIDA: cas du village de Mindourou dans l'Est-Cameroun,' *Annales de l'IFORD*, 16, 1–2 (December 1993), 33.

27 J.L. Lesbordes, G. Baquillon, and others, 'La tuberculose au cours de l'infection par le virus de l'immunodéficience humaine (VIH) à Bangui,' *Médecine Tropicale*, 48 (1988), 21–5; J.L. Lesbordes, J.B. McCormick, and others, 'Aspects cliniques du SIDA en République Centrafricaine,' *ibid.*, 45 (1985), 405–11; D. Tarantola and B. Schwartländer, 'HIV/AIDS epidemics in sub-Saharan Africa: dynamism, diversity and discrete declines?' *AIDS*, 11 (1997), supplement B, s7.

28 G. Gresenguet, L. Belec, and others, 'Connaissance, attitudes et croyances sur le SIDA,' *Médecine d'Afrique Noire*, 36 (1989), 48–53; G. Remy, 'Paysage épidémiologique de l'infection à VIH 1 parmi les prostituées africaines,' *ibid.*, 45 (1998), 287–8; Lesbordes and others, 'Aspects cliniques,' p. 406; J.L. Lesbordes, B. Couland, and A.J. Georges, 'Malnutrition et virus de l'immunodéficience humaine (VIH) à Bangui,' *Médecine Tropicale*, 50 (1990), 163; 'La tuberculose au cours de l'infection par le virus de l'immunodéficience humaine (VIH) à Bangui,' *Bulletin de l'OCEAC*, 88 (April 1989), 74.

29 République Centrafricaine, 'Première conférence nationale sur le sida à l'intention des leaders de l'Union Démocratique des Femmes Centrafricaines du 3 au 8 Décembre 1990' (duplicated), annexe 9, p. 2; G. Remy, C. M'Biaga, and others, 'Dynamique socio-géographique de l'infection à VIH-1 en Afrique Centrale: régions de Batouri (Cameroun)-Berberati (Centrafrique),' *Médecine d'Afrique Noire*, 43 (1996), 452–7; R. Chambon, F. J. Louis, and others, 'Enquête C.A.P.C. et de séro-prévalence VIH-1 à Mbaimboum,' *Bulletin de l'OCEAC*, 27, 3 (September 1994), 141; J. Burdon, 'Another deadly Zairian disease,' *BMJ*, 313 (1996), 58.

30 Makala-Lizumu and Mwana Elas, 'Modernization and urban poverty: a case study of Kinshasa,' in G. Gran (ed.), *Zaire: the political economy of underdevelopment* (New York, 1979), p. 112; J. MacGaffey, *Entrepreneurs and parasites: the struggle for indigenous capitalism in Zaire* (Cambridge, 1987), p. 115; B.G. Schoepf, 'AIDS action-research with women in Kinshasa, Zaire,' *SSM*, 37 (1993), 1402.

31 T. de Herdt and L.L. Luzolele Lola Nkakala, *La pauvreté urbaine en Afrique subsaharienne: le cas de Kinshasa* (3 parts, Antwerp, 1997), part 3, p. 90; J.S. La Fontaine, 'The free women of Kinshasa: prostitution in a city in Zaire,' in J. Davis (ed.), *Choice and change* (London, 1974), ch. 6.

32 A. Buvé, M. Caraël, and others, 'Variations in HIV prevalence between urban areas in sub-Saharan Africa: do we understand them?' *AIDS*, 9 (1995), supplement A, s105; Remy, 'Paysage épidémiologique,' pp. 287–8; Mengistu Mehret, L. Khodakevich, and others, 'Sexual behaviours and some social features of female sex workers in the city of Addis Ababa,' *EJHD*, 4 (1990), 136.

33 M. Caraël, 'En Afrique: une maladie culturelle,' in E. Hirsch (ed.), *Le sida: rumeurs et faits* (Paris, 1987), pp. 57–8.

34 V. Batter, Baangi Matela, and others, 'High HIV-1 incidence in young women masked by stable overall seroprevalence among childbearing women in Kinshasa, Zaire,' *AIDS*, 8 (1994), 816; L. Corey, A. Wald, and others, 'The effects of herpes simplex virus-2 on HIV-1 acquisition and transmission,' *Journal of AIDS*, 35 (2004), 435–45; B. Auvert, A. Buvé, and others, 'Ecological and individual level analysis of risk factors for HIV infection in four urban populations in sub-Saharan Africa with different levels of HIV infection,' *AIDS*, 15 (2001), supplement 4, s19–21.

35 G. Pictet, S. Le Coeur, and others, 'Contributions of AIDS to the general mortality in central Africa: evidence from a morgue-based study in Brazzaville, Congo,' *AIDS*, 12 (1998), 2218; UNAIDS, 'AIDS epidemic update, December 2004,' p. 29, http://www.unaids.org (accessed 28 November 2004).

36 *AAA*, February 1998.

37 M. Makuwa, S. Souquière, and others, 'HIV prevalence and strain diversity in Gabon: the end of a paradox,' *AIDS*, 14 (2000), 1275; UNAIDS, *Report on the global AIDS epidemic 2004* (Geneva, 2004), pp. 191–2.

38 T. Barnett and A. Whiteside, *AIDS in the twenty-first century: disease and globalization* (Basing-

stoke, 2002), p. 142.

39   C. Mulanga-Kabeya, Nzila Nzilambi, and others, 'Evidence of stable HIV seroprevalence in selected populations in the Democratic Republic of the Congo,' *AIDS*, 12 (1998), 908.

40   P.W. Ewald, *Evolution of infectious disease* (Oxford, 1994), pp. 141–2; Mulanga-Kabeya and others, 'Evidence,' p. 909.

41   Batter and others, 'High HIV-1 incidence,' pp. 811, 815; Tarantola and Schwartländer, 'HIV/AIDS epidemics,' p. s8.

42   L. Walker, G. Reid, and M. Cornell, *Waiting to happen: HIV/AIDS in South Africa – the bigger picture* (Boulder, 2004), p. 85.

43   http://www.hst.org.za/news/20040592 (accessed 14 December 2004).

44   N. Vidal, M. Peeters, and others, 'Unprecedented degree of human immunodeficiency virus type 1 (HIV-1) group M genetic diversity in the Democratic Republic of Congo suggests that the HIV-1 pandemic originated in central Africa,' *Journal of Virology*, 74 (2000), 10505; N. Vidal, G. Mulanga-Kabeya, and others, 'Identification of a complex *env* subtype E HIV type 1 virus from the Democratic Republic of Congo,' *ARHR*, 16 (2000), 2059.

45   F.E. McCutchan, 'Understanding the genetic diversity of HIV-1,' *AIDS*, 14 (2000), supplement 3, s33; F.A.J. Konings, Ping Zhong, and others, 'Protease mutations in HIV-1 non-B strains infecting drug-naive villagers of Cameroon,' *ARHR*, 20 (2004), 106; F.E. McCutchan, J.-L. Sankale, and others, 'HIV type 1 circulating recombinant form CRF09_cpx from West Africa combines subtypes A, F, G, and may share ancestors with CRF02_AG and Z231,' *ARHR*, 20 (2004), 824; M. Peeters, C. Toure-Kane, and others, 'Genetic diversity of HIV in Africa: impact on diagnosis, treatment, vaccine development and trials,' *AIDS*, 17 (2003), 2551; Y. Tamiguchi, Jun Takehisa, and others, 'Genetic subtypes of HIV type 1 based on the *vpu/env* sequences in the Republic of Congo,' *ARHR*, 18 (2002), 82–3.

46   McCutchan, 'Understanding,' p. s32; Vidal and others, 'Unprecedented degree,' pp. 10498, 10501.

47   Vidal and others, 'Unprecedented degree,' pp. 10500–1. A later survey found subtype C to be uncommon in the southern town of Likasi: Kayoko Kita, Nicaise Ndembi, and others, 'Genetic diversity of HIV type 1 in Likasi, southeast of the Democratic Republic of Congo,' *ARHR*, 20 (2004), 1352–3.

4 *The Drive to the East* (pages 19–32)

1   M.A. Rayfield, R.G. Downing, and others, 'A molecular epidemiologic survey of HIV in Uganda,' *AIDS*, 12 (1998), 524.

2   T. Jonckheer, I. Dab, and others, 'Cluster of HTLV-III/LAV infection in an African family,' *Lancet*, 1985/i, 400–1. E. Hooper, *The river: a journey back to the source of HIV and AIDS* (reprinted, London, 2000), p. 91, mentions another possible case.

3   M. Caraël, 'Women, AIDS, and STDs in sub-Saharan Africa: the impact of marriage change,' in G. Cabrera, D. Pitt, and P. Staugård (eds), *AIDS and the grassroots: problems, challenges and opportunities* (Gaborone, 1996), p.64; P. Van de Perre, D. Rouvroy, and others, 'Acquired immunodeficiency syndrome in Rwanda,' *Lancet*, 1984/ii, 62.

4   J. Morvan, B. Carterton, and others, 'Enquête séro-épidémiologique sur les infections à HIV au Burundi entre 1980 et 1981,' *Bulletin de la Société de Pathologie Exotique*, 82 (1989), 130–3; R. Laroche, J.J. Floch, and others, 'Principaux aspects du syndrome d'immuno-dépression acquise (SIDA) de l'adulte au Burundi,' *Médecine Tropicale*, 48 (1988), 359, 363.

5   B. Standaert, P. Kocheleff, and others, 'Acquired immunodeficiency syndrome and human immunodeficiency virus infection in Bujumbura, Burundi,' *TRSTMH*, 82 (1988), 902–3; M. de Loenzien, *Connaissances et attitudes face au VIH/sida* (Paris, 2002), p. 35.

6   B. Standaert, F. Niragira, and others, 'The association of tuberculosis and HIV infection in Burundi,' *ARHR*, 5 (1989), 247; G. Charmot and R. Laroche, 'L'apparition et l'évolution de l'épidémie par le virus de l'immunodéficience humaine en Afrique sub-Saharienne,' *Médecine Tropicale*, 54 (1994), 209; de Loenzien, *Connaissances*, p. 35.

7   C. Bizimungu and others, 'Nationwide community-based serological survey of HIV-1 and other human retrovirus infections in a central African country,' *Lancet*, 1989/i, 941–3; V. Leroy, P. Van de Perre, and others, 'Seroincidence of HIV-1 infection in African women of reproductive age: a prospective cohort study in Kigali, Rwanda, 1988–1992,' *AIDS*, 8 (1994), 983.

8   M. Caraël, 'Sexual behaviour,' in J. Cleland and B. Ferry (eds), *Sexual behaviour and AIDS in*

the developing world (London, 1995), p. 80. The table appears to have exchanged the figures between the Central African Republic and Guinea-Bissau.

9   P. Van de Perre, M. Caraël, and others, 'Female prostitutes: a risk group for infection with human T-cell lymphotropic virus type III,' *Lancet*, 1985/ii, 524; Caraël in Cabrera and others, *AIDS*, p. 67; P. Aubry, F. Bigirimana, and others, 'Les aspects actuels du syndrome d'immunodéficience acquise de l'adulte à Bujumbura,' *Médecine d'Afrique Noire*, 37 (1990), 569.

10 Panos Institute, *The hidden cost of AIDS: the challenge of HIV to development* (London, 1992), p. 6; M. Vandersypen, 'Femmes libres de Kigali,' *Cahiers d'Etudes Africaines*, 17 (1977), 118.

11 M. Caraël, 'En Afrique: une maladie culturelle,' in B. Hirsch (ed.), *Le sida: rumeurs et faits* (Paris, 1987), p. 57; N. Meda, *La surveillance épidémiologique des maladies sexuellement transmises (MST), de l'infection à VIH et du SIDA au Rwanda* (Brazzaville, 2000); A. van der Straten, R. King, and others, 'Couple communication, sexual coercion and HIV risk reduction in Kigali, Rwanda,' *AIDS*, 9 (1995), 935–44.

12 S. Allen, J. Tice, and others, 'Effect of serotesting with counselling on condom use and seroconversion among HIV discordant couples in Africa,' *BMJ*, 304 (1992), 1609.

13 Meda, *La surveillance*, p. 6; de Loenzien, *Connaissances*, p. 35.

14 M. Bulterys, A. Chao, and others, 'Incident HIV-1 infection in a cohort of young women in Butare, Rwanda,' *AIDS*, 8 (1994), 1588.

15 D. Serwadda, N.K. Sewankambo, and others, 'Slim disease: a new disease in Uganda and its association with HTLV-III infection,' *Lancet*, 1985/ii, 851; J. Cook, 'Kaposi's sarcoma in Uganda,' MS thesis, Edinburgh University, 1963, p. 36; A.C. Bayley, R. Cheingsong-Popov, and others, 'HTLV-III serology distinguishes atypical and endemic Kaposi's sarcoma in Africa,' *Lancet*, 1985/i, 359–61; J. Goudsmit, *Viral sex: the nature of AIDS* (New York, 1997), p. 67.

16 S.I. Okware, 'Towards a national AIDS-control program in Uganda', *Western Journal of Medicine*, 147 (1987), 726.

17 F.S. Mhalu, A Dahoma, and others, 'Some aspects of the epidemiology of AIDS and infections with the human immunodeficiency virus in the United Republic of Tanzania,' in G. Giraldo, E. Beth-Giraldo, and others (eds), *AIDS and associated cancers in Africa* (Basel, 1988), p. 50; *New Vision* (Kampala), 9 April 1991; A Shomatoff, *African madness* (New York, 1988), p. 192; Hooper, *River*, pp. 37–8. See also R. Stoneburner, M Carballo, and others, 'Simulation of HIV incidence dynamics in the Rakai population-based cohort, Uganda,' *AIDS*, 12 (1998), 227.

18 A.M.T. Lwegaba, 'Preliminary report of "an unusual wasting disease" complex nicknamed "Slim" a slow epidemic of Rakai District, Uganda,' November 1984, photocopy of typescript, UMOH library.

19 J. Appleton, '"At my age I should be sitting under that tree": the impact of AIDS on Tanzanian lakeshore communities,' *Gender and Development*, 8, 2 (2000), 19–27.

20 H. Pickering, M. Okongo, and others, 'Sexual behaviour in a fishing community on Lake Victoria, Uganda,' *HTR*, 7 (1997), 13–20; A. Kamali, M. Quigley, and others, 'Syndromic management of sexually-transmitted infections and behaviour change interventions on transmission of HIV-1 in rural Uganda: a community randomised trial,' *Lancet*, 361 (2003), 649; C. Obbo, 'HIV transmission: men are the solution,' *Population and Environment*, 14 (1992–3), 219.

21 H. Pickering, M. Okongo, and others, 'Sexual mixing patterns in Uganda: small-time urban/rural traders,' *AIDS*, 10 (1996), 535–6.

22 F.J. Kaijage, 'AIDS control and the burden of history in northwestern Tanzania,' *Population and Environment*, 14 (1992–3), 297; J. Killewo, L. Dahlgren, and A. Sandström, 'Socio-geographical patterns of HIV-1 transmission in Kagera region, Tanzania,' *SSM*, 38 (1994), 129–30.

23 G.H.R. Rugalema, *Adult mortality as entitlement failure: AIDS and the crisis of rural livelihoods in a Tanzanian village* (PhD thesis, Institute of Social Studies, The Hague, 1999: published in Maastricht), pp. 73–4.

24 Stoneburner and others, 'Simulation,' p. 227.

25 D. Serwadda, M.J. Wawer, and others, 'HIV risk factors in three geographic strata of rural Rakai district,' *AIDS*, 6 (1992), 985; F. Nalugoda, R.H. Gray, and others, 'Burden of infection among heads and non-heads of rural households in Rakai, Uganda,' *AIDS Care*, 16 (2004), 112; Hooper, *River*, p. 48.

26 J.W. Carswell, 'HIV infection in healthy persons in Uganda,' *AIDS*, 1 (1987), 225; M.

Hierholzer, R.R. Graham, and others, 'HIV type 1 strains from East and West Africa are intermixed in Sudan,' *ARHR*, 18 (2002), 1163–4.

27   Hooper, *River*, pp. 43–5; D. Low-Beer, 'The diffusion of AIDS in East Africa: from emergence to decline?' PhD thesis, University of Cambridge, 1997, pp. 137, 163; G.C. Bond and J. Vincent, 'AIDS in Uganda: the first decade,' in G.C. Bond, J. Kreniske, and others (eds), *AIDS in Africa and the Caribbean* (Boulder, 1997), p. 94.

28   J.W. Carswell, G. Lloyd, and J. Howells, 'Prevalence of HIV-1 in East African lorry drivers,' *AIDS*, 3 (1989), 759.

29   D. Ndagij'Imana and others, 'St Francis Hospital, Mutolere, 1989–1991,' duplicated, UMOH library.

30   Hooper, *River*, pp. 37–8; D. Serwadda and J.W. Carswell, 'Generalised Kaposi's sarcoma in Uganda,' in *The proceedings of the Association of Surgeons of East Africa*, 8 (1985), 55; N. Sewankambo, R.D. Mugerwa, and others, 'Enteropathic AIDS in Uganda: an endoscopic, histological and microbiological study,' *AIDS*, 1 (1987), 9.

31   Quoted in *New Vision*, 4 September 1993.

32   Carswell, 'HIV infection,' p. 225; R.L. Stoneburner and D. Low-Beer, 'Population-level HIV decline and behavioural risk avoidance in Uganda,' *Science*, 304 (2004), 717.

33   P. Nsubuga, R. Mugerwa, and others, 'The association of genital ulcer disease and HIV infection at a dermatology-STD clinic in Uganda,' *Journal of AIDS*, 3 (1990), 1005; C.J. Bakwesegha, *Profiles of urban prostitution: a case study from Uganda* (Nairobi, 1982).

34   S. Wallman and V. Pons, 'Where have all the young men gone? Evidence and explanations of changing age-sex ratios in Kampala,' *Africa*, 71 (2001), 113–27; A. Larson, 'Social context of human immunodeficiency virus transmission in Africa,' *Review of Infectious Diseases*, 11 (1989), 719; Uganda: Ministry of Health, *Uganda: demographic and health survey 1988/1989: summary report* (Entebbe, 1990), pp. 10–11; O.I. Morrow, 'Sexual cultures and vulnerability to HIV infection among Baganda youth in Mpigi, Uganda,' PhD thesis, Johns Hopkins University, 2000, pp. 20–3, 142, 324, 389.

35   Serwadda and others,'Slim disease,' pp. 849–52; J.W. Carswell, R. Mugerwa, and others, 'AIDS in Uganda: a special report by the Clinical Committee on AIDS,' *Health Information Quarterly* (Entebbe), 2, 1 (February 1986), 11–20.

36   Stoneburner and Low-Beer, 'Population-level HIV decline,' p. 715; *AAA*, September 1991, p. 5.

37   Hooper, *River*, p. 39; G. Haukenes, J. Shao, and others, 'The AIDS epidemic in Tanzania,' *Scandinavian Journal of Infectious Diseases*, 24 (1992), 701; E.J.N. Urassa, F.J. Mhalu, and others, 'Prevalence of HIV infection among pregnant women in Dar es Salaam,' *Tanzania Medical Journal*, 5, 2 (September 1990), 15; R.S. Katapa, 'Caretakers of AIDS patients in rural Tanzania,' *IJSA*, 15 (2004), 673.

38   Hooper, *River*, p. 45; Kaijage, 'AIDS control,' pp. 279–300; F. Mhalu, U. Bredberg-Rädén, and others, 'Prevalence of HIV infection in healthy subjects and groups of patients in Tanzania,' *AIDS*, 1 (1987), 217–19; A.K. Tibaijuka, 'AIDS and economic welfare in peasant agriculture: case studies from Kagabiro village, Kagera region, Tanzania,' *World Development*, 25 (1997), 964; F.S. Mhalu, 'AIDS and infections with the human immunodeficiency virus in Tanzania,' *Tanzania Medical Journal*, 4, 1 (June 1989), 1.

39   S.H. Kapiga, J.F. Shao, and others, 'Risk factors for HIV infection among women in Dar es Salaam, Tanzania,' *Journal of AIDS*, 7 (1994), 301–9.

40   P.B. Hiza, 'International co-operation in the national AIDS control programme,' in A.F. Fleming, M. Carballo, and others (eds), *The global impact of AIDS* (New York, 1988), p. 234; R.D. Swai, 'Epidemiology of AIDS in Tanzania,' in J.Z.J. Killewo, G.K. Lwihula, and others (eds), *Behavioural and epidemiological aspects of AIDS research in Tanzania* (Stockholm, 1992), p. 14.

41   B. Jordan-Harder, Y.A. Koshuma, and others, 'Hope for Tanzania: lessons learned from a decade of comprehensive AIDS control in Mbeya region: part 1' (2000), p. 15, http://www.gtz.de/aids/download/heft_1.pdf (accessed 9 September 2004); R. Hoelscher, Bokye Kim, and others, 'High proportion of unrelated HIV-1 intersubtype recombinants in the Mbeya region of southwest Tanzania,' *AIDS*, 15 (2001), 1468.

42   P.W. Setel, *A plague of paradoxes: AIDS, culture, and demography in northern Tanzania* (Chicago, 1999), pp. 3, 84, 148, 210; K.S. Mnyika, K.-I. Klepp, and others, 'Prevalence of HIV-1 infection in urban, semi-urban and rural areas in Arusha region, Tanzania,' *AIDS*, 8 (1994), 1479.

43   B. Renjifo, P. Gilbert, and others, 'Preferential in-utero transmission of HIV-1 subtype C as

compared to HIV-1 subtype A or D,' *AIDS*, 18 (2004), 1629–33.

44 *Weekly Review* (Nairobi), 24 March 1989; P. Piot, F.A. Plummer, and others, 'Retrospective epidemiology of AIDS virus infection in Nairobi populations,' *Journal of Infectious Diseases*, 155 (1987), 1108–12; J.N. Simonsen, F.A. Plummer, and others, 'HIV infection among lower socioeconomic strata prostitutes in Nairobi,' *AIDS*, 4 (1990), 139.

45 Piot and others, 'Retrospective epidemiology,' p. 1108; D.W. Cameron, L.J. D'Costa, and others, 'Female to male transmission of human immunodeficiency virus type 1: risk factors for seroconversion in men,' *Lancet*, 1989/ii, 404.

46 A. O'Connor, *The African city* (London, 1983), p. 93; M.H. Dawson, 'AIDS in Africa: historical roots,' in N. Miller and R.C. Rockwell (eds), *AIDS in Africa: the social and policy impact* (Lewiston, 1988), p. 62.

47 J.K. Kreiss, D. Koech, and others, 'AIDS virus infection in Nairobi prostitutes: spread of the epidemic to East Africa,' *NEJM*, 314 (1986), 414–15; F.A. Plummer, E.N. Ngugi, and S. Moses, 'The Pumwani experience: evolution of a partnership in disease control,' in Network of AIDS Researchers of Eastern and Southern Africa, *Focusing interventions among vulnerable groups for HIV infection: experiences from eastern and southern Africa* (Nairobi, 1994), p. 75; E. Hooper, *Slim: a reporter's own story of AIDS in East Africa* (London, 1990), p. 310.

48 Cameron and others, 'Female to male transmission,' p. 403; S. Moses, E. Muia, and others, 'Sexual behaviour in Kenya: implications for sexually transmitted disease transmission and control,' *SSM*, 39 (1994), 1654; UNAIDS, *Consultation on STD interventions for preventing HIV* (Geneva, 2000), p. 32; E. Pisani, G.P. Garnett, and others, 'Back to basics in HIV prevention: focus on exposure,' *BMJ*, 326 (2003), 1385.

49 UNAIDS, *Consultation on HIV interventions*, p. 32; O.A. Anzala, N.J.D. Nagelkerke, and others, 'Rapid progression to disease in African sex workers with human immunodeficiency virus type 1 infection,' *Journal of Infectious Diseases*, 171 (1995), 686–9.

50 Plummer, Ngugi, and Moses, 'The Pumwani experience,' and F.A. Plummer and E.N. Ngugi, 'Elements of targeted interventions,' in Network of AIDS Researchers, *Focusing interventions*, pp. 77–8, 12.

51 *AAA*, January 1992; J.M. Baeten, B.A. Richardson, and others, 'Trends in HIV-1 incidence in a cohort of prostitutes in Kenya,' *Journal of AIDS*, 24 (2000), 459; M.P. Hawken, R.D.J. Melis, and others, 'Opportunity for prevention of HIV and sexually transmitted infections in Kenyan youth: results of a population-based survey,' *ibid.*, 31 (2002), 529.

52 T.M. Okeyo, G.M. Baltazar, and others, *AIDS in Kenya: background, projections, impact and interventions* (3rd edn, Nairobi, 1996), p. 7; M. Aliber, C. Walker, and others, 'The impact of HIV/AIDS on land rights: case studies from Kenya' (2004), pp. 27–8, 72–3, http://www.fao.org/ed/dim_pe3/ docs/pe3_040902d1_en.pdf (accessed 28 December 2004); R.K. Nyaga, D.N. Kimani, and others, 'HIV/AIDS in Kenya: a review of research and policy issues' (2004), p. 13, http://www.kippra.org/Download/DPN038.pdf (accessed 21 March 2005); UNAIDS, *Report on the global AIDS epidemic 2004* (Geneva, 2004), pp. 24, 191–2.

53 *Daily Nation* (Nairobi), 28 July 1994; Okeyo, Baltazar, and others, *AIDS in Kenya*, p. 7.

54 C. Bishop-Sambrook, 'Labour constraints and the impact of HIV/AIDS on rural livelihoods in Bondo and Busia districts, western Kenya' (2003), pp. 6, iv, http://www.fao.org/ag/AGS/subjects/en/farmpower/pdf/labour.pdf (accessed 28 December 2004).

55 P. W. Geissler, '"Are we still together here?" Negotiations about relatedness and time in the everyday life of a modern Kenyan village,' PhD thesis, University of Cambridge, 2003, p. 16; D.J. Jackson, E.N. Ngugi, and others, 'Stable antenatal HIV-1 seroprevalence with high population mobility and marked seroprevalence variation among sentinel sites within Nairobi, Kenya,' *AIDS*, 13 (1999), 585.

56 R.C. Bailey, R. Muga, and others, 'The acceptability of male circumcision to reduce HIV infections in Nyanza province, Kenya,' *AIDS Care*, 14 (2002), 28.

57 J.E. Volk and C. Koopman, 'Factors associated with condom use in Kenya,' *AIDS Education and Prevention*, 13 (2001), 502; A. Buvé, M. Caraël, and others, 'Multicentre study on factors determining differences in rate of spread of HIV in sub-Saharan Africa: methods and prevalence of HIV infection,' *AIDS*, 15 (2001), supplement 4, s11.

58 Geissler, '"Are we still together here?",' esp. chs 1 and 5; *Standard* (Nairobi), 15 December 2004; UNAIDS, *Report on the global HIV/AIDS epidemic, June 2000* (Geneva, 2000), p. 58.

59 UNDP, *Botswana human development report 2000* (Gaborone, 2000), p. 27; Buvé and others, 'Multicentre study,' p. s5.

60 UNAIDS, *Report on the global AIDS epidemic 2004*, pp. 191–2.

61 Almaz Abebe, V.V. Lukashov, and others, 'Timing of the HIV-1 subtype C epidemic in

Ethiopia based on early virus strains and subsequent virus diversification,' *AIDS*, 15 (2001), 1555–61; A. Fontanet and Tilahun W/Michael, 'The Ethio-Netherlands AIDS Research Project (ENARP): description and major findings after four years of activities,' *Ethiopian Medical Journal*, 37 (1999), supplement 1, p. 12.

62   Laketch Dirasse, 'The socio-economic position of women in Addis Ababa: the case of prostitution,' PhD thesis, Boston University, 1978, p. 50; C. Clapham, *Transformation and continuity in revolutionary Ethiopia* (Cambridge, 1988), p. 140; Mengistu Mehret, L. Khodakevich, and others, 'Sexual behaviours and some social features of female sex workers in the city of Addis Ababa,' *EJHD*, 4 (1990), 134–5.

63   D.N. Levine, *Wax and gold: tradition and innovation in Ethiopian culture* (Chicago, 1965), p. 100; R. Lucas, 'Sex, sexuality, and the meaning of AIDS in Addis Ababa, Ethiopia,' PhD thesis, University of Michigan, 2001, pp. 55, 110, 159, 199; L. Garbus, 'HIV/AIDS in Ethiopia' (2003), pp. 32, 56, http://ari.ucsf.edu/policy/profiles/Ethiopia.pdf (accessed 8 February 2005); Mathias Aklilu, Tsehaynesh Messele, and others, 'Factors associated with HIV-1 infection among sex workers of Addis Ababa,' *AIDS*, 15 (2001), 94; Mengistu Mehret, L. Khodakevich, and others, 'Pregnancy/STD protective means used by HIV female sex workers in Ethiopia,' *EJHD*, 4 (1990), 139–42.

64   M.E. Duncan, G. Tibaux, and others, 'A socioeconomic, clinical and serological study in an African city of prostitutes and women still married to their first husband,' *SSM*, 39 (1994), 323, 328; Zewdu Woubalem, 'HIV/AIDS in Ethiopia: knowledge, practice, and attitudes,' PhD thesis, Brown University, 2003, p. 10; H. Kloos and Damien Haile Mariam, 'HIV/AIDS in Ethiopia: an overview,' *Northeast African Studies*, NS, 7, 1 (2000), 17.

65   Center for International Health Information, *Ethiopia: country health profile, 1996* (Arlington, n.d.), p. 43; Mengistu Mehret, L. Khodakevich, and others, 'HIV-1 infection and some related risk factors among female sex workers in Addis Ababa,' *EJHD*, 4 (1990), 175; Ethiopia, 'AIDS in Ethiopia' (4th edn, 2002), p. 11, http://www.policyproject.com/pubs/countryreports/ETH_AIM_2002.pdf (accessed 15 July 2004).

66   Mengistu Mehret, L. Khodakevich, and others, 'HIV-infection and related risk factors among female sex workers in urban areas of Ethiopia,' *EJHD*, 4 (1990), 163–5; Solomon Gebre, 'Sexual behaviour and knowledge of AIDS and other STDs: a survey of senior high school students,' *EJHD*, 4 (1990), 123.

67   Ethiopia: Federal Ministry of Health, 'AIDS in Ethiopia' (5th edn, 2004), pp. 9, 25, http://www.etharc.org/spotlight/AIDSinEth5th.pdf (accessed 9 February 2005).

68   A.L. Fontanet, Tsehaynesh Messele, and others, 'Age- and sex-specific HIV-1 prevalence in the urban community setting of Addis Ababa, Ethiopia,' *AIDS*, 12 (1998), 320; Fontanet and Tilahun W/Michael, 'Ethio-Netherlands Project,' p. 13; 'Update on HIV/AIDS: age-specific prevalence of HIV infection among women attending antenatal care clinics by health centre, Addis Ababa, Ethiopia, 1995–2003,' *Ethiopian Medical Journal*, 41 (2003), supplement 1, p. 89; Derege Kebele, Mathias Aklilu, and E. Sanders, 'The HIV epidemic and the state of its surveillance in Ethiopia,' *ibid.*, 38 (2000), 287.

69   Ethiopia, 'AIDS in Ethiopia' (2004), pp. v, 6, 9, 26; World Bank, *World development report 2000/2001* (New York, 2000), p. 276; Woubalem, 'HIV/AIDS,' p. 93; *Daily Monitor* (Addis Ababa), 21 December 2004, in http://allafrica.com/stories (accessed 29 December 2004).

70   Quoted in J. Lydall, 'The threat of the HIV/AIDS epidemic in South Omo Zone, southern Ethiopia,' *Northeast African Studies*, NS, 7, 1 (2000), 52.

71   Ethiopia: National AIDS Control Programme, 'Second medium term plan 1992–1996 and workplan and budget for 1992–1993,' duplicated, p. 7, Library of Congress, Washington; Shabbir Ismail, Fasil H/Giorgis, and others, 'Knowledge, attitude and practice on high risk factors pertaining to HIV/AIDS in a rural community,' *Ethiopian Medical Journal*, 33 (1995), 3–4; I. Shabbir and C.P. Larson, 'Urban to rural routes of HIV infection spread in Ethiopia,' *Journal of Tropical Medicine and Hygiene*, 98 (1995), 338–42; Gegu Degu Alene, 'Knowledge and practice of condom in preventing HIV/AIDS infection among commercial sex workers in three small towns of northwestern Ethiopia,' *EJHD*, 16 (2002), 277–80.

72   C. Bishop-Sambrook, 'The challenge of the HIV/AIDS epidemic in rural Ethiopia: averting the crisis in low AIDS-impacted communities: findings from fieldwork in Kersa Woreda, Eastern Hararghe Zone, Oromiya Region' (2004), http://www.fao.org/sd/dim_pe3/docs/pe3_040402d1_en.doc (accessed 6 September 2004).

5 *The Conquest of the South* (pages 33–47)

1 This account is based on J.R. Glynn, J. Pönninghaus, and others,'The development of the HIV epidemic in Karonga district, Malawi,' *AIDS*, 15 (2001), 2025–9; G.P. McCormack, J.R. Glynn, and others, 'Early evolution of the human immunodeficiency virus type 1 subtype C epidemic in rural Malawi,' *Journal of Virology*, 76 (2002), 12890–9, and 'Highly divergent HIV type 1 group M sequences evident in Karonga district, Malawi in the early 1980s,' *ARHR*, 19 (2003), 441–5; A.C. Crampin, S. Floyd, and others, 'Long-term follow-up of HIV-positive and HIV-negative individuals in rural Malawi,' *AIDS*, 16 (2002), 1545–50.

2 S. Osmanov, C. Pattou, and others, 'Estimated global distribution and regional spread of HIV-1 genetic subtypes in the year 2000,' *Journal of AIDS*, 29 (2002), 186.

3 See p. 18.

4 J.R. Dyer. P. Kazembe, and others, 'High levels of human immunodeficiency virus type 1 in blood and semen of seropositive men in sub-Saharan Africa,' *Journal of Infectious Diseases*, 177 (1998), 1742–6.

5 R. Sher, S. Antunes, and others, 'Seroepidemiology of human immunodeficiency virus in Africa from 1970 to 1974,' *NEJM*, 317 (1987), 450–1; Malawi: National AIDS Control Programme, *AIDS cases surveillance 1997 report* (Lilongwe, n.d.), figure 2; M. King and E. King, *The great rift: Africa surgery Aids aid* (Cambridge, n.d.), pp. 31–2; B. Brink and L. Clausen, 'The acquired immune deficiency syndrome,' *Journal of the Mine Medical Officers' Association of South Africa* (Marshalltown), 63 (April 1987), 14–15; S.C. Watkins, 'Navigating the AIDS epidemic in rural Malawi,' *Population and Development Review*, 30 (2004), 680.

6 A.C. Bayley, 'Aggressive Kaposi's sarcoma in Zambia,' *Lancet*, 1984/i, 1318–20; A.C. Bayley, R. Cheingsong-Popov, and others, 'HTLV-III serology distinguishes atypical and endemic Kaposi's sarcoma in Africa,' *Lancet*, 1985/i, 360; E. Hooper, *The river: a journey back to the source of HIV and AIDS* (reprinted, London, 2000), pp. 89–90; A. Bayley, *One new humanity: the challenge of AIDS* (London, 1996), pp. 35, 37.

7 O.O. Simooya, M.N. Maboshe, and others, 'HIV infection in early diagnosed tuberculosis patients in Ndola, Zambia,' *Central African Journal of Medicine*, 37 (1991), 5; D.J. Buchanan, R.G. Downing, and R.S. Tedder, 'HTLV-III antibody positivity in Zambian Copperbelt,' *Lancet*, 1986/i, 155; *Times of Zambia* (Ndola), 13 August 1987.

8 Bayley, *One new humanity*, p. 5; *Times of Zambia*, 5 March 1986.

9 M. Pitts and H. Jackson, 'Press coverage of AIDS in Zimbabwe: a five-year review,' *AIDS Care*, 5 (1993), 224; M.T. Bassett and M. Mhloyi, 'Women and AIDS in Zimbabwe: the making of an epidemic,' *International Journal of Health Services*, 21 (1991), 143–56; K. Dehne, D. Dhlakama, and others, 'Pattern of HIV-infection in Hurungwe district, Mashonaland West, Zimbabwe,' *Central African Journal of Medicine*, 38 (1992), 139; S. Gregson, 'The early socio-demographic impact of the HIV-1 epidemic in rural Zimbabwe,' DPhil thesis, 2 vols, University of Oxford, 1996, vol. 1, p. 197; A. Whiteside, 'Zimbabwe: a country profile,' *AAA*, September 1991, p. 6.

10 *Times of Zambia*, 22 March 1986; P. Ubomba-Jaswa, *Mass media and AIDS in Botswana: what the newspapers say and their implications* (Gaborone, 1993), pp. 13–14.

11 *Times of Zambia*, 22 March 1986; Ubomba-Jaswa, *Mass media*, pp. 20, 23; S. Tlou, 'Empowering older women in AIDS prevention: the case of Botswana,' *Southern African Journal of Gerontology*, 5, 2 (1996), 27.

12 T.E. Taha, G.A. Dallabetta, and others, 'Trends of HIV-1 and sexually transmitted diseases among pregnant and postpartum women in urban Malawi,' *AIDS*, 12 (1998), 199–200; *AAA*, April 1996; World Bank, *World development report 1992* (New York, 1992), p. 278.

13 N. Walker, N.C. Grassly, and others,'Estimating the global burden of HIV/AIDS,' *Lancet*, 363 (2004), 2183; K. Fylkesnes, R. Mubanga Musonda, and others, 'HIV infection among antenatal women in Zambia, 1990–1993,' *AIDS*, 10 (1996), 556; World Bank, *World development report 1992*, p. 278; Zambia: Ministry of Health, *HIV/AIDS in Zambia: background, projections, impacts and interventions* (Lusaka, 1999), p. 12.

14 Zimbabwe, *Working document for National AIDS Council strategic framework for a national response to HIV/AIDS (2000–2004)* (Harare, 1999), p. 4; M.T. Bassett, W.G. McFarland, and others, 'Risk factors for HIV infection at enrollment in an urban male factory cohort in Harare, Zimbabwe,' *Journal of AIDS*, 13 (1996), 287; World Bank, *World development report 1992*, p. 278.

15 Zimbabwe, *Working document*, p. 5; *AAA*, April 2001.

16 *AAA*, June 2002, p. 4.

17 S. Gregson, R.M. Anderson, and others, 'Recent upturn in mortality in rural Zimbabwe: evidence for an early demographic impact of HIV-1 infection?' *AIDS*, 11 (1997), 1273; P.L.N. Sikosana, D. Hlabangana, and I. Moyo, 'Quantifying morbidity in pregnant women in a rural population in Tsholotsho district in Zimbabwe,' *Central African Journal of Medicine*, 43 (1997), 93.

18 Botswana, *Botswana HIV and AIDS: second medium term plan 1997–2002* (Gaborone, 1997), p. 8; UNDP, *Botswana human development report 2000* (Gaborone, 2000), p. 10.

19 T. Barnett and A. Whiteside, *AIDS in the twenty-first century: disease and globalization* (Basingstoke, 2002), p. 120.

20 *AAA*, April 2000; Botswana: National AIDS Coordinating Agency, 'Status of the 2002 national response to the UNGASS declaration of commitment on HIV/AIDS,' March 2003, pp. 14, 12, http://www.unaids.org (accessed 21 November 2003).

21 D.S. Macdonald, 'Notes on the socio-economic and cultural factors influencing the transmission of HIV in Botswana,' *SSM*, 42 (1996), 1325.

22 *AAA*, March 1992; T. Campbell and M. Kelly, 'Women and AIDS in Zambia: a review of the psychological factors implicated in the transmission of HIV,' *AIDS Care*, 7 (1995), 366.

23 D. Wilson, P. Chiroro, and others, 'Sex workers, client sex behaviour and condom use in Harare, Zimbabwe,' *AIDS Care*, 1 (1989), 277; J. Decosas and N. Padian, 'The profile and context of the epidemics of sexually transmitted infections including HIV in Zimbabwe,' *Sexually Transmitted Infections*, 78 (2002), supplement 1, p. i44; *Sowetan*, 28 November 1990; E.W. Perkins, 'The spatial dynamics of internal migration: implications for the diffusion of HIV,' PhD thesis, University of Cambridge, 2000, p. 101; A. Buvé, M. Caraël and others, 'Multicentre study on factors determining differences in rate of spread of HIV in sub-Saharan Africa: methods and prevalence of HIV infections,' *AIDS*, 15 (2001), supplement 4, s5.

24 Wilson and others, 'Sex workers,' pp. 269, 277; P. Kishindo, 'Sexual behaviour in the face of risk: the case of bar girls in Malawi's major cities,' *HTR*, 5 (1995), supplement, 158; Zambia: Ministry of Health, *HIV/AIDS in Zambia*, p. 21.

25 S. Ray, A. Latif, and others, 'Sexual behaviour and risk assessment of HIV seroconvertors among urban male factory workers in Zimbabwe,' *SSM*, 47 (1998), 1431–43; S. Gregson, R. Machekano, and others, 'Estimating HIV incidence from age-specific prevalence data: comparison with concurrent cohort estimates in a study of male factory workers, Harare, Zimbabwe,' *AIDS*, 12 (1998), 2049, 2058; K. Mapemba, 'The Zimbabwe HIV prevention program for truck drivers and commercial sex workers,' in J.C. Caldwell, P. Caldwell, and others (eds), *Resistances to behavioural change to reduce HIV/AIDS infection in predominantly heterosexual epidemics in Third World countries* (Canberra, 1999), p. 134.

26 Andsen Jojo, quoted in *Mail and Guardian* (Johannesburg), 8 August 2003.

27 S.K. Hira, B.M. Nkowane, and others, 'Epidemiology of human immunodeficiency virus in families in Lusaka, Zambia,' *Journal of AIDS*, 3 (1990), 84; Gregson and others, 'Recent upturn,' p. 1279; S. Gregson, P.R. Mason, and others, 'A rural HIV epidemic in Zimbabwe? Finding from a population-based survey,' *IJSA*, 12 (2001), 191–3.

28 Malawi, *Knowledge, attitudes and practices in health survey 1996* (Zomba, 1997), pp. 81–3; Gregson and others, 'Recent upturn,' p. 1273.

29 Botswana, *Botswana AIDS impact survey 2001* (Gaborone, 2002), p. 55; D. Meekers and G. Ahmed, 'Contemporary patterns of adolescent sexuality in urban Botswana,' *Journal of Biosocial Science*, 32 (2000), 468, 473; D. Meekers, G. Ahmed, and M.T. Molatlhegi, 'Understanding constraints to adolescent condom procurement: the case of urban Botswana,' *AIDS Care*, 13 (2001), 298; M. Dynowski Smith, *Profile of youth in Botswana* (Gaborone, 1989), p. 120; G. Letamo and K. Bainame, 'The socio-economic and cultural context of the spread of HIV/AIDS in Botswana,' *HTR*, 7 (1997), supplement 3, p. 98.

30 J. Helle-Valle, 'Sexual mores, promiscuity and "prostitution" in Botswana,' *Ethnos*, 64 (1999), 375; Dynowski Smith, *Profile*, p. 5.

31 This is clear from I. Schapera, *Married life in an African tribe* (London, 1940), and Dynowski Smith, *Profile*.

32 N.I. Kumwenda, T.E. Taha, and others, 'HIV-1 incidence among male workers at a sugar estate in rural Malawi,' *Journal of AIDS*, 27 (2001), 202; *AAA*, January 2002, pp. 1, 4.

33 Botswana, *Second medium term plan*, pp. 4–5, 14–16; S. Gregson, B. Zaba, and others, 'Projections of the magnitude of the HIV/AIDS epidemic in southern Africa,' in A. Whiteside

(ed.), *Implications of AIDS for demography and policy in southern Africa* (Pietermaritzburg, 1998), p. 46.

34 Perkins, 'Spatial dynamics,' pp. 13, 235, 413, 586–7, 600–1.

35 J.S. Solway, 'Reaching the limits of universal citizenship: "minority" struggles in Botswana,' in B. Berman, D. Eyoh, and others (eds), *Ethnicity and democracy in Africa* (Oxford, 2004), p. 140; Botswana, *Second medium term plan*, p. 5; Botswana: National AIDS Co-ordinating Agency, 'National HIV/AIDS strategic framework 2003–2009,' p. 17, http://www.naca.gov.bw/documents/NSF%20final2.pdf (accessed 6 September 2004).

36 UNAIDS, 'AIDS epidemic update, December 2004,' p. 26, http://www.unaids.org (accessed 28 November 2004).

37 P. Mwaba, M. Maboshe, and others, 'The relentless spread of tuberculosis in Zambia – trends over the past 37 years (1964–2000),' *SAMJ*, 93 (2003), 150–1; B.C. Pazvakavambwa, 'The Zimbabwe mother-to-child HIV transmission prevention project: situation analysis,' March 1998, p. 15, http://www.unaids.org (accessed 24 November 2003); *SAfAids News*, March 2001, p. 16, http://www.safaids.org.zw/publications (accessed 31 December 2004).

38 Taha and others, 'Trends,' pp. 197–200; B. Auvert, A. Buvé, and others, 'Ecological and individual level analysis of risk factors for HIV infection in four urban populations in sub-Saharan Africa with different levels of HIV infection,' *AIDS*, 15 (2001), supplement 4, s19–21; Gregson and others,'Rural HIV epidemic,' p. 193; C.L. Mattson, R.C. Bailey, and others, 'Acceptability of male circumcision and predictors of circumcision preference among men and women in Nyanza province, Kenya,' *AIDS Care*, 17 (2005), 184.

39 J. Barreto, J. Liljestrand, and others, 'HIV-1 and HIV-2 antibodies in pregnant women in the city of Maputo, Mozambique: a comparative study between 1982/1983 and 1990,' *Scandinavian Journal of Infectious Diseases*, 25 (1993), 685–8.

40 Namibia, 'The national strategic plan on HIV/AIDS (medium term plan II) 1990–2004,' p. 4 and enclosure, http://www.unaids.org (accessed 21 November 2003); D. Webb and D. Simon, *Migrants, money and the military: the social epidemiology of HIV/AIDS in Ovambo, northern Namibia*, CEDAR research paper no. 8 (Egham, 1993), pp. 2–3, 7–13, 33–5; *AAA*, March 1994; UNAIDS, *Report on the global AIDS epidemic 2004* (Geneva, 2004), pp. 191–2.

41 G. Liotta, L. Palombi, and others, 'HIV infection in northern Mozambique,' *SAMJ*, 92 (2002), 12; *AAA*, April 2003, p. 9; L.M. Newman, F. Miguel, and others, 'HIV seroprevalence among military blood donors in Manica province, Mozambique,' *IJSA*, 12 (2001), 226; UNAIDS, *Accelerating action against AIDS in Africa* (Geneva, 2003), p. 10.

42 UNAIDS, 'AIDS epidemic update, December 2004,' p. 23. For a lower estimate (4.68 million) see T.M. Rehle and O. Shisana, 'Epidemiological and demographic HIV/AIDS projections: South Africa,' *African Journal of AIDS Research* (Grahamstown), 2 (2003), 5.

43 A. Buvé, K. Bishikwabo-Nsarhaza, and G. Mutangadura, 'The spread and effect of HIV-1 infection in sub-Saharan Africa,' *Lancet*, 359 (2002), 2013.

44 B.G. Weniger, Khanchit Limpakarnjanarat, and others, 'The epidemiology of HIV infection and AIDS in Thailand,' *AIDS*, 5 (1991), supplement 2, s71–85.

45 *Epidemiological Comments* (Pretoria), January 1983, p. 5; *The Star*, 8 January 1983.

46 R. Sher, 'HIV infection in South Africa, 1982–1988 – a review,' *SAMJ*, 76 (1989), 315; D.S. de Miranda, R. Sher, and others, 'Lack of evidence of HIV infection in drug abusers at present,' *SAMJ*, 70 (1986), 776; 'Working in the gay community,' *Critical Health*, 22 (April 1988), 34–9; *Epidemiological Comments*, November 1991, p. 256; B.D. Schoub, A.N. Smith, and others, 'Considerations on the further expansion of the HIV epidemic in South Africa – 1990,' *SAMJ*, 77 (1990), 614.

47 J. van Harmelen, R. Wood, and others, 'An association between HIV-1 subtypes and mode of transmission in Cape Town, South Africa,' *AIDS*, 11 (1997) 81–7; O. Shisana, L. Simbayi, and others, *Nelson Mandela/HSRC study of HIV/AIDS: South African national HIV prevalence, behavioural risks and news media: household survey 2002: executive summary* (Cape Town, 2002), p. 8.

48 N. O'Farrell, 'South African AIDS,' *SAMJ*, 72 (1987), 436; R. Sher, 'AIDS in Johannesburg,' *SAMJ*, 68 (1985), 137; S.F. Lyons, B.D. Schoub, and others, 'Lack of evidence of HTLV-III endemicity in southern Africa,' *NEJM*, 312 (1985), 1257.

49 Brink and Clausen, 'The acquired immune deficiency syndrome,' pp. 13–16; W.C. Chirwa, 'Migrant labour, sexual networking and multi-partnered sex in Malawi,' *HTR*, 7 (1997), supplement 3, pp. 6, 11; L. Grundlingh, 'HIV/AIDS in South Africa: a case of failed responses because of stigmatisation, discrimination and morality, 1983–1994,' *New Contree*, 46 (November 1999), 76–7.

50 M.C. Botha. F.A. Neethling, and others, 'Two black South Africans with AIDS,' *SAMJ*, 73 (1988), 132–4; B.D. Schoub, S.F. Lyons, and others, 'Absence of HIV infection in prostitutes and women attending sexually-transmitted disease clinics in South Africa,' *TRSTMH*, 81 (1987), 874–5; South African Institute for Medical Research, *Annual report 1986*, p. 66; *AIDS Bulletin* (Tygerberg), December 1996, p. 29.

51 D. van Rensburg, I. Friedman, and others, *Strengthening local government and civic responses to the HIV/AIDS epidemic in South* Africa (Bloemfontein, 2002), p. 31; G. Ramjee and E. Gouws, 'Targeting HIV-prevention efforts on truck drivers and sex workers,' *AIDS Bulletin*, April 2001, p. 14; Schoub and others, 'Absence of HIV infection,' pp. 874–5; South African Institute for Medical Research, *Annual report 1990*, p. 50; N. O'Farrell, A.A. Hoosen, and others, 'Sexual behaviour in Zulu men and women with genital ulcer disease,' *Genitourinary Medicine*, 68 (1992), 247; K.L. Dunkle, R.H. Jewkes, and others, 'Transactional sex among women in Soweto, South Africa,' *SSM*, 59 (2004), 1582, 1588.

52 *Epidemiological Comments*, April 1987, p. 43; R. Shapiro, R.L. Crookes, and E. O'Sullivan, 'Screening antenatal blood samples for anti-human immunodeficiency virus antibodies by a large-pool enzyme-linked immunosorbent assay system,' *SAMJ*, 76 (1989), 246.

53 M. Gordon, T. De Oliveira, and others, 'Molecular characteristics of human immunodeficiency virus type 1 subtype C viruses from KwaZulu-Natal, South Africa,' *Journal of Virology*, 77 (2003), 2587–99; *Sowetan*, 29 May 1991; H.G.V. Küstner, J.P. Swanevelder, and A. van Middelkoop, 'National HIV surveillance – South Africa, 1990–1992,' *SAMJ*, 84 (1994), 198.

54 Q. Abdool Karim, S.S. Abdool Karim, and others, 'Seroprevalence of HIV infection in rural South Africa,' *AIDS*, 6 (1992), 1535–9; M.N. Lurie, B.G. Williams, and others, 'Who infects whom? HIV-1 concordance and discordance among migrant and non-migrant couples in South Africa,' *AIDS*, 17 (2003), 2245–52; V. Hosegood, A.-M. Vanneste,and I.M. Timaeus, 'Levels and causes of adult mortality in rural South Africa: the impact of AIDS,' *AIDS*, 18 (2004), 669; L. Gilbert and L. Walker, 'Treading the path of least resistance: HIV/AIDS and social inequalities – a South African case study,' *SSM*, 54 (2002), 1104–5.

55 E. Gouws, B.G. Williams, and others, 'High incidence of HIV-1 in South Africa using a standardized algorithm for recent HIV seroconversion,' *Journal of AIDS*, 29 (2002), 531–5; S.S. Abdool Karim, Q. Abdool Karim, and others, 'Implementing antiretroviral therapy in resource-constrained settings,' *AIDS*, 18 (2004), 978; *AAA*, February 1999.

56 D. Bradshaw, A. Pettifor, and others, 'Trends in youth risk for HIV,' in P. Ijumba and A. Ntuli (eds), 'South African health review 2003/04' (2004), p. 136, http://www.hst.org.za/uploads/files/pdf (accessed 14 December 2004).

57 Lesotho, 'Monitoring the UNGASS declaration of commitment on HIV/AIDS: country report, January–December 2002,' http://www.unaids.org (accessed 21 November 2003); SAfAIDS, *Men and HIV in Lesotho* (Maseru, 2000), p. 4.

58 UNDP, *Swaziland human development report 2000* (Mbabane, 2001), pp. 37–8; UNAIDS, *Report on the global AIDS epidemic 2004*, pp. 191–2.

59 Shisana and others, *Nelson Mandela/HSRC study: executive summary*, p. 6.

60 O. Shisana, L. Simbayi, and others, *Nelson Mandela/HSRC study of HIV/AIDS: South African national HIV prevalence, behavioural risks and mass media: household survey 2002* (Cape Town, 2002), p. 56; B. Auvert, R. Ballard, and others, 'HIV infection in a South African mining town is associated with herpes simplex virus-2 seropositivity and sexual behaviour,' *AIDS*, 15 (2001), 889; B.G. Williams and E. Gouws, 'The epidemiology of human immunodeficiency virus in South Africa,' *Phil. Trans. R. Soc. Lond. B*, 356 (2001), 1082.

61 Shisana and others, *Nelson Mandela/HSRC study*, p. 70.

62 See P. Delius and C. Glaser, 'Sexual socialisation in South Africa: a historical perspective,' *African Studies*, 61 (2002), 27–54; K. Kelly and P. Ntlabati, 'Early adolescent sex in South Africa: HIV intervention challenges,' *Social Dynamics*, 28, 1 (2002), 56; M. Hunter, 'Masculinities, multiple sexual-partners, and AIDS: the making and unmaking of Isoka in KwaZulu-Natal,' *Transformation*, 54 (2004), 123–53.

63 Hunter, 'Masculinities', p. 141; T.-A. Selikow, B. Zulu, and E. Cedras, 'The *ingagara*, the *regte* and the *cherry*: HIV/AIDS and youth culture in contemporary urban townships,' *Agenda*, 53 (2002), 24–6; C. Campbell, *Townships, families and youth identity: the family's influence on the social identity of township youth in a rapidly changing South Africa* (Pretoria, 1994), p. 75.

64 L. Eaton, A.J. Flisher, and L.E. Aarø, 'Unsafe sexual behaviour in South African youth,' *SSM*, 56 (2003), 149; S. Abdool Karim, Q. Abdool Karim, and others, 'Reasons for lack of condom use among high school students, *SAMJ*, 82 (1992), 107–10; A.E. Pettifor, H.U. Rees, and

others, 'HIV and sexual behaviour among young South Africans: a national survey of 15–24 year-olds' (2004), p. 10, http://search:netscape.com (accessed 2 January 2005); S. Leclerc-Madlala, 'Infect one, infect all: Zulu youth response to the AIDS epidemic in South Africa,' *Medical Anthropology*, 17 (1996–7), 363.

65 Auvert and others, 'HIV infection,' p. 889; R. Jewkes and N. Abrahams, 'The epidemiology of rape and sexual coercion in South Africa: an overview,' *SSM*, 55 (2002), 1231; K. Kelly and W. Parker, *Communities of practice: contextual mediators of youth response to HIV/AIDS* (Pretoria, 2000), p. 37.

66 Dunkle and others, 'Transactional sex,' p. 1588; S. Leclerc-Madlala, 'Transactional sex and the pursuit of modernity,' *Social Dynamics*, 29, 2 (2003), 220.

67 Selikow and others, 'The *ingagara*,' pp. 27–8; K. Wood, F. Maforah, and R. Jewkes, '"He forced me to love him": putting violence on adolescent sexual health agendas,' *SSM*, 47 (1998), 233; Pettifor and others, 'HIV and sexual behaviour,' p. 30.

6 *The Penetration of the West* (pages 48–57)

1 B.H. Hahn, G.M. Shaw, and others, 'AIDS as a zoonosis: scientific and public health implications,' *Science*, 287 (2000), 610; T.C. Quinn, 'Population migration and the spread of types 1 and 2 human immunodeficiency viruses,' *Proc. Natl. Acad. Sci. USA*, 91 (1994), 2409; Feng Gao, Ling Yue, and others, 'Human infection by genetically diverse SIVsm-related HIV-2 in West Africa,' *Nature*, 358 (1992), 496; Zhiwei Chen, P. Telfer, and others, 'Genetic characterization of new West African simian immunodeficiency virus SIVsm,' *Journal of Virology*, 70 (1996), 3617.

2 M. Peeters, C. Toure-Kane, and others, 'Genetic diversity of HIV in Africa: impact on diagnosis, treatment, vaccine development and trials,' *AIDS*, 17 (2003), 2549; F. Damond, R. Worobey, and others, 'Identification of a highly divergent HIV type 2 and proposal for a change in HIV type 2 classification,' *ARHR*, 20 (2004), 666–72.

3 P. Lemey, O.G. Pybus and others, 'Tracing the origin and history of the HIV-2 epidemic,' *Proc. Natl. Acad. Sci. USA*, 100 (2003), 6588.

4 J. Goudsmit, *Viral sex: the nature of AIDS* (New York, 1997), p. 127; R. Marlink, 'Lessons from the second AIDS virus, HIV-2,' *AIDS*, 10 (1996), 691.

5 J.D. Reeves and R.W. Doms, 'Human immunodeficiency virus type 2,' *Journal of General Virology*, 83 (2002), 1255; M.F. Schim van der Loeff, S. Jaffer, and others, 'Mortality of HIV-1, HIV-2 and HIV-1/HIV-2 dually infected patients in a clinic-based cohort in The Gambia,' *AIDS*, 16 (2002), 1781.

6 F. Barin, F. Denis, and others, 'Serological evidence for virus related to simian T-lymphotropic retrovirus III in residents of West Africa,' *Lancet*, 1985/ii, 1387–8.

7 For early cases of HIV-2, see E. Hooper, *The river: a journey back to the source of HIV and AIDS* (reprinted, London, 2000), ch. 47.

8 Lemey and others, 'Tracing the origin,' pp. 6590–1; P. Gomes, A. Abecasis, and others, 'Transmission of HIV-2,' *Lancet Infectious Diseases*, 3 (2003), 683–4; A.J. Venter, *Portugal's guerrilla war* (Cape Town, 1973), pp. 132–4.

9 A. Mota-Miranda, H. Gomes, and others, 'Transmission of HIV-2: another perspective,' *Lancet Infectious Diseases*, 4 (2004), 265; A.-G. Poulsen, P. Aaby, and others, 'Risk factors for HIV-2 seropositivity among older people in Guinea-Bissau: a search for the early history of HIV-2 infection,' *Scandinavian Journal of Infectious Diseases*, 32 (2000), 169–75; L.H. Harrison, A.P. José da Silva, and others, 'Risk factors for HIV-2 infection in Guinea-Bissau,' *Journal of AIDS*, 4 (1991), 1159; A. Nauclér. P.-A. Andreasson, and others, 'HIV-2-associated AIDS and HIV-2 seroprevalence in Bissau,' *ibid.*, 2 (1989), 88.

10 E. Holmgren, Z. da Silva, and others, 'Dual infection with HIV-1, HIV-2 and HTLV-1 are more common in older women than in men in Guinea-Bissau,' *AIDS*, 17 (2003), 241; A. Wilkins, D. Ricard, and others, 'The epidemiology of HIV infection in a rural area of Guinea-Bissau,' *AIDS*, 7 (1993), 1119–22; P. Kanki, S. M'Boup, and others, 'Prevalence and risk determinants of human immunodeficiency virus type 2 (HIV-2) and human immunodeficiency virus type 1 (HIV-1) in West African female prostitutes,' *American Journal of Epidemiology*, 136 (1992), 895–907; A. Wilkins, R. Hayes, and others, 'Risk factors for HIV-2 infection in The Gambia,' *AIDS*, 5 (1991), 1127–32.

11 Hooper, *River*, p. 105; D. Vittecoq and J. Modai, 'AIDS in a black Malian,' *Lancet*, 1983/ii,1023; J. Hampton, *Meeting AIDS with compassion: AIDS care and prevention in Agomanya*,

Ghana (London, 1991), p. 2.

12   F. Denis, G. Gershy-Damet, and others, 'Prevalence of human T-lymphotropic retroviruses type III (HIV) and type IV in Ivory Coast,' *Lancet*, 1987/i, 408–11; I. Wendler, J. Schneider, and others, 'Seroepidemiology of human immunodeficiency virus in Africa,' *BMJ*, 293 (1986), 783; M. Garenne, M. Madison, and others, *Conséquences démographiques du SIDA en Abidjan: 1986–1992* (Paris, 1995), pp. xxi, 14, 117–18; S.A. Ouattara, J. Chotard, and others, 'Retrovirus infections (LAV/HTLV-III and HTLV-I) in Ivory Coast,' *Annales de l'Institut Pasteur/ Virologie*, 137E (1986), 304–8.

13   M. Peeters, B. Koumara, and others, 'Genetic subtypes of HIV type 1 and HIV type 2 strains in commercial sex workers from Bamako, Mali,' *ARHR*, 14 (1998), 51–8; J.N. Nkengasong, Chi-Cheng Luo, and others, 'Distribution of HIV-1 subtypes among HIV-seropositive patients in the interior of Côte d'Ivoire,' *Journal of AIDS*, 23 (2000), 430–6; F.E. McCutchan, 'Understanding the genetic diversity of HIV-1,' *AIDS*, 14 (2000), supplement 3, s33.

14   M. Peeters, E. Esu-Williams, and others, 'Predominance of subtype A and G HIV type 1 in Nigeria, with geographical differences in their distribution,' *ARHR*, 16 (2000), 315; Peeters and others, 'Genetic diversity,' pp. 2551–2.

15   World Bank, *World development report 1990* (New York, 1990), p. 180.

16   D. Vangroenweghe, *Sida et sexualité en Afrique* (trans. J.-M. Flémal, Brussels, 2000), pp. 333–4; P. Antoine and C. Henry, 'La population d'Abidjan dans ses murs,' in P. Haeringer (ed.), *Abidjan au coin de la rue: éléments de la vie citadine dans la métropole ivoirienne* (Paris, 1983), p. 372.

17   Vinh-Kim Nguyen, 'Epidemics, interzones and biosocial change: retroviruses and biologies of globalisation in West Africa,' PhD thesis, McGill University, 2001.

18   Dédy Séry and Tapé Gojé, 'Jeunesse, sexualité et sida en Côte d'Ivoire,' in J.-P. Dozon and L. Vidal (eds), *Les sciences sociales face au SIDA: cas africains autour de l'exemple ivoirien* (Paris, 1995), p. 84.

19   G. Williams, A.D. Blibolo, and D. Kerouedan, *Filling the gaps: care and support for people with HIV/AIDS in Côte d'Ivoire* (London, 1995), p. 7.

20   *Fraternité Matin* (Abidjan), 14 November 1990.

21   K.M. De Cock. K. Odehouri, and others, 'Rapid emergence of AIDS in Abidjan, Ivory Coast,' *Lancet*, 1989/ii, 410; Garenne and others, *Conséquences*, p. xxi.

22   K. Koffi, G.M. Gershy-Damet, and others. 'Rapid spread of HIV infections in Abidjan, Ivory Coast, 1987–1990,' *European Journal of Clinical Microbiology and Infectious Diseases*, 11 (1992), 272; G. Djomand, A.E. Greenberg, and others, 'The epidemic of HIV/AIDS in Abidjan, Côte d'Ivoire: a review of data collected by Projet RETRO-CI from 1987 to 1993,' *Journal of AIDS*, 10 (1995), 360, 363; De Cock and others, 'Rapid emergence,' p. 408; M.L. Garenne, M. Madison, and others, 'Mortality impact of AIDS in Abidjan, 1986–1992,' *AIDS*, 10 (1996), 1283; Garenne and others, *Conséquences*, pp. 88, 90.

23   *Fraternité Matin*, 4 May 1991; D. Tarantola and B. Schwartländer, 'HIV/AIDS epidemics in sub-Saharan Africa: dynamism, diversity and discrete declines?' *AIDS*, 11 (1997), supplement B, s17; Djomand and others, 'Epidemic,' p. 363.

24   Koffi and others, 'Rapid spread,' p. 272; Djomand and others, 'Epidemic,' p. 360; Tarantola and Schwartländer, 'HIV/AIDS epidemics,' pp. s6-7; Côte d'Ivoire, *Enquête démographigue et de santé, Côte d'Ivoire, 1994* (Abidjan, 1995), p. 167.

25   P.D. Ghys, M.O. Diallo, and others, 'Increase in condom use and decline in HIV and sexually transmitted diseases among female sex workers in Abidjan, Côte d'Ivoire, 1991–1998,' *AIDS*, 16 (2002), 253–7.

26   A.R. Neequaye, J.A.A. Mingle, and others, 'Human immune deficiency virus infection in Ghana,' in G. Giraldo, E. Beth-Giraldo, and others (eds), *AIDS and associated cancers in Africa* (Basel, 1988), p. 86; A.R. Neequaye, L. Osei, and others, 'Dynamics of human immune deficiency virus (HIV) epidemic – the Ghanaian experience,' in A.F. Fleming, M. Carballo, and others (eds), *The global impact of AIDS* (New York, 1988), p. 10; S. Agyei-Mensah, 'Twelve years of HIV/AIDS in Ghana: puzzles of interpretation,' *Canadian Journal of African Studies*, 35 (2001), 457–8; Hampton, *Meeting AIDS*, p. 25.

27   R.W. Porter, 'AIDS in Ghana: priorities and practices,' in D.A. Feldman (ed.), *Global AIDS policy* (Westport, 1994), pp. 98–103; Ghana: National AIDS/STI Control Programme, 'HIV sentinel survey report 2003,' http://www.ghanaids.gov.gh/docs (accessed 22 March 2005); A.-M. Coté, F. Sobela, and others, 'Transactional sex is the driving force in the dynamics of HIV in Accra, Ghana,' *AIDS*, 18 (2004), 917, 921.

28   C.M. Lowndes, M. Alary, and others, 'Role of core and bridging groups in the transmission

dynamics of HIV and STIs in Cotonou, Benin,' *Sexually Transmitted Infections*, 78 (2000), supplement 1, i70, i73; A. Buvé, M. Caraël, and others, 'Multicentre study on factors determining differences in rate of spread of HIV in sub-Saharan Africa: methods and prevalence of HIV infection', *AIDS*, 15 (2001), supplement 4, s5, s11; M. Alary and C. Lowndes, 'The central role of clients of female sex workers in the dynamics of heterosexual HIV transmission in sub-Saharan Africa', *AIDS*, 18 (2004), 945; Benin, 'Cadre stratégique national de lutte contre le VIH/SIDA/IST au Bénin 2001–2005,' http://www.unaids.org (accessed 30 November 2003).

29   Lowndes and others, 'Role,' i73–6; Coté and others, 'Transactional sex,' p. 917.

30   R. Lalou and V. Piché, *Migration et sida en Afrique de l'Ouest: un état des connaissances* (Paris, 1994), p. 14n17; A.Y. Sawadogo, *Le sida autour de moi* (Paris, 2003), p. 70.

31   M. Cros, 'Participer autrement: de l'ethnographie en temps de pandémie,' in Dozon and Vidal, *Les sciences sociales*, p. 259.

32   *L'Hebdomadaire du Burkina* (Ouagadougou), 8 March 2002; 'Présentation de la délégation du Burkina Faso,' in Organisation de Coordination et de Coopération pour la Lutte contre les grandes Endémies, *Premier plan concerté pour l'information, la surveillance épidémiologique et la lutte contre le sida dans les états membres de l'OCCGE* (Bobo Dioulasso, 1990), p. 6; N. Nagot, N. Meda, and others, 'Review of STI and HIV epidemiological data from 1990 to 2001 in urban Burkina Faso,' *Sexually Transmitted Infections*, 80 (2004), 127.

33   'Présentation de la délégation du Niger,' in OCCGE, *Premier plan*, p. 23; UNAIDS, 'AIDS epidemic update, December 2004,' p. 27, http://www.unaids.org (accessed 28 November 2004).

34   J.T. Boerma, P.D. Ghys, and N. Walker, 'Estimates of HIV-1 prevalence from national population-based surveys as a new gold standard,' *Lancet*, 362 (2003), 1929; Mali, 'Plan stratégique national de lutte contre le VIH/SIDA 2001–2005,' http://www.unaids.org (accessed 4 December 2003).

35   Mauritania, 'Cadre stratégique national de lutte contre les IST/VIH/SIDA 2003–2007,' http://www.unaids.org (accessed 3 December 2003); K. Wyss, G. Hulton, and Y. N'Diekhor, 'Costs attributable to AIDS at household level in Chad,' *AIDS Care*, 16 (2004), 809.

36   P. Boisier, O.N. Ouwe Missi Oukem-Boyer, and others, 'Nationwide HIV prevalence survey in general population in Niger,' *Tropical Medicine and International Health*, 9 (2004), 1164; Mali, 'Plan stratégique 2001–2005'; Niger, *Enquête démographique et de santé, Niger, 1998* (Niamey, 1999), pp. 190, 193; J.G. Cleland, M.M. Ali, and V. Capo-Chichi, 'Post-partum sexual abstinence in West Africa: implications for AIDS-control and family planning programmes,' *AIDS*, 13 (1999), 126.

37   UNAIDS, *Report on the global AIDS epidemic 2004* (Geneva, 2004), pp. 34, 202; UNAIDS, 'AIDS in Africa: three scenarios to 2025' (2005), p. 28, http://www.unaids.org (accessed 7 March 2005); A. Dialmy, *Jeunesse, sida et Islam au Maroc: les comportements sexuels des Marocains* (Casablanca, 2000).

38   Nigeria: National HIV/AIDS/STD Control Programme, '1993/94 sentinel sero-prevalence surveillance report, June 1995' (duplicated), p. 110; J.O. Chikwem, I. Mohammed, and others, 'Prevalence of human immunodeficiency virus (HIV) infection in Borno state of Nigeria,' *East African Medical Journal*, 65 (1988), 342–6; E. Williams, N. Lamson, and others, 'Implementation of an AIDS prevention program among prostitutes in the Cross River state of Nigeria,' *AIDS*, 6 (1992), 229–30.

39   Nigeria: National Action Committee on HIV/AIDS, 'HIV/AIDS emergency action plan (HEAP), January 2001,' http://www.unaids.org (accessed 30 November 2003); O. Alubo, A. Zwandor, and others, 'Acceptance and stigmatization of PLWA in Nigeria,' *AIDS Care*, 14 (2002), 118, 120, 123; S.C. Ogbuagu and J.O. Charles, 'Survey of sexual networking in Calabar,' *HTR*, 3 (1993), supplement, 105–19.

40   Nigeria, 'A report on the UNGASS indicators in Nigeria: a follow-up to the declaration of commitment on HIV/AIDS' (2002), p. 4, http://www.unaids.org (accessed 30 November 2003); G. Remy, 'Paysage épidémiologique de l'infection à VIH 1 parmi les prostituées africaines,' *Médecine d'Afrique Noire*, 45 (1998), 287–8, 290; Nigeria, 'HIV/AIDS emergency action plan.'

41   E.P. Renne, *Population and progress in a Yoruba town* (London, 2003), pp. 71–8; I.O. Orubuloye, 'Behavioural research as a tool in the prevention and control of HIV/AIDS,' in Nigeria, 'Proceedings of the National Conference on HIV/AIDS, Abuja, 15–17 December 1998' (duplicated), pp. 251–3.

42   Nigeria, '1993/94 sentinel report,' p. 16; *Newswatch* (Lagos), 28 February 2005.

43 Nigeria, '1993/94 sentinel report,' p. 17.
44 *Rapport sur le fonctionnement technique de l'Institut Pasteur de Dakar, 1987,* p. 51; P. Lemardeley, 'Compte-rendu sur la VIe Conférence Internationale sur le Syndrome d'Immuno-dépression Acquise,' *Médecine Tropicale,* 52 (1992), 201; Senegal, 'Bulletin séro-épidémiologique no. 10 de surveillance du VIH,' July 2003, p. 17, http://www.fhi.org/ NL/rdonlyres (accessed 6 September 2004); *Le Soleil* (Dakar), 3 December 2004.
45 Senegal, 'Bulletin séro-épidémiologique no. 10,' p. 16.
46 J.V. Millen, 'The evolution of vulnerability: ethnomedicine and social change in the context of HIV/AIDS among the Jola of southwestern Senegal,' PhD thesis, University of Connecticut, 2003, ch. 13; E. Lagarde, G. Pison, and C. Enel, 'A study of sexual behavior change in rural Senegal,' *Journal of AIDS,* 11 (1996), 282–7.
47 E.C. Green, *Rethinking AIDS prevention: learning from successes in developing countries* (Westport, 2003), pp. 227–37.

7 *Causation: a Synthesis* (pages 58–64)

1 See J.C. Caldwell, P. Caldwell, and P. Quiggin, 'The social context of AIDS in sub-Saharan Africa,' *Population and Development Review,* 15 (1989), 185–234; E. Stillwaggon, 'HIV/AIDS in Africa: fertile terrain,' *Journal of Development Studies,* 38, 6 (August 2002), 1–22.
2 S. Sontag, *AIDS and its metaphors* (reprinted, London, 1990), p. 89.
3 For reading on earlier African epidemics, see p. 204.
4 For the American epidemic, see R. Shilts, *And the band played on: politics, people, and the AIDS epidemic* (reprinted, London, 1988); E.J. Sobo, *Choosing unsafe sex: AIDS-risk denial among disadvantaged women* (Philadelphia, 1995).
5 J.M. Garcia Calleja, N. Walker, and others, 'Status of the HIV/AIDS epidemic and methods to counter it in the Latin American and Caribbean region,' *AIDS,* 16 (2002), supplement 3, s3–12.
6 B.G. Weniger, Khanchit Limpakarnjanarat, and others, 'The epidemiology of HIV infection and AIDS in Thailand,' *AIDS,* 5 (1991), supplement 2, s71–85.
7 J.G. Cooke (ed.), *The second wave of the HIV/AIDS pandemic: China, India, Russia, Ethiopia, Nigeria* (Washington, 2002).
8 J. Cohen, 'Asia and Africa: on different trajectories?' *Science,* 304 (2004), 1932–8.
9 World Bank, *Confronting AIDS: public priorities in a global epidemic* (Oxford, 1997), p. 2.
10 See J. Iliffe, *Africans: the history of a continent* (Cambridge, 1995).
11 World Bank, *World development report 1997* (New York, 1997), p. 231.
12 K.-I. Klepp, P.M. Biswalo, and A. Talle (eds), *Young people at risk: fighting AIDS in northern Tanzania* (Oslo, 1995), p. xxii.
13 M.R. Grmek, *History of AIDS* (trans. R.C. Maulitz and J. Duffin, Princeton, 1990), p. 161.
14 World Bank, *World development report 1993* (New York, 1993), p. 29.
15 *Ibid.,* 1990, p. 233; 1993, p. 293.
16 R. Gallo, *Virus hunting: AIDS, cancer, and the human retrovirus* (New York. 1991), p. 320.
17 Grmek, *History of AIDS,* p. xi.
18 The following data are from M. Caraël, 'Sexual behaviour,' in J. Cleland and B. Ferry (eds), *Sexual behaviour and AIDS in the developing world* (London, 1995), ch. 4.
19 J. Cleland, B. Ferry, and M. Caraël, 'Summary and conclusion,' in *ibid.,* p. 212.
20 J.R. Goody, *Production and reproduction: a comparative study of the domestic domain* (Cambridge, 1976), pp. 14–21; Caldwell and others, 'Social context,' pp. 185–234.
21 L. Corey, A. Wall, and others, 'The effects of herpes simplex virus-2 on HIV-1 acquisition and transmission: a review of two overlapping epidemics,' *Journal of AIDS,* 35 (2004), 435–45; WHO, 'Herpes simplex virus 2: report of a WHO/UNAIDS/LSHTM workshop (London, 14–16 February 2001),' http://www.who.int/hiv/pub/sti/en/hiv_aids_2001,05.pdf (accessed 22 March 2005).
22 N. Siegfried, M. Muller, and others, 'HIV and male circumcision – a systematic review with assessment of the quality of studies,' *Lancet Infectious Diseases,* 5 (2005), 165–73.
23 R.M. Anderson and R.M. May, *Infectious diseases of humans: dynamics and control* (Oxford, 1991), p. 360.
24 Goody, *Production,* pp. 102–4.
25 A. Katz, 'AIDS, individual behaviour and the unexplained remaining variation,' *African Journal of AIDS Research,* 1 (2002), 125.

26 N. Kaleeba, *We miss you all* (Harare, 1991), p. 80.

27 A. Kilian, 'HIV/AIDS control in Kabarole district, Uganda' (2002), p. 26, http://www.afronets-org/files/gtz-aids-brochure-uganda.pdf (accessed 20 July 2004); J.A. Seeley, S.S. Malamba, and others, 'Socioeconomic status, gender and risk of HIV-1 infection in a rural community in south west Uganda,' *Medical Anthropology Quarterly*, 8 (1994), 78.

28 J.R. Hargreaves, L.M. Morison, and others, 'Socioeconomic status and risk of HIV infection in an urban population in Kenya,' *Tropical Medicine and International Health*, 7 (2002), 793–802.

29 O. Shisana, L. Simbayi, and others, *Nelson Mandela/HSRC study of HIV/AIDS: South African national HIV prevalence, behavioural risks and mass media: household survey 2002* (Cape Town, 2002), pp. 46, 54.

30 N. Nattrass, 'AIDS and human security in southern Africa,' *Social Dynamics*, 28, 1 (2002), 4; Stillwaggon, 'HIV/AIDS,' pp. 1–22.

31 N. French, A. Mujugira, and others, 'Immunologic and clinical stages in HIV-1-infected Ugandan adults are comparable and provide no evidence of rapid progression but poor survival with advanced disease,' *Journal of AIDS*, 22 (1999), 509–16.

32 World Bank, *World development report 1992* (New York, 1992), p. 221.

33 V. van der Vliet, *The politics of AIDS* (London, 1996), p. 23.

34 A.L. Martin, 'The costs of health care,' in J.M. Mann and D.J.M. Tarantola (eds), *AIDS in the world II* (New York, 1996), p. 404.

8 *Responses from Above* (pages 65–79)

1 V. Berridge, *AIDS in the UK: the making of policy, 1981–1994* (Oxford, 1996), pp. 4, 55, 112, 152; M. Steffen, 'AIDS policies in France,' in V. Berridge and P. Strong (eds), *AIDS and contemporary history* (Cambridge, 1993), pp. 252–62.

2 S. Epstein, *Impure science: Aids, activism, and the politics of knowledge* (Berkeley, 1996).

3 M.P. Mandara, 'Health services in Tanzania: a historical overview,' in G.M.P. Mwaluko, W.L. Kilama, and others (eds), *Health and disease in Tanzania* (London, 1991), p. 5.

4 E. Silla, *People are not the same: leprosy and identity in twentieth-century Mali* (Portsmouth NH, 1998), p. 172.

5 I.R. Friedland, K.P. Klugman, and others, 'AIDS – the Baragwanath experience,' *SAMJ*, 82 (1992), 99; N. Kaleeba, *We miss you all* (Harare, 1991), p. 6.

6 E.g. *Daily News* (Dar es Salaam), 8 August 1986.

7 Quoted in J. Manchester, 'The HIV epidemic in South Africa: personal views of positive people,' MA (Education) thesis, University of London, 2000, p. 7.

8 Botswana, *Family health survey II, 1988* (Gaborone, 1989), p. 97; Zimbabwe, *Demographic and health survey 1988* (Harare, 1989); B.A. Ogot, *Politics and the Aids epidemic in Kenya 1983–2003* (Kisumu, 2004), p. 42.

9 *Daily News*, 7 August 1989.

10 Okware, 'Brief report and policy considerations on AIDS Control Programme,' 15 April 1989, UMOH unnumbered file; World Health Assembly resolution, May 1987, in WHO, *Handbook of resolutions and decisions of the World Health Assembly and the Executive Board: volume III: third edition (1985–1992)* (Geneva, 1993), p. 121.

11 See esp. D. Fassin, *Les enjeux politiques de la santé: études sénégalaises, équatoriennes et françaises* (Paris, 1994), ch. 19.

12 J. Cohen, 'The rise and fall of Projet SIDA,' *Science*, 278 (1997), 1566.

13 *Weekly Review*, 11 October 1985.

14 M. Heywood, 'The price of denial' (2004), http://www.tac.org.za (accessed 7 March 2005).

15 R. Caputo, 'Uganda: land beyond sorrow', *National Geographic*, 173 (1988), 482.

16 *Epidemiological Comments*, January 1983, p. 5, and April 1985, pp. 12–13; P.M'Pele, A. Itoua-Ngaporo, and others, 'Prise en charge de l'infection à HIV à Brazzaville (Congo),' *Médecine d'Afrique Noire*, 34 (1987), 1059–61; F. Eboko, 'L'état camerounais et les cadets sociaux face à la pandémie du sida,' *Politique Africaine*, 64 (1996), 136.

17 R.G. Choto, 'Foreword,' in H. Jackson, *AIDS: action now: information, prevention and support in Zimbabwe* (Harare, 1988); L. Garrett, *The coming plague* (reprinted, New York, 1995), pp. 347–8; S. Allen, C. Lindau, and others, 'Human immunodeficiency virus infection in urban Rwanda,' *JAMA*, 266 (1991), 1657.

18 J. Iliffe, *East African doctors: a history of the modern profession* (Cambridge, 1998), pp. 223, 230–1.

19 Quoted in J.M. Mann, D.J.M. Tarantola, and T.W. Netter (eds), *AIDS in the world* (Cambridge, Mass.,1992), p. 567.

20 *Times of Zambia,* 11 September 1985.

21 See B.D. Schoub, 'Report back: international symposium on African AIDS: Brussels, 22 and 23 November 1985,' *Southern African Journal of Epidemiology and Infection,* 1 (1986), 25–9, 52–6.

22 Executive Board resolution, January 1986, in WHO, *Handbook,* vol. 3, pp. 119–20; WHO, *Weekly Epidemiological Record,* 28 March 1986, p. 93; J.M. Mann and K. Kay, 'Confronting the pandemic: the World Health Organization's Global Programme on AIDS, 1986–1989,' *AIDS,* 5 (1991), supplement 2, s221.

23 See M. Carballo, 'Jonathan Mann (1947–1998),' *SSM,* 48 (1999), 573–4.

24 J.M. Mann, 'The global picture of AIDS,' *Journal of AIDS,* 1 (1988), 216.

25 UNAIDS, *Report on the global AIDS epidemic 2004* (Geneva, 2004), p. 90.

26 *La Semaine Africaine* (Brazzaville), 29 December 1988.

27 Mann, 'Global picture,' p. 215.

28 World Health Assembly resolution, May 1992, in WHO, *Handbook,* vol. 3, p. 127; J.M. Mann and D.J.M. Tarantola (eds), *AIDS in the world II* (New York, 1996), p. 433. The chief document on human rights was WHO, *Social aspects of AIDS prevention and control programmes* (Geneva, 1987).

29 See p. 78 and K.M. Booth, 'National mother, global whore, and transnational femocrats: the politics of Aids and the construction of women at the World Health Organization,' *Feminist Studies,* 24 (1998), 115–39.

30 Mann and others, *AIDS in the world,* p. 542.

31 Mann, 'Global picture,' pp. 212–13.

32 WHO: Special Programme on AIDS, 'Strategies and structure: projected needs' (WHO/SPA/GEN/87.1), March 1987, pp. 10–13; Mann and others, *AIDS in the world,* p. 300.

33 F.A. Plummer, N.J.D. Nagelkerke, and others, 'The importance of core groups in the epidemiology and control of HIV-1 infection,' *AIDS,* 5 (1991), supplement 1, s169–76; UNAIDS, *Consultation on STD interventions for preventing HIV* (Geneva, 2000), p. 32.

34 'First supplementary memorandum submitted by the Department for International Development,' in Great Britain: House of Commons (Session 2000–01): International Development Committee: Third Report, *HIV/AIDS: the impact on social and economic development,* vol. II (HC 354-II), p. 70.

35 The best account is N. Meda, I. Ndoye, and others, 'Low and stable HIV infection rates in Senegal: natural course of the epidemic or evidence for success of prevention?' *AIDS,* 13 (1999), 1397–1405.

36 'Meeting of interested participating parties in support of the "AIDS Control Programme" (ACP) in Uganda,' 21–22 May 1987, UMOH unnumbered file; S.I. Okware, 'Towards a national AIDS-control program in Uganda,' *Western Journal of Medicine,* 147 (1987), 728.

37 *New Vision,* 2 December 1988; E.C. Green, *Rethinking AIDS prevention: learning from successes in developing countries* (Westport, 2003), pp. 152–3, 183.

38 J.O. Parkhurst, 'HIV prevention policy in sub-Saharan Africa: the Ugandan experience,' DPhil thesis, University of Oxford, 2000, chs 3 and 5; Iliffe, *East African doctors,* pp. 232–3. See also pp. 128–30.

39 Tanzania: National AIDS Control Programme, 'Strategic framework for the third medium term plan (MTP-III) for prevention and control of HIV/AIDS/STDs,' July 1998, p. vi; F. Eboko, 'Introduction à la question du sida en Afrique: politique publique et dynamiques sociales,' in D. Kerouedan and F. Eboko, *Politiques publiques du sida en Afrique* (Bordeaux, 1999), p. 47.

40 M.-E. Gruénais,'Communautés et état dans les systèmes de santé en Afrique,' in B. Hours (eds), *Systèmes et politiques de santé: de la santé publique à l'anthropologie* (Paris, 2001), pp. 67–8, 77; D.A. Eaton Jr, 'Men's lives and the politics of AIDS in the Republic of Congo,' PhD thesis, University of California at Berkeley, 2001, p. 65.

41 J.T. Boerma, M. Urassa, and others,'Sociodemographic context of the AIDS epidemic in a rural area in Tanzania with a focus on people's mobility and marriage,' *Sexually Transmitted Infections,* 78 (2002), supplement 1, i99.

42 I.O. Orubuloye and F. Oguntimehin, 'Death is pre-ordained, it will come when it is due: attitudes of men to death in the presence of AIDS in Nigeria,' in J.C. Caldwell, P. Caldwell, and others (eds), *Resistances to behavioural change to reduce HIV/AIDS infection in predominantly heterosexual epidemics in Third World countries* (Canberra, 1999), pp. 101–2; Great Britain, *HIV/AIDS: the impact,* vol. 1, p. lxix; *Nigeria AIDS Monitor* (Lagos), May 1993; M.A.S. Safana,

'How adequate is the Nigerian policy on HIV/AIDS?' in Nigeria, 'Proceedings of the National Conference on HIV/AIDS, Abuja, 15–17 December 1998' (duplicated), p. 283.

43 For accounts of this period, see L. Grundlingh, 'HIV/AIDS in South Africa: a case of failed responses because of stigmatization, discrimination and morality,' *New Contree*, 46 (November 1999), 55–81; H. Phillips, 'AIDS in the context of South Africa's epidemic history: preliminary historical thoughts,' *South African Historical Journal*, 45 (2001), 11–26.

44 'Health and welfare in transition: a report on the Maputo Conference April 1990,' *Critical Health*, 31 (August 1990), 50–1.

45 NACOSA, *A national AIDS plan for South Africa 1994–1995* (Sunnyside, 1994).

46 African National Congress, *A national health plan for South Africa* (Johannesburg, 1994),p. 7; Q. Abdool Karim, 'The HIV/AIDS epidemic,' in Health Systems Trust, *South African health review 1995* (Durban, 1995), p. 176.

47 Bosenge N'Galy, R.W. Ryder, and others, 'Human immunodeficiency virus infection among employees in an African hospital,' *NEJM*, 319 (1988), 1123–7; O. Shisana, E.J. Hall, and others, 'HIV/AIDS prevalence among South African health workers,' *SAMJ*, 94 (2004), 849; B. Gumodoko, I. Favot, and others, 'Occupational exposure to the risks of HIV infection among health care workers in Mwanza region,' *Bulletin of the WHO*, 75 (1997), 133–40.

48 M.-E. Gruénais, 'Dire ou ne pas dire: enjeux de l'annonce de la séropositivité au Congo,' in J.-P. Dozon and L. Vidal (eds), *Les sciences sociales face au SIDA: cas africaines autour de l'exemple ivoirien* (Paris, 1995), p. 165.

49 UNAIDS, *Report on the global AIDS epidemic 2004*, p. 126.

50 Naamara to Permanent Secretary, minute, 9 January 1992, UMOH GCD 2/1/30.

51 *SAMJ*, 89 (1999), 563, 583, 609–11; *ibid.*, 90 (2000), 95.

52 P. Modiba. L. Gilson, and H. Schneider, 'Voices of service users,' in Health Systems Trust, *South African health review 2001* (Durban, 2001), p. 195; A. Shomatoff, *African madness* (New York, 1988), p. 186.

53 F. Jabot, A. van den Dries, and others, 'Attitudes, opinions et pratiques de practiciens de santé relatives à l'annonce de résultat sérologique VIH,' *Bulletin de l'OCEAC*, 26, 1 (May 1993), 15–16.

54 Kenya: Ministry of Health, *National guidelines on counselling for HIV infection, December 1988* (Nairobi, 1988), p. 10; '15th NCPA [National Council for the Prevention of AIDS] meeting, 28 October 1987,' UMOH unnumbered file; G.T. Lie and P.M. Biswalo, 'HIV-positive patients' choice of a significant other to be informed about the HIV-test result,' *AIDS Care*, 8 (1996), 286.

55 NACOSA, 'National AIDS plan,' p. 29.

56 WHO: Global Programme on AIDS and Programme of STD, 'Consensus statement from consultation on partner notification for preventing HIV transmission, Geneva, 11-13 January 1989' (WHO/GPA/INF/89.3), p. 3n1; *SAMJ*, 92 (2002), 189–90; Tanzania: Prime Minister's Office, 'National policy on HIV/AIDS' (November 2001), pp. 23–4, http://www.tzonline.org/pdf/nationalaidspolicy.pdf (accessed 17 July 2004).

57 K. Awusabo-Asare and C. Marfo, 'Attitudes to and management of HIV/AIDS among health workers in Ghana: the case of Cape Coast municipality,' *HTR*, 7 (1997), supplement, 278.

58 G. Seidel, 'Confidentiality and HIV status in Kwazulu-Natal, South Africa,' *Health Policy and Planning*, 11 (1996), 423.

59 A.F. Chimwaza, 'A descriptive study of the experience of primary caregivers of patients with symptoms of AIDS in resource poor communities: the case of Malawi,' PhD thesis, University of Pennsylvania, 2002, pp. 26, 188–9.

60 Seidel, 'Confidentiality,' p. 419.

61 R. Goodgame in *New Vision*, 13 July 1988; C.B.K. Nzioka, 'The social construction and management of HIV and AIDS among low-income patients in Nairobi,' PhD thesis, University of London, 1994, p. 119.

62 R. Kasirye, 'Community response to AIDS affected households: a case study of Kamwokya,' BA thesis, Makerere University, 1992, p. 36.

63 S.B. Adebajo, A.D. Bamgbala, and M.A. Oyediran, 'Attitudes of health care providers to persons living with HIV/AIDS in Lagos state, Nigeria,' *African Journal of Reproductive Health*, 7, 1 (April 2003), 103. For a sympathetic analysis of the role of nurses, see K.M. Booth. *Local women, global science: fighting AIDS in Kenya* (Bloomington, 2004), chs 2 and 5.

64 S.D. Foster, 'The socioeconomic impact of HIV/AIDS in Monze district. Zambia,' PhD thesis, University of London, 1996, p. 90; Clacherty and Associates, *The role of stigma and discrimination in increasing the vulnerability of children and youth affected by HIV/AIDS: report on*

participatory workshops (Arcadia, South Africa, 2001), p. 62.

65   'Kitovu complex: annual report, 1993' (duplicated) UMOH library.

66   M.-J. DelVecchio Good, 'Clinical realities and moral dilemmas: contrasting perspectives from academic medicine in Kenya, Tanzania, and America,' *Daedalus*, 128, 4 (Fall 1999), 170, 172.

67   Garrett, *Coming plague*, p. 343.

68   Dr Athenase Kiromera of Namitete, Malawi, in *Africa Today*, May 2003, p. 33.

69   G. Raviola, M. Machoki, and others, 'HIV, disease plague, demoralization and "burnout": resident experience of the medical profession in Nairobi, Kenya,' *Culture, Medicine and Psychiatry*, 26 (2002), 55, 60, 64.

70   J. Hampton, *Living positively with AIDS: The Aids Support Organisation (TASO), Uganda* (London, 1990), p. 10.

71   E.T. Katabira, 'Looking after AIDS patients,' *Health Information Quarterly*, 4, 4 (December 1988), 25.

72   M. Schoofs, 'Use what you have,' *Village Voice*, 4 January 2000, p. 54.

73   J. Decosas in *AAA*, February 2000; Fassin, *Les enjeux politiques*, p. 288; Eboko, 'Introduction,' in Kerouedan and Eboko, *Politiques publiques*, pp. 41–6; Booth, *Local women*, pp. 66, 77; K.A. Hartwig, E. Eng, and others, 'AIDS and "shared sovereignty" in Tanzania from 1987 to 2000,' *SSM*, 60 (2005), 1613, 1617.

74   R. Mattes and R. Manning, *The impact of HIV/AIDS on democracy in southern Africa* (Cape Town, 2003), p. 11; Burkina Faso, 'Cadre stratégique de lutte contre le VIH/SIDA 2001–2005,' p. 15, http://www.unaids.org (accessed 3 December 2003); UNAIDS, *Accelerating action against AIDS in Africa* (Geneva, 2003), p. 49.

75   Mann and others, *AIDS in the world*, p. 505; Great Britain, *HIV/AIDS: the impact*, vol. 1, p. lxv, and vol 2, p. 103; WHO, *1991 progress report: Global Programme on AIDS* (Geneva, 1992), pp. 15–16.

76   P. Selby, 'Mann overboard,' *BMJ*, 300 (1990), 831; *Fraternité Matin*, 22 March and 6 August 1990; Mann and Kay, 'Confronting the pandemic,' p. s228; Booth, *Local women*, p. 55.

77   Mann and others, *AIDS in the world*, pp. xiii, 330, 6.

78   World Health Assembly resolutions, May 1989 and May 1990, in WHO, *Handbook*, vol. 3, pp. 124–5; *Global AIDSNews*, 1992, no. 3.

79   P. Lemardeley, 'Compte-rendu sur la VIe Conférence Internationale sur le Syndrome d'Immunodépression Acquise,' *Médecine Tropicale*, 52 (1992), 202; C. O'Manique, *Neoliberalism and AIDS crisis in sub-Saharan Africa: globalization's pandemic* (Basingstoke, 2004), pp. 59, 62.

9 *Views from Below* (pages 80–97)

1   O.I. Morrow, 'Sexual cultures and vulnerability to HIV infection among Baganda youth in Mpigi, Uganda,' PhD thesis, Johns Hopkins University, 2000, p. 218.

2   P. Boggio, 'L'épidémie de SIDA à Kinshasa,' *Le Monde*, 24 December 1986; M. Cros, 'Participer autrement: de l'ethnographie en temps de pandémie,' in J.-P. Dozon and L. Vidal (eds), *Les sciences sociales face au SIDA: cas africaines autour de l'exemple ivoirien* (Paris, 1995), p. 259.

3   V. van der Vliet, 'South Africa divided against AIDS: a crisis of leadership,' in K.D. Kauffman and D.L. Lindauer (eds), *AIDS and South Africa: the social expression of a pandemic* (Basingstoke, 2004), pp. 50–1.

4   M. Lyons, 'The point of view: perspectives on AIDS in Uganda,' in G.C. Bond, J. Kreniske, and others (eds), *AIDS in Africa and the Caribbean* (Boulder, 1997), p. 138.

5   K.J.J. Meursing, *A world of silence: living with HIV in Matabeleland, Zimbabwe* (Amsterdam, 1997), p. 119.

6   G.K. Amofah, 'AIDS in Ghana: profile, strategies and challenges,' *AAA*, September 1992.

7   Boggio, 'L'épidémie'; *New Vision*, 25 November 2000; *Daily News* (Dar es Salaam), 28 September 1987; *Sunday News*, 6 March 1988.

8   M.K. Mutembei, *Poetry and AIDS in Tanzania: changing metaphors and metonymies in Haya oral traditions* (Leiden, 2001), p. 144; S. Ayoubzadeh, T. Ben Abdallah, and others, 'Sida et tiers monde,' *Environnement Africain*, 118 (1987), 21.

9   E. Hooper, 'AIDS in Uganda,' *African Affairs*, 86 (1987), 471.

10   B.G. Schoepf, 'AIDS, history, and struggles over meaning,' in E. Kalipeni, S. Craddock, and others (eds), *HIV and AIDS in Africa: beyond epidemiology* (Malden MA, 2004), pp. 20–2; *Jeune Afrique*, 13 April 1988, p. 75.
11   J.J. Stadler, 'The young, the rich, and the beautiful: secrecy, suspicion and discourses of AIDS in the South African lowveld,' *African Journal of AIDS Research*, 2 (2003), 130; UNAIDS, *Stepping back from the edge: the pursuit of antiretroviral therapy in Botswana, South Africa and Uganda* (revised edition, Geneva, 2004), p. 53.
12   M. Schoofs, 'A tale of two brothers,' *Village Voice*, 16 November 1999, pp. 51–2.
13   D. Vangroenweghe, *Sida et sexualité en Afrique* (trans. J.M. Flémal, Brussels, 2000), p. 12.
14   Mutembei, *Poetry and AIDS*, pp. 54–7, 60, 196–7.
15   J. Lwanda, 'The [in]visibility of HIV/AIDS in the Malawi public sphere,' *African Journal of AIDS Research*, 2 (2003), 117–18.
16   M.G. Magezi, 'Against a sea of troubles: AIDS control in Uganda,' *World Health Forum*, 12 (1991), 304.
17   Tanzania, *Demographic and health survey 1991/1992* (Dar es Salaam, 1993), p. 147; S. Panda, A. Chatterjee, and A.S. Abdul-Quader (eds), *Living with the AIDS virus: the epidemic and the response in India* (New Delhi, 2002), pp. 19, 53.
18   J. Killewo, A. Sandström, and others, 'Communicating with the people about HIV infection risk as a basis for planning interventions: lessons from the Kagera region of Tanzania,' *SSM*, 45 (1997), 324; Nigeria, *Demographic and health survey 1999* (Abuja, 2000), pp. 142–3.
19   Ethiopia, *Demographic and health survey 2000* (Addis Ababa, 2001), pp. 161–2; Uganda, *Demographic and health survey 1995* (Entebbe, 1996), pp. 147–8.
20   Tanzania, *Reproductive and child health survey 1999* (Dar es Salaam, 2000), p. 130; L. Vidal, 'La transmission: le sida et ses savoirs,' *L'Homme*, 150 (1999), 59–84; K.P. Smith and S.C. Watkins, 'Perceptions of risk and strategies for prevention: responses to HIV/AIDS in rural Malawi,' *SSM*, 60 (2005), 654; K. Irwin, J. Bertrand, and others, 'Knowledge, attitudes and beliefs about HIV infection and AIDS among healthy factory workers and their wives, Kinshasa, Zaire,' *SSM*, 32 (1991), 921; A. Nicoll, U. Laukamm-Josten, and others, 'Lay health beliefs concerning HIV and AIDS – a barrier for control programmes,' *AIDS Care*, 5 (1993), 234; *New Vision*, 18 January 1999; C. Larson, Mekonnen Asefa, and others, 'Risk factors for HIV infection: their occurrence and determinants in Jima-town, southwestern Ethiopia,' *Ethiopian Medical Journal*, 29 (1991), 129.
21   *Lesotho Epidemiological Bulletin*, 4, 3 (1989), 2; Ethiopia, *Demographic and health survey 2000*, p. 166; Uganda, *Demographic and health survey 2000–2001* (Entebbe, 2001), pp. 171–2; S.C. Watkins, 'Navigating the AIDS epidemic in rural Malawi,' *Population and Development Review*, 30 (2004), 681.
22   E. Ratsma, E.P. Manjolo, and J. Simon, 'Voices from the epidemic,' *Malawi Medical Journal*, 8 (1992), 64.
23   WHO, *TASO Uganda – the inside story: participatory evaluation of HIV/AIDS counselling, medical and social services 1993–1994* (WHO/GPA/TCO/HCS/95.1: Geneva, 1995), p. 46; C. Els, W. Boshoff, and others, 'Psychiatric co-morbidity in South African HIV/AIDS patients,' *SAMJ*, 89 (1999), 992; M.F. Chimwaza and S.C. Watkins, 'Giving care to people with symptoms of AIDS in rural sub-Saharan Africa,' *AIDS Care*, 16 (2004), 803.
24   *New Vision*, 7 April 2000.
25   N. Kaleeba, *We miss you all* (Harare, 1991), pp. 38–40.
26   J.K. Konde-Lule, M. Musagara, and S. Musgrave, 'Focus group interviews about AIDS in Rakai district of Uganda,' *SSM*, 37 (1993), 683; A.C. Crampin, J.R. Glynn, and others, 'Trends and measurement of HIV prevalence in northern Malawi,' *AIDS*, 17 (2003), 1819.
27   J.M. Wojcicki and J. Malala, 'Condom use, power and HIV/AIDS risk: sex-workers bargain for survival in Hillbrow/Joubert Park/Berea, Johannesburg,' *SSM*, 53 (2001), 114.
28   Great Britain: House of Commons (Session 2000–01): International Development Committee: Third Report, *HIV/AIDS: the impact on social and economic development* (London, 2001), vol. 2 (HC 354-II), p. 236 (evidence of P. Piot).
29   M.G. Alwano-Edyegu and E. Marcum, *Knowledge is power: voluntary HIV counselling and testing in Uganda* (Geneva, 1999), pp. 18–22.
30   M. Dlamini in *AIDS Bulletin*, March 1993, p. 4; Meursing, *World of silence*, p. 272; *New Vision*, 7 October 1994.
31   C. Kennedy, *From the coalface: a study of the response of a South African colliery to the threat of AIDS* (Cape Town, 2002), p. 9; Christian Medical Board of Tanzania, *Participatory action research on AIDS and the community as a source of care and healing* (Uganda, 1993), p. 18; N.K.

Ndosi and M.C. Waziri, 'The nature of parasuicide in Dar es Salaam,' *SSM*, 44 (1997), 59; *Mail and Guardian*, 31 October 2003; *Lancet*, 356 (2000), 840.

32 M.G. Sangiwa, A. van der Straten, and others,'Clients' perspective of the role of voluntary counselling and testing in HIV/AIDS prevention and care in Dar es Salaam, Tanzania,' *AIDS and Behavior*, 4 (2000), 35–48.

33 Meursing, *World of silence*, p. 273; A.G. Kidan, F. Belete, and H. Negassa, 'Response to counselling of HIV carriers and AIDS patients in Ethiopia,' *EJHD*, 4 (1990), 245–7.

34 A.O. Ndonji, 'Living positively,' *AIDS Watch*, 11 (1990), 5–6.

35 J. Manchester, 'The HIV epidemic in South Africa: personal views of positive people,' MA (Education) thesis, University of London, 2000, p. 54.

36 B. Joinet and T. Mugolola, *Survivre face au sida en Afrique* (Paris, 1994), p. 147.

37 M.-C. Samba-Lefebvre, 'Le sida et la société congolaise,' *Etudes*, 380 (1994), 350.

38 F. Kazahura, 'The impact of counselling on the behaviour of AIDS victims: a case study of TASO Mbarara branch,' BA thesis, Makerere University, 1992, pp. 44–5; I. Clarke, *The man with the key has gone!* (Chichester, 1993), p. 274; *Mail and Guardian*, 29 November 1996.

39 S. Maman, J. Mbwambo, and others, 'Women's barriers to HIV-1 testing and disclosure,' *AIDS Care*, 13 (2001), 596; C. Killewo, A. Massawe, and others, 'HIV counselling and testing of pregnant women in sub-Saharan Africa: experiences from a study on prevention of mother-to-child transmission in Dar es Salaam,' *Journal of AIDS*, 28 (2001), 458; P. Keogh, S. Allen, and others, 'The social impact of HIV infection on women in Kigali, Rwanda,' *SSM*, 38 (1994), 1047; S. Maman, J.K. Mbwambo, and others, 'High rates and positive outcomes of HIV-serostatus disclosure to sexual partners: reasons for cautious optimism from a voluntary counseling and testing clinic in Dar es Salaam,' *AIDS and Behavior*, 7 (2003), 378.

40 M. Schoofs, 'South Africa acts up,' *Village Voice*, 28 December 2000, p. 67.

41 Botswana, *Botswana AIDS impact survey 2001* (Gaborone, 2002), p. 35.

42 Anannia Admasou, 'Coping with the challenges of AIDS: the experience of persons living with HIV/AIDS in Addis Ababa,' *Northeast African Studies*, NS, 7, 2 (2000), 95–6.

43 Smith and Watkins, 'Perceptions,' p. 656.

44 Many of these complexities are illustrated in Meursing, *World of silence*.

45 C. Obbo, 'Social science research: understanding and action,' in C. Becker, J.-P. Dozon, and others (eds), *Vivre et penser le sida en Afrique* (Paris, 1999), p. 76.

46 Melody Kunene, in J. Hall, *Testimonies of hope from people with HIV and AIDS* (Johannesburg, 2002), pp. 114–16.

47 C. Bungener, N. Marchand-Gonod, and R. Jouvent, 'African and European HIV-positive women: psychological and psychosocial differences,' *AIDS Care*, 12 (2000), 545.

48 D.A. Eaton Jr, 'Men's lives and the politics of AIDS in the Republic of Congo,' PhD thesis, University of California at Berkeley, 2001, pp. 103–4.

49 Clacherty and Associates, *The role of stigma and discrimination in increasing the vulnerability of children and youth affected by HIV/AIDS: report on participatory workshops* (Arcadia, South Africa, 2001), pp. 29–30.

50 Yemisrach Kifle, in *Addis Tribune*, 26 July 2002.

51 UNDP, *HIV/AIDS and human development: South Africa 1998* (n.p., n.d.), p. 55.

52 J. Bujra, 'Risk and trust: unsafe sex, gender and AIDS in Tanzania,' in P. Caplan (ed.), *Risk revisited* (London, 2000), p. 77.

53 Quoted in Vinh-Kim Nguyen, 'Epidemics, interzones and biosocial change: retroviruses and biologies of globalisation in West Africa,' PhD thesis, McGill University, 2001, p. 232.

54 *Express* (Dar es Salaam), 8 January 2004.

55 Quoted in C.B. Rwabukwali, 'Gender, poverty, and AIDS in Kabarole, Western Uganda: the sociocultural context of risk and prevention behaviors,' PhD thesis, Case Western Reserve University, 1997, p. 165.

56 Quoted in Clacherty and Associates, *Role of stigma*, p. 45.

57 Konde-Lule and others, 'Focus group interviews,' p. 681; R. Kasirye, 'Community response to AIDS affected households: a case study of Kamwokya,' BA thesis, Makerere University, 1992, p. 26.

58 Meursing, *World of silence*, pp. 226, 231–2; S.D. Foster, 'The socioeconomic impact of HIV/AIDS in Monze district, Zambia,' PhD thesis, University of London, 1996, p. 24.

59 A. Desgrées du Loû and N. de Béchon, 'Attitudes par rapport au sida, accès au dépistage et connaissances des traitements du VIH à Abidjan dans le contexte de l'Initiative,' in P. Msellati, L. Vidal, and J.-P. Moatti (eds), *L'accès aux traitements du VIH/sida en Côte d'Ivoire* (Paris, 2001), p. 257; O. Shisana, L. Simbayi, and others, *Nelson Mandela/HSRC study of*

HIV/AIDS: *South African national HIV prevalence, behavioural risks and mass media: household survey 2002* (Cape Town, 2002), pp. 86, 89.

60   Killewo and others, 'Communicating,' p. 319; S. Leclerc-Madlala, 'Demonising women in the era of AIDS,' *Society in Transition*, 32 (2001), 44.

61   A. Williams, *Ageing and poverty in Africa: Ugandan livelihoods in a time of HIV/AIDS* (Aldershot, 2003), p. 167; S.M. Monico, E.O. Tanga, and A. Nawagaba, 'Uganda and AIDS-related discrimination, stigmatization and denial' (2001), http://www.unaids.org (accessed 28 November 2003); Mutembei, *Poetry and AIDS*, p. 57.

62   E. Guest, *Children of AIDS: Africa's orphan crisis* (2nd edn, London, 2003), p. 22; O. Alubo, A. Zwandor, and others, 'Acceptance and stigmatization of PLWA in Nigeria,' *AIDS Care*, 14 (2002), 117–26.

63   L. Nyblade, R. Pande, and others, 'Disentangling HIV and AIDS stigma in Ethiopia, Tanzania and Zambia' (2003), p. 33, http://www.icrw.org/docs/stigmareportO93003.pdf (accessed 15 July 2004); S. Fox, W. Parker. and M. Mundawarara, *Living openly: HIV positive South Africans tell their stories* (Pretoria, 2004), pp. 5, 9.

64   Manchester, 'HIV epidemic,' pp. 41, 45, 91; Hall, *Testimonies*, p. 119.

65   Horizons (Population Council), 'Positive, engaged, involved: the participation of people living with HIV/AIDS (PLHA) in community-based organizations' (1999), http://www.popcouncil.org/horizons/ressum/plha_ burkina.html (accessed 19 July 2004).

66   Malawi Network of People Living with HIV/AIDS, 'Voices for equality and dignity: qualitative research on stigma and discrimination issues as they affect PLWHA in Malawi' (2003), http://www.policyproject.com/pubs/countryreports/MALA_MANET_FGD.pdf (accessed 20 July 2004); *Le Soleil*, 4 November 2003; UNIRIN, 10 December 2004, in http://allafrica.com/stories (accessed 29 December 2004); *Lancet*, 353 (1999), 130.

67   AAA, September 1992; L. Vidal, *Le silence et le sens: essai d'anthropologie du sida en Afrique* (Paris, 1996), ch. 1; Kaleeba, *We miss you all*, p. 34.

68   *Fraternité Matin*, 7 February 1991; *Times of Zambia*, 14 November 1989.

69   *New Vision*, 5 April 2000 and 22 January 1995; *Africa Today*, December 2000, p. 15.

70   *La Semaine Africaine*, 26 November 1987, quoted in D. Fassin, *Les enjeux politiques de la santé: études sénégalaises, équatoriennes et françaises* (Paris, 2000), p. 255. For Abalaka, see *Lancet*, 356 (2000), 493.

71   C.E. Rosenberg, *The cholera years: the United States in 1832, 1849, and 1866* (Chicago, 1962).

72   See p. 146; M.-E. Gruénais, F.M. Mbambi, and J. Tonda, 'Messies, fétiches et lutte de pouvoirs entre les "grands hommes" du Congo démocratique,' *Cahiers d'Etudes Africaines*, 35 (1995), 186.

73   Benin, 'Cadre stratégique national de lutte contre le VIH/SIDA/IST au Bénin 2001–2005,' http://www.unaids.org (accessed 30 November 2003).

74   *New Vision*, 7 March 1989 and 6 December 1988; A. Byashera, 'Field experiences and lessons gained for future research from the HIV serosurvey in the Kagera region, Tanzania,' in J.Z.J. Killewo, G.K. Lwihula, and others (eds), *Behavioural and epidemiological aspects of AIDS research in Tanzania* (Stockholm, 1992), p. 66; P. Probst, 'Danser le sida: spectacles du *nyau* et culture populaire chewa dans le centre du Malawi,' *Autrepart*, 1 (1997), 91–112.

75   S. Sontag, *AIDS and its metaphors* (reprinted, London, 1990), p. 34.

76   H. Schneider, 'On the fault-line: the politics of AIDS policy in contemporary South Africa,' *African Studies*, 61 (2002), 160.

77   This account is based on S. Heald, 'It's never as easy as ABC: understandings of AIDS in Botswana,' *African Journal of AIDS Research*, 1 (2002), 1–10.

78   H.O. Mogensen, 'The narrative of AIDS among the Tonga of Zambia,' *SSM*, 44 (1997), 431–9; A. Wolf. 'AIDS, morality and indigenous concepts of sexually transmitted disease in southern Africa,' *Afrika Spectrum*, 36 (2001), 97–107; F. Hagenbucher-Sacripanti, *Représentations du sida et médecines traditionnelles dans la région de Pointe-Noire (Congo)* (Paris, 1994); P.W. Geissler, '"Are we still together here?" Negotiations about relatedness and time in the everyday life of a modern Kenyan village,' PhD thesis, University of Cambridge, 2003, pp. 127–34, 172–3, 282; Feiruz Surur and Mirgissa Kaba, 'The role of religious leaders in HIV/AIDS prevention, control, and patient care and support: a pilot project in Jimma Zone,' *Northeast African Studies*, NS, 7, 2 (2000), 65.

79   Basuakuamba wa Bashipayi, Mbu Mputu, and others, *Croyances populaires concernant les épidémies (Rép. Zaire)* (Bandundu, 1995), pp. 59–60, 78–9, 93–6.

80   E.M. Ankrah, 'AIDS: methodological problems in studying its prevention and spread,' *SSM*, 29 (1989), 266–7; Mutembei, *Poetry and AIDS*, pp. 196–7; *New Vision*, 24 February 1995.

81 Samba-Lefebvre, 'Le sida,' p. 349; C.B. Yamba, 'Cosmologies in turmoil: witchfinding and AIDS in Chiawa, Zambia,' *Africa*, 67 (1997), 200–23; *Times of Zambia*, 17 April 2004; R. Tuju, *AIDS: understanding the challenge* (Nairobi, 1996), pp. 25–7.

82 J. Seeley, U. Wagner, and others, 'The development of a community-based HIV/AIDS counselling service in a rural area in Uganda,' *AIDS Care*, 3 (1991), 209.

83 J.R.S. Malungo, 'Challenges for sexual behavioural changes in the era of AIDS: sexual cleansing and levirate marriage in Zambia,' in J.C. Caldwell, P. Caldwell, and others (eds), *Resistances to behavioural change to reduce HIV/AIDS infection in predominantly heterosexual epidemics in Third World countries* (Canberra, 1999), p. 47.

84 African National Congress, *A national health plan for South Africa* (Johannesburg, 1994), p. 32.

85 Wiseman Thabede, quoted in G. Mendel, *A broken landscape: HIV and AIDS in Africa* (Auckland Park, 2001), p. 22.

86 J.-P. Dozon, 'Médecines traditionnelles et sida: les modalités de sa prise en charge par un tradipracticien ivoirien,' in Dozon and Vidal (eds), *Les sciences sociales*, p. 193.

87 S. Feierman, 'Struggles for control: the social roots of health and healing in modern Africa,' *African Studies Review*, 28, 2 (June 1985), 126.

88 Y.K. Museveni, *What is Africa's problem?* (Kampala, 1992), p. 277; Nigeria, 'National policy on HIV/AIDS 2003,' p. 31, http://hivaidsclearinghouse.unesco.org/file_download.php (accessed 21 March 2005).

89 Traditional Health Practitioners Act 2004, Section 49(1) (g) (i).

90 R. King and J. Homsy, 'HIV/AIDS: the role of traditional healers in "counselling",' *Medical News* (Brussels), 7, 1 (June 1998), 5, 7; *New Vision*, 21 December 2004.

91 Malungo, 'Challenges,' in Caldwell and others (eds), *Resistances*, ch. 4; Geiseler, '"Are we still together here?",' ch. 5 and appendix; B. Taverne, 'Stratégie de communication et stigmatisation des femmes: lévirat et sida au Burkina Faso,' *Sciences Sociales et Santé*, 14, 2 (June 1996), 88–106.

92 H. Muyinda, J. Nakuya, and others, 'Harnessing the *senga* institution of adolescent sex education for the control of HIV and STDs in rural Uganda,' *AIDS Care*, 15 (2003), 159–67; F. Scorgie, 'Virginity testing and the politics of sexual responsibility: implications for AIDS intervention,' *African Studies*, 61 (2002), 55–75.

93 See S. Ellis and G. ter Haar, *Worlds of power: religious thought and political practice in Africa* (London, 2004), p. 2.

94 R. Smart and R. Fincham (eds), 'Study tour of AIDS programmes in Zambia, Uganda and Kenya, 3–17 October 1993' (duplicated), pp. 49, 55–6; C.M. Fombad, 'The crisis of confidentiality in the control of the HIV/AIDS pandemic in Botswana,' *International Social Science Journal*, 53 (2001), 649; M. Mbilinyi and N. Kaihula, 'Sinners and outsiders: the drama of AIDS in Rungwe,' in C. Baylies, J. Bujra, and others, *AIDS, sexuality and gender in Africa: collective strategies and struggles in Tanzania and Zambia* (London, 2000), pp. 77–8, 87.

95 Heald, 'It's never as easy,' p. 4; R.O. Garner, 'Safe sects? Dynamic religion and AIDS in South Africa,' *Journal of Modern African Studies*, 38 (2000), 41.

96 Christian Churches in Zambia, *Choose to live: reflections on the AIDS crisis* (n.p., 1988), p. 10.

97 Information from Professor R. Werbner.

98 S. Waldorf, 'Mchape: a wake-up call for AIDS control programmes in Africa (a case history from Malawi),' *AIDS and Public Policy Journal*, 12 (1997), 141.

99 Feiruz Surur and Mirgissa Kaba, 'The role of religious leaders,' p. 69; M. al-Ahnaf, B. Botiveau, and F. Frégosi. *L'Algérie par ses islamistes* (Paris, 1991), p. 78.

100 *Newswatch*, 28 February 2005; Senegal, 'Plan strategique 2002–2006 de lutte contre le SIDA,' p. 18, http://www.unaids.org (accessed 3 December 2003); UNAIDS, *Report on the global AIDS epidemic 2004* (Geneva, 2004), p. 157; Islamic Medical Association of Uganda, *AIDS education through Imams: a spiritually motivated community effort in Uganda* (Geneva, 1998), p. 12.

101 Bamar Guèye, in *Le Quotidien* (Dakar), 22 January 2003.

102 H. Kloos, Tadesse Wuhib, and others, 'Community-based organizations in HIV/AIDS prevention, patient care and control in Ethiopia,' *EJHD*, 17 (2003), special issue, 13; Hailegnaw Eshete and Tefera Sahlu, 'The progression of HIV/AIDS in Ethiopia,' *EJHD*, 10, 3 (December 1996), 186; *Addis Tribune*, 9 May 2003.

103 G. Byamugisha, L.Y. Steinitz, and others, *Journeys of faith: church-based responses to HIV and AIDS in three southern African countries* (Pietermaritzburg, 2002), ch. 3.

104 *AAA*, April 1996.

105 *Sunday Vision*, 25 August 1996.

106 World Bank, *Confronting AIDS: public priorities in a global epidemic* (New York, 1997), p. 167; Great Britain, *HIV/AIDS: the impact*, vol. I, pp. lxx–lxxi; *Times of Zambia*, 17 January 2004.
107 *AAA*, June 1995.
108 *West Africa*, 4 May 1987, p. 886; *Standard* (Nairobi), 12 June 2004; J.G. Cooke (ed.), *The second wave of the HIV/AIDS pandemic* (Washington, 2002), p. 53.
109 B.G. Schoepf, 'Women at risk: case studies from Zaire,' in G. Herdt and S. Lindenbaum (eds), *The time of AIDS: social analysis, theory, and method* (Newbury Park, 1992), p. 275; C. Lindan, S. Allen, and others, 'Knowledge, attitudes, and perceived risk of AIDS among urban Rwandan women,' *AIDS*, 5 (1991), 1001; K. Dowling in Byamugisha and others, *Journeys of faith*, pp. 95–6.
110 UNAIDS, *Report on the global AIDS epidemic 2004*, p. 70.
111 M. Mwangi, *The last plague* (Nairobi, 2000); G. Rugalema, 'Understanding the African HIV pandemic: an appraisal of the contexts and lay explanation of the HIV/AIDS pandemic with examples from Tanzania and Kenya,' in E. Kalipeni, S. Craddock, and others (eds), *HIV and AIDS in Africa: beyond epidemiology* (Malden MA, 2004), p. 198.
112 Kapita M. Bila, *Sida en Afrique: maladie et phénomène social* (Kinshasa, 1988), p. 58.

10 *NGOs & the Evolution of Care* (pages 98–111)

1 D. Altman, *Power and community: organizational and cultural responses to AIDS* (London, 1994), p. 6.
2 Uganda: Ministry of Health, 'The report of the joint evaluation of the Uganda Aids Commission and Secretariat' (typescript final draft, 1992), p. 11, UMOH library; *Lancet*, 361 (2003), 319; *Daily Nation* (Nairobi), 30 March 1999.
3 *Le Soleil*, 4 December 2004; UNIRIN, 16 December 2004, http://allafrica.com/stories (accessed 17 December 2004); H. Phillips, 'AIDS in the context of South Africa's epidemic history: preliminary historical thoughts,' *South African Historical Journal*, 45 (2001), 22; J.G. Cooke (ed.), *The second wave of the HIV/AIDS pandemic* (Washington, 2002), p. 51.
4 *New Vision*, 7 November 2000.
5 UNAIDS, *Accelerating action against AIDS in Africa* (Geneva, 2003), p. 35.
6 N. Kaleeba, *We miss you all* (Harare, 1991), p. 79. See also TASO, *TASO 10th anniversary compendium* (Kampala [1997]), pp. 4, 33. I am indebted to Dr S.D. Doyle for TASO documents.
7 TASO, *1999 annual report*, p. 25.
8 TASO, *2003 annual report*, pp. 3, 45; TASO, *Strategic plan for the period 2003–2007* (Kampala, n.d.), p. 18.
9 C. Cornu, S. Mbodj, and S. Kanouté, 'The care and support cellule: an integrated and decentralised approach to care and support for people living with HIV/AIDS in Senegal' (2003), http://www.aidsalliance.org/_res/reports (accessed 15 July 2004).
10 R. Baggaley, J. Sulwe, and others, 'HIV counsellors' knowledge, attitudes and vulnerabilities to HIV in Lusaka, Zambia, 1994,' *AIDS Care*, 8 (1996), 155; *AAA*, September 1994.
11 V.C. Mouli, *All against AIDS: the Copperbelt Health Education Project, Zambia* (London, 1992), p. 4.
12 G. Williams, A. Milligan, and T. Odemwingie, *A common cause: young people, sexuality, HIV and AIDS in three African countries* (2nd edn, London, 1998), pp. 7–19.
13 Zambia, *Strategic framework 2001–2003: National HIV/AIDS/STD/TB Council* (n.p., 2000), pp. 24–5.
14 *New Vision*, 25 May and 1 June 1999.
15 *Global AIDSNews*, 1995 no. 2; C.F. Ndiaye, 'Women and AIDS in Africa: the experience of the Society for Women and AIDS in Africa,' *South African Journal of International Affairs*, 7, 2 (Winter 2000), 59–66.
16 *AAA*, February 1996; *Standard*, 6 December 2003; F. Eboko, 'L'organisation de la lutte contre le sida au Cameroun: de la verticalité à la dispersion,' in M.-E. Gruénais (ed.), *Un systéme de santé en mutation: le cas du Cameroun* (Hamburg, 2001), p. 63.
17 A.W. Logie, 'Africa revisited: a distressing experience,' *BMJ*, 322 (2001), 59; J.O. Parkhurst, 'HIV prevention policy in sub-Saharan Africa: the Ugandan experience,' DPhil thesis, University of Oxford, 2002, pp. 253–77; K. Delaunay, 'Des ONG et des associations: concurrences et dépendances sur un "marché du sida" emergent: cas ivoirien et sénégalais,' in J.-P. Deler, Y.A. Fauré, and others (eds), *ONG et développement: société, économie, politique*

186 *NGOs & the Evolution of Care* (pages 98–111)

(Paris, 1998), ch. 9.
18 H. Marais, *To the edge: AIDS review 2000* (Pretoria, 2000), pp. 31–2; Mali, 'Suivi de la déclaration d'engagement sur le VIH/SIDA (UNGASS)' (2003), http://www.unaids.org (accessed 4 December 2003).
19 UNAIDS, 'AIDS epidemic update, December 2004,' p. 15, http://www.unaids.org (accessed 28 November 2004).
20 M.M. Mtika, 'The AIDS epidemic in Malawi and its threat to household food security,' *Human Organization*, 60 (2001), 184; S. Nnko, B. Chiduo, and others, 'Tanzania: AIDS care – learning from experience,' *Review of African Political Economy*, 86 (2000), 553; A.F. Chimwaza, 'A descriptive study of the experience of primary caregivers of patients with symptoms of AIDS in resource poor communities: the case of Malawi,' PhD thesis, University of Pennsylvania, 2002, p. 212.
21 J.K. Anarfi, *HIV/AIDS in sub-Saharan Africa: its demographic and socio-economic implications* (Nairobi, 1994), p. 23.
22 J.K. Anarfi, 'The condition and care of AIDS victims in Ghana: AIDS sufferers and their relations,' *HTR*, 5 (1995), supplement, 254.
23 K. Awusabo-Asare, 'Living with AIDS: perceptions, attitudes and post-diagnosis behaviour of HIV/AIDS patients in Ghana,' *ibid.*, 272.
24 M. Radstake, *Secrecy and ambiguity: home care for people living with HIV/AIDS in Ghana* (Leiden, 1997), p. 26.
25 O. Alubo, A. Zwandor, and others, 'Acceptance and stigmatization of PLWA in Nigeria,' *AIDS Care*, 14 (2002), 117–26.
26 Chimwaza, 'Descriptive study,' p. 72.
27 A.F. Chimwaza and S.C. Watkins, 'Giving care to people with symptoms of AIDS in rural sub-Saharan Africa,' *AIDS Care*, 16 (2004), 805.
28 E. Ratsma, E.P. Manjolo, and J. Simon, 'Voices from the epidemic,' *Malawi Medical Journal*, 8 (1992), 64.
29 J. Seeley, E. Kajura, and others, 'The extended family and support for people with AIDS in a rural population in south west Uganda: a safety net with holes?' *AIDS Care*, 5 (1993), 117–22.
30 G. Rugalema, 'It is not only the loss of labour: HIV/AIDS, loss of household assets and household livelihood in Bukoba district, Tanzania,' in G. Mutangadura, H. Jackson, and D. Mukurazita (eds), *AIDS and African smallholder agriculture* (Harare, 1999), p. 44.
31 C. Obbo, 'The language of AIDS in rural and urban Uganda,' *African Urban Quarterly*, 6 (1991), 83–92; J.M. Olenja, 'Assessing community attitudes towards home-based care for people with AIDS (PWAs) in Kenya,' *Journal of Community Health*, 24 (1999), 187–99; Ethiopia, *Demographic and health survey 2000* (Addis Ababa, 2001), p. 168.
32 Clacherty and Associates, *The role of stigma and discrimination in increasing the vulnerability of children and youth affected by HIV/AIDS: report on participatory workshops* (Arcadia, South Africa, 2001), pp. 21–2; M. Steinberg, S. Johnson, and others, *Hitting home: how households cope with the impact of the HIV/AIDS epidemic* (Durban, 2002), p. 23.
33 R.J. Earickson, 'International behavioural responses to a health hazard: AIDS,' *SSM*, 21 (1990), 953; Uganda: Ministry of Health, 'AIDS Control Programme: proposals for a five year action plan (1987–1991)' (duplicated, 1987), p. 35; Mafama Oluba Ngandu, 'Health workers, the community and AIDS,' in WHO, *AIDS prevention and control* (Oxford, 1988), p. 109.
34 G. Williams, A.D. Blibolo, and D. Kerouedan, *Filling the gaps: care and support for people with HIV/AIDS in Côte d'Ivoire* (London, 1995), pp. 17–20; T. Tran-Minh, L. Astel, and others, 'Dix ans de prise en charge du VIH/SIDA dans les centres de traitement ambulatoire (CTA) de l'OPALS et de la Croix-Rouge Française,' *Médecine Tropicale*, 64 (2004), 109–14.
35 Ethiopia, 'AIDS in Ethiopia' (5th edn, 2004), p. 10, http://www.etharc.org/spotlight/AIDSinEth5th.pdf (accessed 9 February 2005).
36 WHO: GPA, *Review of six HIV/AIDS home care programmes in Uganda and Zambia* (GPA/IDS/HCS/91.3: Geneva, 1991), pp. 3–4; T. Chaava, 'Approach to HIV counselling in a Zambian rural community,' *AIDS Care*, 2 (1990), 83; D. Wilson and S. Lavelle, 'HIV/AIDS in Africa,' *AIDS Care*, 2 (1990), 372.
37 R. Smart and R. Fincham (eds), 'Study tour of AIDS programmes in Zambia, Uganda and Kenya, 3–17 October 1993' (duplicated), pp. 50–1.
38 M. Duggan, 'Project – Assistance with "Aids" cases: Mobile Unit – Clinic – Home Nursing,' 17 February 1987, UMOH GCC.42/AIDS/IV/28; WHO:GPA, *Review*, pp. 8–9.

39 M. Mensah, 'Home-based care for people with HIV/AIDS: Agomanya, Ghana,' *Development in Practice*, 4 (1994), 58–62; J. Stuart, 'Evaluation of home-based care in KwaZulu,' *AIDS Bulletin*, April 1994, pp. 10–11.

40 K. Hansen, G. Woelk, and others, 'The cost of home-based care for HIV/AIDS patients in Zimbabwe,' *AIDS Care*, 10 (1998), 751; G. Mutangadura, D, Mukurazita, and H. Jackson, *A review of household and community responses to the HIV/AIDS epidemic in the rural areas of sub-Saharan Africa* (Geneva, 1999), p. 42; G. Woelk, H. Jackson, and others, *Do we care? The cost and quality of community home based care for HIV/AIDS patients and their communities in Zimbabwe* (Harare, 1997), p. 8.

41 Quoted in S. Armstrong, *Caring for carers: managing stress in those who care for people with HIV and AIDS* (Geneva, 2000), p. 10.

42 World Bank, *Confronting AIDS: public priorities in a global epidemic* (New York, 1997), p. 182.

43 UNAIDS, *Report on the global HIV/AIDS epidemic, July 2002* (Geneva, 2002), p. 51.

44 H. Jackson and K. Mhambi, *AIDS home care: a baseline survey in Zimbabwe* (Harare, 1992), p. 13.

45 *AAA*, September 1992. See also Smart and Fincham, 'Study tour,' p. 29.

46 UNAIDS, *AIDS: palliative care* (Geneva, 2000), p. 13.

47 G. Foster, 'HIV in youth and children in Zimbabwe,' in B. Gannon (ed.), *Children and youth at risk: HIV/AIDS issues, residential care and community perspectives* (Cape Town, 1994), pp. 102–6.

48 Woelk and others, *Do we care?* p. 1; C. Baylies, J. Bujra, and others, *AIDS, sexuality and gender in Africa: collective strategies and struggles in Tanzania and Zambia* (London, 2000), p. 35; World Bank, *Malawi AIDS assessment study* (2 vols, n.p., 1998), vol. 2, p. 80.

49 UNDP, *Botswana human development report 2000* (Gaborone, 2000), p. 45.

50 G. Byamugisha, L.Y. Steinitz, and others, *Journeys of faith: church-based response to HIV and AIDS in three southern African countries* (Pietermaritzburg, 2002), p. 61.

51 Smart and Fincham, 'Study tour,' pp. 29–31.

52 A. Ssennyonga, 'Caring for AIDS affected children in Rakai-Masaka districts, Uganda,' in Gannon (ed.), *Children*, pp. 85–6.

53 J. Bujra and S.N. Mokalu, 'AIDS activism in Dar es Salaam: many struggles; a single goal,' in Baylies and others, *AIDS, sexuality and gender*, ch.8.

54 UNAIDS, *Reaching out, scaling up: eight case studies of home and community care for and by people with HIV/AIDS* (Geneva, 2001), ch. 6.

55 Y. Berhane and D. Zakus, 'Home care for persons with AIDS: community attitude in a neighbourhood of Addis Ababa, Ethiopia,' *East African Medical Journal*, 72 (1995), 628; H. Kloos, Tadesse Wuhib, and others, 'Community-based organizations in HIV/AIDS prevention, patient care and control in Ethiopia,' *EJHD*, 17 (2003), 15–16.

56 South Africa: Department of Health, 'Strategic priorities for the national health system 2004–2009' (2004), p. 9, http://www.doh.gov.za/docs/reports-f.html (accessed 2 January 2005).

57 M. Russell and H. Schneider, *A rapid appraisal of community based HIV/AIDS care and support programme in South Africa* (Durban, 2000), pp. 22–3, 32; South Africa: Department of Social Development, *HIV/AIDS case studies in South Africa: volume 1* (Pretoria, 2002), pp. 134–46; UNAIDS, *Comfort and hope: six case studies on mobilizing family and community care for and by people with HIV/AIDS* (Geneva, 1999), pp. 53–63.

58 South Africa, *HIV/AIDS case studies*, pp. 123–4.

59 Byamugisha and others, *Journeys of faith*, ch. 3.

60 Ghana, 'Ghana HIV/AIDS strategic framework 2001–2005,' http://www.unaids.org (accessed 30 November 2003); Nigeria, 'Proceedings of the National Conference on HIV/AIDS, Abuja, 15–17 December 1998' (duplicated), pp. 140–1, 144, 307–8; J. Gruber and M. Caffrey, 'HIV/AIDS and community conflict in Nigeria: implications and challenges,' *SSM*, 60 (2005), 1209–18.

61 *Le Soleil*, 8 December 2003.

62 R.S. Katapa, 'Caretakers of AIDS patients in rural Tanzania,' *IJSA*, 15 (2004), 673–8; R.P. Mushonga, 'Social support, coping and perceived burden of female caregivers of HIV/AIDS patients in rural Zimbabwe,' PhD thesis, Case Western Reserve University, 2001; G. Stegling, 'Human rights and ethics in the context of home-based care in Botswana,' *Pula*, 15 (2001), 241–8.

63 W.D. Myslik, A. Freeman, and J. Slawski, 'Implications of AIDS for the South African population age profile,' *Southern African Journal of Gerontology*, 6, 2 (1997), 6.

64 H. Jackson and K. Mhambi, *Family coping and AIDS in Zimbabwe: a study* (Harare, 1994), p. 57.

65 Chimwaza and Watkins, 'Giving care,' p. 795.
66 Quoted in Obbo, 'Language of AIDS,' p. 87.
67 C. Obbo, 'Who cares for the carers? AIDS and women in Uganda,' in H.B. Hansen and M. Twaddle (eds), *Developing Uganda* (Oxford, 1998), p. 214.
68 Woelk and others, *Do we care?* p. 55.
69 Malawi Network of People Living with HIV/AIDS, 'Voices for equality and dignity: qualitative research on stigma and discrimination issues as they affect PLWHA in Malawi' (2003), p. 15, http://www.policyproject.com/pubs/countryreports/MALA_MANET_FGD.pdf (accessed 19 July 2004); R.B. Cheek, 'Playing God with HIV: rationing HIV treatment in southern Africa,' *African Security Review*, 10, 4 (2001), 21; Woelk and others, *Do we care?* p. 2.
70 *SAfAids News*, March 2003, p. 5, http://www.safaids.org.zw/ publications (accessed 31 December 2004).
71 J.F.K. Mutikani, 'The lived experience of family caregivers of AIDS orphans and other orphans in rural Zimbabwe,' PhD thesis, Case Western Reserve University, 2002, p. 165; Botswana: Ministry of Health, *Baseline study for the community home based care programme for terminally ill HIV/AIDS patients in Botswana* (Gaborone, 1996), p. 28; Steinberg and others, *Hitting home*, pp. ii–iii, 16.
72 E.F. Nsutebu, J.D. Walley, and others, 'Scaling up HIV/AIDS and TB home-based care: lessons from Zambia,' *Health Policy and Planning*, 16 (2001), 240; H. Jackson and R. Kerkhoven, 'Developing AIDS care in Zimbabwe: a case for residential community centres?' *AIDS Care*, 7 (1995), 665; G. Mutangadura, *The socio-economic impact of adult morbidity and mortality on households in Kafue district, Zambia* (Harare, 1999), p. 6; Botswana, 'Status of the 2002 national response to the UNGASS declaration of commitment on HIV/AIDS' (2003), p. 11, http://www.unaids.org (accessed 21 November 2003); UNAIDS, *Report on the global AIDS epidemic 2004* (Geneva, 2004), p. 102.
73 KwaZulu-Natal Department of Health, *Annual report 1999*, p. 22; *ANC Today*, 19 April 2002; C. Kenyon, M. Heywood, and S. Conway, 'Mainstreaming HIV/AIDS: progress and challenges,' in Health Systems Trust, *South African health review 2001* (Durban, 2001), p. 175.
74 E. Kikule, 'A good death in Uganda: survey of needs for palliative care for terminally ill people in urban areas,' *BMJ*, 327 (2003), 193.
75 UNAIDS, *Report on the global AIDS epidemic, June 2000* (Geneva, 2000), p. 89.
76 B. Dworzanowski, 'Caring for people dying of AIDS: lessons learnt from hospices,' *Society in Transition*, 33 (2002), 420–31.
77 K. Munk, 'Traditional healers, traditional hospitals and HIV/AIDS: a case study in KwaZulu-Natal,' *AAA*, December 1997.
78 S. Ramsay, 'Leading the way in African home-based palliative care,' *Lancet*, 362 (2003), 1812–13.

11 *Death & the Household* (pages 112–25)

1 W. Blackman in *Mission Field*, 67 (1922), 215.
2 P. Boggio, 'L'épidémie de SIDA à Kinshasa,' *Le Monde*, 24 December 1986; F. Klaits, 'Housing the spirit, hearing the voice: care and kinship in an apostolic church during Botswana's time of AIDS,' PhD thesis, Johns Hopkins University, 2002, pp. 13–14; R. Dorrington, D. Bourne, and others, *The impact of HIV/AIDS on adult mortality in South Africa* (Tygerberg, 2001), pp. 27, 35.
3 D.W. Mulder and others, *MRC/ODA/UVRI programme: annual report 1993* (Entebbe, 1994), p. 4; UNAIDS, *The UNAIDS report* (Geneva, 1999), p. 17; UNAIDS, 'AIDS in Africa: three scenarios to 2025' (2005), p. 28, http://www.unaids.org/unaids_resources/HomePage/images (accessed 7 March 2005); UNAIDS, *Report on the global AIDS epidemic 2004* (Geneva, 2004), p. 30.
4 UNIRIN, 10 June 2004, http://allafrica.com/stories (accessed 12 June 2004).
5 *Mail and Guardian*, 4 February 2005; G. Mendel, *A broken landscape: HIV and AIDS in Africa* (Auckland Park, 2001), p. 90.
6 S.D. Foster, 'The socioeconomic impact of HIV/AIDS in Monze district, Zambia,' PhD thesis, University of London, 1996, p. 153; F. Davachi, P, Baudoux, and others, 'The economic impact on families of children with AIDS in Kinshasa, Zaire,' in A.F. Fleming, M. Carballo, and others (eds), *The global impact of AIDS* (New York, 1988), p. 169; *Mail and Guardian*, 3 May 2002.

7   Klaits, 'Housing the spirit,' p. 265.
8   *The Star* (Johannesburg), 7 October 2003.
9   M. Ayieko, 'From single parents to child-headed households: the case of children orphaned by AIDS in Kisumu and Siaya districts, Kenya' (duplicated, Champaign IL, 1997), p. 45; D. Durham and F. Klaits, 'Funerals and the public space of sentiment in Botswana,' *Journal of Southern African Studies*, 28 (2002), 783.
10 Basuakuamba wa Bashipayi, Mbu Mputu, and others, *Croyances populaires concernant les épidémies (Rép. Zaire)* (Bandundu, 1995), pp. 63, 74, 92.
11 C. Nzioka, 'The social meanings of death from HIV/AIDS: an African interpretative view,' *Culture, health and sexuality*, 2 (2000), 2, 10–11; Kenya, *Demographic and health survey 1993* (Nairobi, 1994), p. 130; H. Muyinda, J. Seeley, and others, 'Social aspects of AIDS-related stigma in rural Uganda,' *Health and Place*, 3 (1997), 146.
12 J. Mukiza-Gapere and J.P.M. Ntozi, 'Impact of AIDS on the family and mortality in Uganda,' *HTR*, 5 (1995), 191–200; G.H.R. Rugalema, *Adult mortality as entitlement failure: AIDS and the crisis of rural livelihoods in a Tanzanian village* (PhD thesis, Institute of Social Studies, The Hague, 1999: published in Maastricht), pp. 72, 130–5.
13 *Times of Zambia*, 5 October 1991.
14 *Sowetan*, 6 October 2003.
15 T.K. Biaya, 'La "mort" et ses métaphores au Congo-Zaire, 1990–1995,' in J.-L. Grootaers (ed.), *Mort et maladie au Zaire* (Tervuren, 1998), p. 108; *Daily Nation*, 9 March 1999; *AAA*, April 1999; N. Nattrass, 'AIDS and human security in southern Africa,' *Social Dynamics*, 28, 1 (2002), 12.
16 Rugalema, *Adult mortality*, passim. See also G. Rugalema, 'Coping or struggling? A journey into the impact of HIV/AIDS in southern Africa,' *Review of African Political Economy*, 86 (2000), 537–45.
17 D Mather, C. Donovan, and others, 'A cross-country analysis of household responses to adult mortality in rural sub-Saharan Africa' (2004), pp. 2, 9, 15, 43, http://www.aec.msu.edu/agecon/fsz/papers/idwp82forreview.pdf (accessed 28 March 2005).
18 Rugalema, *Adult mortality*, ch. 5; A.K. Tibaijuka, 'AIDS and economic welfare in peasant agriculture: case studies from Kagabiro village, Kagera region, Tanzania,' *World Development*, 25 (1997), 968, 972.
19 K. Wyss, G. Hulton, and Y. N'Diekhor, 'Costs attributable to AIDS at household level in Chad,' *AIDS Care*, 16 (2004), 808–16; C. Bishop-Sambrook, 'The challenge of the HIV/AIDS epidemic in rural Ethiopia: averting the crisis in low AIDS impacted communities: findings from fieldwork in Kersa Woreda, Eastern Hararghe Zone, Oromiya Region' (2004), http://www.fao.org/sd/dim_pe3/docs/pe3_040402d1_en.doc (accessed 6 September 2004); M. Steinberg, S. Johnson, and others, *Hitting home: how households cope with the impact of the HIV/AIDS epidemic: a survey of households affected by HIV/AIDS in South Africa* (Durban, 2002), p. 18.
20 Rugalema, *Adult mortality*, pp. 131–3; World Bank, *Confronting AIDS: public priorities in a global epidemic* (New York, 1997), p. 209.
21 Steinberg and others, *Hitting home*, p. 19.
22 Rugalema, *Adult mortality*, p. 133; Mukiza-Gapere and Ntozi, 'Impact of AIDS,' p. 197; A. Pankhurst and Damen Haile Mariam, 'The *iddir* in Ethiopia: historical development, social function, and potential role in HIV/AIDS prevention and control,' *Northeast African Studies*, NS, 7, 2 (2000), 36, 48–53.
23 World Bank, *Confronting AIDS*, p. 222; M. Lundberg, M. Over, and P. Mujinja, *Sources of financial assistance for households suffering an adult death in Kagera, Tanzania*, World Bank policy research working paper 2508 (Washington, 2000), pp. 13–14; C. Cross, 'Sinking deeper down: HIV/AIDS as an economic shock to rural households,' *Society in Transition*, 32 (2001), 141–3.
24 K. Beegle, *Labor effects of adult mortality in Tanzanian households*, World Bank policy research working paper 3062 (Washington, 2003), pp. 21–4; Rugalema, *Adult mortality*, pp. 79–84.
25 Mather and others, 'Cross-country analysis,' pp. iv–v; A. Whiteside, 'Poverty and HIV/AIDS in Africa,' in N.K. Poku and A. Whiteside (eds), *Global health and governance: HIV/AIDS* (Basingstoke, 2004), p. 132.
26 TASO, *Strategic plan for the period 2003–2007* (Kampala, n.d.), p. 28.
27 F. Kaijage, 'Social exclusion and the social history of disease: the impact of HIV/AIDS and the changing concept of the family in northwestern Tanzania,' in S. McGrath, C. Jedrej, and others (eds), *Rethinking African history* (Edinburgh, 1997), pp. 343–50; N. Kaleeba, *We miss*

you all (Harare, 1991), p. 66; *Le Quotidien*, 29 May 2004.

28 Rugalema, *Adult mortality*, pp. 161, 169; Zambia: Ministry of Health, *HIV/AIDS in Zambia: background, projections, impacts and interventions* (Lusaka, 1999), p. 51; UNAIDS, *Report on the global AIDS epidemic 2004*, p. 47.

29 UNAIDS, 'AIDS in Africa: three scenarios,' p. 28; Great Britain: House of Commons (Session 2000–01): International Development Committee: Third Report, *HIV/AIDS: the impact on social and economic development* (2 vols, London, 2001), vol. 2 (HSC 354-II), p. 101.

30 A. Dunn, 'The social consequences of HIV/AIDS in Uganda,' Save the Children Fund Overseas Department working paper no. 2 (1992), p. 6; TASO, 'Strategic plan,' p. v.

31 E. Guest, *Children of AIDS: Africa's orphan crisis* (2nd edn, London, 2003), p. 42.

32 L. Garbus, 'HIV/AIDS in Ethiopia' (2003), p. 67, http://ari.ucsf.edu/policy/profiles/Ethiopia.pdf (accessed 8 February 2005).

33 S.S. Hunter, 'Orphans as a window on the AIDS epidemic in sub-Saharan Africa: initial results and implications of a study in Uganda,' *SSM*, 31 (1990), 681.

34 *New Vision*, 1 December 2000; African Medical and Research Foundation, 'Strengthening community structures to support Orphans in Luwero, Uganda' (c.2002), http://www.aidsconsortium.org.uk (accessed 28 December 2004); C. Bishop-Sambrook, 'Labor constraints and the impact of HIV/AIDS on rural livelihoods in Bondo and Busia districts, western Kenya' (2003), p. 50, http://www.fao.org/ag/AGS/subjects/en/farmpower/pdf/labour.pdf (accessed 28 December 2004); World Food Programme, 'Widening the "window of hope": using food aid to improve access to education for orphans and vulnerable children in sub-Saharan Africa' (2003), p. 3, http:/www.wfp.org/index.asp?section=1 (accessed 27 December 2004); L. Guarcello, S. Lyon, and others, 'The influence of orphanhood on children's schooling and labour: evidence from sub-Saharan Africa' (2004), p. 8, http://www.ucw-project.org/pdf/publications/orphans (accessed 17 March 2005).

35 G. Foster, C. Makufa, and others, 'Factors leading to the establishment of child-headed households: the case of Zimbabwe,' *HTR*, 7 (1997), supplement 2, 164–5; C. Obbo, 'Reflections on the AIDS orphans problem in Uganda,' in M. Berer (ed.), *Women and HIV/AIDS* (London, 1993), p. 109; T. Barnett and P. Blaikie, *AIDS in Africa: the present and future impact* (London, 1992), p. 116.

36 R. Smart and R. Fincham (eds), 'Study tour of AIDS programmes in Zambia, Uganda and Kenya, 3–17 October 1993' (duplicated), p. 24.

37 Guest, *Children of AIDS*, p. 146; R. Bray, 'Predicting the social consequences of orphanhood in South Africa,' *African Journal of AIDS Research*, 2 (2003), 50.

38 D.B.T. Hackland, 'Children affected by HIV/AIDS and affordable care: results of a survey,' in N.H. McKerrow, R.A. Smart, and S.A. Snyman (eds), *AIDS, orphans and affordable care* (Pretoria, 1996), pp. 19–21.

39 G. Foster and J. Williamson. 'A review of current literature on the impact of HIV/AIDS on children in sub-Saharan Africa,' *AIDS*, 14 (2000), supplement 3, s276.

40 H.V. Doctor, 'Parental survival, living arrangements and school enrolment of children in Malawi in the era of HIV/AIDS,' *Journal of Social Development in Africa*, 19, 1 (January 2004), 40; TASO, *Strategic plan*, p. 16; Southern African Development Community, *Towards identifying impacts of HIV/AIDS on food insecurity in southern Africa and implications for response: findings from Malawi, Zambia and Zimbabwe* (Harare, 2003), p. 7.

41 Ayieko, 'From single parents,' p. 31.

42 R. Monasch and J.T. Boerma, 'Orphanhood and childcare patterns in sub-Saharan Africa: an analysis of national surveys from 40 countries,' *AIDS*, 18 (2004), supplement 2, s55; G. Foster, 'The capacity of the extended family safety net for orphans in Africa,' *Psychology, health and medicine*, 5 (2000), 55.

43 G. Foster, C. Makufa, and others, 'Supporting children in need through a community-based orphan visiting programme,' *AIDS Care*, 8 (1996), 399–400; UNAIDS, *Report on the global AIDS epidemic 2004*, p. 65; H. Brookes, O. Shisana, and L. Richter, *The national household HIV prevalence and risk survey of South African children* (Cape Town, 2004), p. 26; J.F.K. Mutikani, 'The lived experience of family caregivers of AIDS orphans and other orphans in rural Zimbabwe,' PhD thesis, Case Western Reserve University, 2002, p. 132.

44 Mendel, *Broken landscape*, p. 24.

45 UNAIDS, 'AIDS epidemic update, December 2004,' p. 16, http://www.unaids.org (accessed 28 November 2004); R. Mupedziswa, 'AIDS and older Zimbabweans: who will care for the carers?' *Southern African Journal of Gerontology*, 6, 2 (1997), 10; M. Ainsworth and D. Filmer, *Poverty, AIDS and children's schooling: a targeting dilemma*, World Bank policy research

working paper 2885 (Washington, 2002), p. 15; Brookes and others, *National household*, p. 20.

46 L. Nyblade, R. Pande, and others, 'Disentangling HIV and AIDS stigma in Ethiopia, Tanzania and Zambia' (2003), p. 35, http://www.icrw.org/docs/stigmareport093003.pdf (accessed 15 July 2004); Guest, *Children of AIDS*, p. 31.

47 Mercy Makhalemele, quoted in S. Fox, W. Parker, and M. Mundawarara, *Living openly: HIV positive South Africans tell their stories* (Pretoria, 2000), p. 3.

48 Clacherty and Associates, *The role of stigma and discrimination in increasing the vulnerability of children and youth affected by HIV/AIDS: report on participatory workshops* (Arcadia, South Africa, 2001), pp. 20, 26, 29–30; Nyblade and others, 'Disentangling,' p. 35.

49 *Mail and Guardian*, 30 May 2003.

50 Klaits, 'Housing the spirit,' p. 131; G. Foster, C. Makufa, and others, 'Perceptions of children and community members concerning the circumstances of orphans in rural Zimbabwe,' *AIDS Care*, 9 (1997), 399; M. Ainsworth and I. Semali, *The impact of adult death on children's health in northwestern Tanzania*, World Bank policy research working paper 2266 (Washington, 2000), pp. 16–29.

51 Guarcello and others, 'Influence of orphanhood,' pp. 14–15; A. Case, C. Paxson, and J. Ableidinger, 'Orphans in Africa: parental death, poverty, and school enrollment,' *Demography*, 41 (2004), 485; C. Nyamukapa and S. Gregson, 'Extended family's and women's roles in safeguarding orphans' education in AIDS-affected rural Zimbabwe,' *SSM*, 60 (2005), 2155; WHO:GPA, 'The care and support of children of HIV-infected parents, May 1991' (WHO/GPA/CNP/IDS/91.1), p. 31.

52 Ayieko, 'From single parents,' p. 79; Kaijage, 'Social exclusion,' in McGrath and others (eds), *Rethinking*, pp. 347–50; UNDP, *Botswana human development report 2000* (Gaborone, 2000), p. 18.

53 *New Vision*, 15 April and 30 November 2000.

54 Smart and Fincham, 'Study tour,' pp. 37–9; A. Ssennyonga, 'Caring for Aids affected children in Rakai-Masaka districts, Uganda,' in B. Gannon (ed.), *Children and youth at risk: HIV/AIDS issues, residential care and community perspectives* (Cape Town, 1994), pp. 85–6; *AAA*, March 1992; J. Muwonge, 'World Vision's experience working with HIV/AIDS orphans in Uganda – 1990–1995' (2002), http://wblu0018.worldbank.org/HDNet/hddocs.ncf (accessed 20 July 2004); *New Vision*, 7 November 2000.

55 Guest, *Children of AIDS*, p. 41; *Fraternité Matin*, 2 November 1994; UNAIDS, *Report on the global AIDS epidemic 2004*, p. 64.

56 *AAA*, June 2001; UNICEF, 'Children orphaned by AIDS: front-line reponses from eastern and southern Africa' (n.d.), p. 12, http://www.unaids.org (accessed 20 November 2003); G. Foster, 'HIV in youth and children in Zimbabwe,' in Gannon (ed.), *Children*, pp. 102–6; S. Fox, 'International strategies for combating HIV/AIDS: a case study of the United Nations in Zimbabwe,' MA thesis, University of the Witwatersrand, 2001, p. 41.

57 *AAA*, January 1994 and August 1995; J. Grinling, 'L'intervention auprès des orphelins dans un système social en crise: le travail d'AMO-Zaire à Kinshasa,' in A. Desclaux and C. Raynaut (eds), *Urgence, précarité, et lutte contre le VIH/SIDA en Afrique* (Paris, 1997), ch. 3; Zambia, *Strategic framework 2001–2003: National HIV/AIDS/STD/TB Council* (n.p., 2000), p. 31; K. Deininger, M. Garcia, and K. Subbarao, 'AIDS-induced orphanhood as a systemic shock: magnitude, impact, and program interventions in Africa,' *World Development*, 31 (2003), 1214.

58 Zambia, *Strategic framework*, p. 30; Cross, 'Sinking deeper,' pp. 133–47.

59 *Le Soleil*, 31 October 2003 and 20 June 2004; *Le Quotidien*, 8 July 2004 and 5 January 2005.

60 Deininger and others, 'AIDS-induced orphanhood,' p. 1202; K. Kober and W. Van Damme, 'Scaling up access to antiretroviral treatment in southern Africa: who will do the job?' *Lancet*, 364 (2004), 103.

61 J.-P. Platteau, 'The food crisis in Africa: a comparative structural analysis,' in J. Drèze and A. Sen (eds), *The political economy of hunger* (3 vols, Oxford, 1990–1), vol. 2. p. 281; K.E. Fritz, 'Women, power, and HIV risk in rural Mbale district, Uganda,' PhD thesis, Yale University, 1998, p. 29.

62 Tibaijuka, 'AIDS and economic welfare,' pp. 970–1.

63 Swaziland, *The impact of HIV/AIDS on agriculture and the private sector in Swaziland* (Mbabane, 2002), pp. 3, 17, 19; FAO, *The effects of HIV/AIDS on farming systems in eastern Africa* (Rome, 1995), pp. 36, 47, 58, 60, 74, 142; Mather and others, 'Cross-country analysis,' pp. vi, 29, 33.

64   T. Barnett, 'HIV/AIDS and the African agrarian crisis: which way forward?' in G. Mutangadura, H. Jackson, and D. Mukurazita (eds), *AIDS and African smallholder agriculture* (Harare, 1999), p. 11; T. Barnett and A. Whiteside, *AIDS in the twenty-first century: disease and globalization* (Basingstoke, 2002), ch. 9.

65   *Mail and Guardian*, 30 October 1998; Hunter, 'Orphans as a window,' p. 686; *New Vision*, 26 January and 6 March 1999.

66   S. Devereux, 'The Malawi famine of 2002,' *IDS Bulletin*, 33, 4 (2002), 70–8; M. Vaughan, 'Poverty and famine: Malawi in 2002,' unpublished paper, 2003; *Herald* (Harare), 25 February and 4 March 2005.

67   UNAIDS, *Report on the global AIDS epidemic 2004*, p. 44; Great Britain: House of Commons (Session 2002–3): International Development Committee: Third Report, *The humanitarian crisis in southern Africa* (HC 116: 2 vols, London, 2003), vol. 1, pp. 20–3, 32–5; vol. 2, pp. 52, 97.

68   A. de Waal and A. Whiteside, 'New variant famine: AIDS and food crisis in southern Africa,' *Lancet*, 362 (2003), 1234–7.

69   Southern African Development Community, *Towards identifying impacts*, pp. v, 10–15; Vaughan, 'Poverty and famine'; Devereux, 'Malawi famine,' p. 71.

70   J.T. Morris and S. Lewis, 'Mission report: Lesotho, Malawi, Zambia, and Zimbabwe, 22–29 January 2003,' p. 4, http://www.unaids.org (accessed 20 November 2003).

71   World Bank, *Confronting AIDS*, p. 34; K. Quattek, 'The economic impact of AIDS in South Africa,' in R. Shell, K. Quattek, and others, *HIV/AIDS: a threat to the African renaissance?* (Johannesburg, 2000), p. 29; UNAIDS, *Report on the global HIV/AIDS epidemic, July 2002* (Geneva, 2002), pp. 56–7.

72   Botswana, *Macro-economic impacts of the HIV/AIDS epidemic in Botswana* ([Gaborone] 2000), p. vi.

73   *Herald* (Port Elizabeth), 22 September 2004; *Standard* (Nairobi), 11 February 2004; *AAA*, October 2002.

74   J.D. Lewis, 'Assessing the demographic and economic impact of HIV/AIDS,' in K.D. Kauffman and D.L. Lindauer (eds), *AIDS and South Africa: the social expression of a pandemic* (Basingstoke, 2004), pp. 105–9; G. George and A. Whiteside, 'AIDS and the private sector,' in Health Systems Trust, *South African health review 2002* (Durban, 2003), ch. 12.

75   *Mail and Guardian*, 26 April and 20 December 2002; Great Britain, *HIV/AIDS: the impact*, vol. 2, p. 172; S. Rosen and J.L. Simon, 'Shifting the burden of HIV/AIDS,' *AAA*, April 2002.

76   *AAA*, January 1993; *EastAfrican*, 11 August 1997; *Daily Nation*, 12 February 1999; Great Britain, *HIV/AIDS: the impact*, vol. 2, p. 162.

77   P.P. Fourie, 'One burden too many: public policy making on HIV/AIDS in South Africa, 1982–2004,' thesis for the Doctorate of Literature and Philosophy, University of Johannesburg, 2004, pp. 116–17; *AAA*, April 2000.

78   *Standard*, 20 March 2004; J. Doherty and H. McLeod, 'Medical schemes,' in Health Systems Trust, *South African health review 2002*, ch. 3; *Namibian*, 25 February 2005.

79   N.K. Poku and F. Cheru, 'The politics of poverty and debt in Africa's AIDS crisis,' *International Relations*, 16, 6 (December 2001), 42.

80   *L'Hebdomadaire du Burkina*, 15 November 2002; Great Britain, *HIV/AIDS: the impact*, vol. 2, p. 220; L. Garbus, 'HIV/AIDS in Malawi' (2003), p. 38, http://ari.ucsf.edu/policy/profiles/Malawi.pdf (accessed 3 March 2005); *Mail and Guardian*, 20 February 2003; O. Shisana, E. Hall, and others, *The impact of HIV/AIDS on the health sector* (Pretoria, 2003), p. xii.

81   *Sowetan*, 31 October 1991.

82   R.M. Anderson, R.M. May, and others, 'The spread of HIV-1 in Africa: sexual contact patterns and the predicted demographic impact of AIDS,' *Nature*, 352 (1991), 584.

83   *Cape Times*, 21 September 2000. For explanation, see J.C. Caldwell, I.O. Orubuloye, and P. Caldwell, 'Fertility decline in Africa: a new type of transition?' *Population and Development Review*, 18 (1992), 211–42; J.C. Caldwell and P. Caldwell, 'The South African fertility decline,' *ibid.*, 19 (1993), 225–62.

84   *AAA*, August 2000; Inter Press Service (Johannesburg), 24 February 2005, http://allafrica.com/stories (accessed 25 February 2005).

85   *L'Hebdomadaire du Burkina*, 22 November 2002.

86   S. Dodwell, 'We cannot afford an AIDS epidemic,' *BMJ*, 301 (1990), 1283; R. Shell, 'Halfway to the holocaust,' in Shell and others, *HIV/AIDS*, p. 19.

87   UNAIDS, *Report on the global HIV/AIDS epidemic, June 2000* (Geneva, 2000), p. 22; *AAA*,

August 1999.

88   D. Chiweza, *HIV and AIDS: the last stand: the total strategy for the annihilation of HIV and AIDS in Zimbabwe and the rest of the world* (Harare [1997]), p. 43; R. Mattes and R. Manning, *The impact of HIV/AIDS on democracy in southern Africa* (Cape Town, 2003), p. 18; A. de, Waal, 'How will HIV/AIDS transform African governance?' *African Affairs*, 102 (2003), 1–23; UNAIDS, *Report on the global HIV/AIDS epidemic, July 2002*, p. 102; *Weekend Argus* (Cape Town), 25 October 2003; W.D. Myslik, A. Freeman, and J. Slawski, 'Implications of AIDS for the South African population age profile,' *Southern African Journal of Gerontology*, 6, 2 (1997), 7.

89   Words attributed to A. de Waal in B. Marchal, V. De Brouwere, and G. Kegels, 'HIV/AIDS and the health workforce crisis: what are the next steps?' *Tropical Medicine and International Health*, 10 (2005), 302.

12 *The Epidemic Matures* (pages 126–37)

1   UNAIDS, 'AIDS epidemic update, December 2004,' p. 2, http://www.unaids.org (accessed 28 November 2004).

2   R. Stoneburner, M. Carballo, and others, 'Simulation of HIV incidence dynamics in the Rakai population-based cohort, Uganda,' *AIDS*, 12 (1998), 226–8.

3   G. Asiimwe-Okiror, A.A. Opio, and others, 'Change in sexual behaviour and decline in HIV infection among young pregnant women in urban Uganda,' *AIDS*, 11 (1997), 1761–2; A.A. Opio, G. Asiimwe-Okiror, and others, *A report on declining trends in HIV infection rates in sentinel surveillance sites in Uganda, October 1996* (Entebbe, 1996), p. 4; J.K. Konde-Lule, 'The declining   HIV seroprevalence in Uganda: what evidence?' *HTR*, 5 (1995), supplement, 27–33; Uganda: Ministry of Health, *STD/AIDS   Control Programme: end of year report 1994 and plan of activity for   1995* (Entebbe, 1995), pp. 16–17; *New Vision*, 28 November 1995.

4   UNAIDS, *Report on the global AIDS epidemic 2004* (Geneva,   2004), p. 32.

5   Uganda: Ministry of Health, 'STD/HIV/AIDS surveillance report, June 2003,' pp. 14–15, http://www.health.go.ug/docs/hiv0603.pdf (accessed 21 July 2004); *New Vision*, 16 July 1999; *Monitor* (Kampala), 9 February 2005; UNAIDS, 'AIDS epidemic update, December 2004,' p. 25.

6   J. Lugalla, M. Emmelin, and others, 'Social, cultural and sexual behavioural determinants of observed decline in HIV infection trends: lessons from the Kagera region, Tanzania,' *SSM*, 59 (2004), 186; G. Kwesigabo, J. Killewo, and others, 'Decline in the prevalence of HIV-1 infection in young women in the Kagera region of Tanzania,' *Journal of AIDS*, 17 (1998), 264.

7   Opio and others, *Report on declining trends*, p. 11; J.O. Parkhurst, 'HIV prevention policy in sub-Saharan Africa: the Ugandan experience,' DPhil thesis, University of Oxford, 2002, pp. 162–4, 218, 221–8; *New Vision*, 13 July 2002.

8   T.E. Mertens and D. Low-Beer, 'HIV and AIDS: where is the epidemic going?' *Bulletin of the WHO*, 74 (1996), 128.

9   M.J. Wawer, D. Serwadda, and others, 'Trends in HIV-1 prevalence may not reflect trends in incidence in mature epidemics: data from the Rakai population-based cohort, Uganda,' *AIDS*, 11 (1997), 1023–4; Konde-Lule, 'Declining HIV seroprevalence,' p. 32.

10   A.H.D. Killian, S. Gregson, and others, 'Reductions in risk behaviour provide the most consistent explanation of declining HIV-1 prevalence in Uganda,' *AIDS*, 13 (1999), 396.

11   S.M. Mbulaiteye, C. Mahe, and others, 'Declining HIV-1 incidence and associated prevalence over 10 years in a rural population in south-west Uganda: a cohort study,' *Lancet*, 360 (2002), 41–6; D. Low-Beer, 'HIV-1 incidence and prevalence trends in Uganda,' *ibid.*, 1788; J.A.G. Whitworth, C. Mahe, and others, 'HIV-1 epidemic trends in rural south-west Uganda over a 10-year period,' *Tropical Medicine and International Health*, 7 (2002), 1051.

12   *EastAfrican*, 21 June 2004. See also D.A. Shuey, B.B. Babishangire, and others, 'Increased sexual abstinence among in-school adolescents as a result of school health education in Soroti district, Uganda,' *Health Education Research*, 14 (1999), 411–19.

13   D. Low-Beer and R.L. Stoneburner, 'Behaviour and communication change in reducing HIV: is Uganda unique?' *African Journal of AIDS Research*, 2 (2003), 9–21; A. de Waal, 'A disaster with no name: the HIV/AIDS pandemic and the limits of governance,' in G. Ellison, M. Parker, and C. Campbell (eds), *Learning from HIV and AIDS* (Cambridge, 2003), p. 260.

14   *Le Soleil*, 16 April 2004.

15   Uganda, 'Follow-up to the declaration of commitment on HIV/AIDS (UNGASS): Uganda country report, January–December 2002,' p. 14, http://www.unaids.org (accessed 28 November 2003); World Bank, *Confronting AIDS: public priorities in a global epidemic* (New York, 1997), p. 93; A. Kamali, L.M. Carpenter, and others, 'Seven-year trends in HIV-1 infection rates, and changes in sexual behaviour, among adults in rural Uganda,' *AIDS*, 14 (2000), 431.

16   FAO, *The effects of HIV/AIDS on farming systems in eastern Africa* (Rome, 1995), p. 86.

17   Uganda, *Demographic and health survey 2000–2001* (Entebbe, 2001), p. 184; E.C. Green, *Rethinking AIDS prevention: learning from successes in developing countries* (Westport, 2003), pp. 11–12; A. Peterson in United States Senate: Foreign Relations Committee, 'Fighting AIDS in Uganda: what went right?' May 19, 2003,' p. 13, http://www.Kaisernetwork.org.doc

18   Uganda, *Demographic and health survey 2000–2001*, p. 184; Green, *Rethinking*, p. 205; Lugalla and others, 'Behavioural determinants,' p. 185.

19   Uganda, *Demographic and health survey 1995* (Entebbe, 1996), p. 153; Zimbabwe, *Demographic and health survey 1994* (Harare, 1995), p. 152; C.B. Rwabukwali, 'Gender, poverty, and AIDS in Kabarole, western Uganda: the sociocultural context of risk and prevention behaviors,' PhD thesis, Case Western Reserve University, 1997, p. 153.

20   Low-Beer and Stoneburner, 'Behaviour and communication change,' pp. 9–21; *Le Soleil*, 15 April 2004.

21   *New Vision*, 15 November 1990 and 21 November 1991; J.A. Hogle (ed.), 'What happened in Uganda? Declining HIV prevalence, behavior change, and the national response' (n.d.), p.8, http://www.usaid.govt/our_work/global_health/aids/Countries/africa/uganda_report.pdf (accessed 24 July 2004).

22   E.C. Green, in U.S. Senate, 'Fighting AIDS in Uganda,' p. 41; M.G. Alwano-Edyegu and E. Marum, *Knowledge is power: voluntary HIV counselling and testing in Uganda* (Geneva, 1999), p. 7; Uganda, *Demographic and health survey 2000–2001*, pp. 188–9; N. Hearst and S. Chen, 'Condom promotion for AIDS prevention in the developing world: is it working?' *Studies in Family Planning*, 35 (2004), 41.

23   UNAIDS, *Report on the global AIDS epidemic 2004*, p. 73.

24   M.J. Wawer, R. Gray, and others, 'Declines in HIV prevalence in Uganda: not as simple as ABC,' Twelfth Conference on Retroviruses and Opportunistic Infections, Boston, 22–25 February 2005, paper 27 LB, http://www.retroconference.org; B. Raehr, 'Abstinence programmes do not reduce HIV prevalence in Uganda,' *BMJ*, 330 (2005), 496.

25   *Standard* (Nairobi), 13 July 2004.

26   *Monitor* (Kampala), 27 February 2005.

27   P. Das, 'Is abstinence-only threatening Uganda's HIV success story?' *Lancet Infectious Diseases*, 5 (2005), 263–4.

28   K. Fylkesnes, R.M. Musonda, and others, 'Declining HIV prevalence and risk behaviours in Zambia: evidence from surveillance and population-based surveys,' *AIDS*, 15 (2001), 907–16; Zambia: Ministry of Health, *HIV/AIDS in Zambia: background, projections, impacts and interventions* (Lusaka, 1999), pp. 13–16; N. Walker, N.C. Grassly, and others, 'Estimating the global burden of HIV/AIDS: what do we really know about the HIV pandemic?' *Lancet*, 363 (2004), 2183; R.L. Stoneburner and D. Low-Beer, 'Population-level HIV decline and behavioral risk avoidance in Uganda,' *Science*, 304 (2004), 717.

29   D.J. Jackson, E.N. Ngugi, and others, 'Stable antenatal HIV-1 seroprevalence with high population mobility and marked seroprevalence variation among sentinel sites within Nairobi, Kenya,' *AIDS*, 13 (1999), 586.

30   R.K. Nyaga, D.N. Kimani, and others, 'HIV/AIDS in Kenya: a review of research and policy issues' (2004), p. 13, http://www.kippra.org/Download/DPNOS8.pdf (accessed 21 March 2005); D.T. Halperin and G.L. Post, 'Global HIV prevalence: the good news might be even better,' *Lancet*, 364 (2004), 1035; *Standard* (Nairobi), 9 January 2004.

31   Asfer Tsegaye, T.F. Rinke de Wit, and others, 'Decline in prevalence of HIV-1 infection and syphilis among young women attending care clinics in Addis Ababa, Ethiopia,' *Journal of AIDS*, 30 (2002), 359–62; UNAIDS, *Report on the global AIDS epidemic 2004*, p. 33; Ethiopia: Federal Ministry of Health, 'AIDS in Ethiopia' (5th edn, 2004), pp. v, 6, 9, 21, 25, http://www.etharc.org/spotlight/AIDSinEth5th.pdf (accessed 9 February 2005).

32   N. Meda, *La surveillance épidémiologique des maladies sexuellement transmises (MST), de l'infection à VIH et du SIDA au Rwanda* ([Brazzaville] 2000), p. 6; S. Babalola, D. Awasun, and B. Quenum-Renaud, 'The correlates of safe sex practices among Rwandan youth,' *African Journal of AIDS Research*, 1 (2002), 11–21; UNAIDS, *Report on the global AIDS epidemic*

2004, pp. 175–6, 191–2; UNAIDS, 'HIV/AIDS and STI prevention and care in Rwandan refugee camps in the United Republic of Tanzania' (2003), p. 21, http://www.unaids.org (accessed 17 November 2003).

33 Tanzania, 'National multi-sectoral strategic framework on HIV/AIDS 2003–2007' (2003), http://www.unaids.org (accessed 25 November 2003).

34 UNAIDS, *Report on the global AIDS epidemic 2004*, pp. 191–2; N. Nagot. N. Meda, and others, 'Review of STI and HIV epidemiological data from 1990 to 2001 in urban Burkina Faso,' *Sexually Transmitted Infections*, 80 (2004), 127–8.

35 Ghana Health Service, 'HIV sentinel survey report 2003,' http://www.ghanaids.gov.gh/docs (accessed 22 March 2005).

36 UNAIDS, 'AIDS epidemic update, December 2004,' p. 24.

37 Malawi, *National HIV prevalence estimates from sentinel surveillance data 2001* (Lilongwe, n.d.), pp. 5–6, 10–18.

38 J. Decosas and N. Padian, 'The profile and context of the epidemics of sexually transmitted infections including HIV in Zimbabwe,' *Sexually Transmitted Infections*, 78 (2002), supplement 1, i44; *New Vision*, 28 November 2000.

39 Botswana National AIDS Co-ordinating Agency, 'National HIV/AIDS strategic framework 2003–2009,' p. 15, http://www.naca.gov.bw/documents (accessed 6 September 2004); UNAIDS, *Report on the global AIDS epidemic 2004*, p. 32.

40 *Namibian*, 2 and 6 December 2004.

41 D. Bradshaw, A. Pettifor, and others, 'Trends in youth risk for HIV,' in P. Ijumba and others (eds), 'South African health review 2003/04,' ch. 10, http://www.hst.org.za/uploads/files; 0. Shisana, L. Simbayi, and others, *Nelson Mandela/HSRC study of HIV/AIDS: South African national HIV prevalence, behavioural risks and mass media: household survey 2002* (Cape Town, 2002), p. 53; *Mail and Guardian*, 24 September 2004; *Cape Times*, 24 September 2004.

42 T.M. Rehle and O. Shisana, 'Epidemiological and demographic HIV/AIDS projections: South Africa,' *African Journal of AIDS Research*, 2 (2003), 1–5; C. Bateman, 'Did we really help break the HIV prevalence wave?' *SAMJ*, 93 (2003), 890.

43 Bradshaw and others, 'Trends,' in Ijumba and others, 'South African health review 2003/04,' pp. 140, 143; L.C. Simbayi, J. Chauveau, and O. Shisana, 'Behavioural responses of South African youth to the HIV/AIDS epidemic: a nationwide survey,' *AIDS Care*, 16 (2004), 605; A.E. Pettifor, H.V. Rees, and others, *HIV and sexual behaviour among young South Africans: a national survey of 15–24 year olds* (Johannesburg, 2004), p. 8.

44 Pettifor and others, *HIV and sexual behaviour*, pp. 9, 52; Ijumba and others, 'South African health review 2003/04,' pp. 143, 202.

45 Pettifor and others, *HIV and sexual behaviour*, pp. 8–10; K. Kelly, *Communicating for action: a contextual evaluation of youth responses to HIV/AIDS* (Pretoria, 2000), p. 31; Bateman, 'Did we really help?' p. 891.

46 Pettifor and others, *HIV and sexual behaviour*, pp. 10, 11, 54, 61; Kelly, *Communicating*, p. 5; K. Kelly and W. Parker, *Communities of practice: contextual mediators of youth response to HIV/AIDS* (Pretoria, 2000), p. 5.

47 M. Hunter, 'Masculinities, multiple sexual-partners, and AIDS: the making and unmaking of Isoka in KwaZulu-Natal,' *Transformation*, 54 (2004), 123, 141. For *isoka*, see p. 46.

48 Kelly, *Communicating*, pp. 24, 27; Simbayi and others, 'Behavioural responses,' p. 612.

49 S. Mapolisa, 'Socio-cultural beliefs concerning sexual relations, sexually transmitted diseases and HIV/AIDS amongst young male clients at a Guguletu STD clinic,' MA thesis, University of Cape Town, 2001, p. 3.

50 C. Campbell, *'Letting them die': why HIV/AIDS intervention programmes fail* (Oxford, 2003), pp. 153, 156.

51 Green, *Rethinking*, pp. 50–1.

52 S.S. Bloom, C. Banda, and others, 'Looking for change in response to the AIDS epidemic: trends in AIDS knowledge and sexual behaviour in Zambia, 1990 through 1998,' *Journal of AIDS*, 25 (2000), 77; Fylkesnes and others, 'Declining HIV prevalence,' pp. 907–16.

53 Derege Kebede, Mathias Aklilu, and E. Sanders, 'The HIV epidemic and the state of its surveillance in Ethiopia,' *Ethiopian Medical Journal*, 38 (2000), 289–90; J.Z.L. Ng'weshemi, J.T. Boerma, and others, 'Changes in male sexual behaviour in response to the AIDS epidemic: evidence from a cohort study in urban Tanzania,' *AIDS*, 10 (1996), 1415.

54 Kenya, *Demographic and health survey 1998* (Nairobi, 1999), p. 130; Malawi, *Demographic and health survey 2000* (Zomba, 2001), p. 166; Tanzania, *Reproductive and child health survey 1999* (Dar es Salaam, 2000), p. 134; A. Kaler, 'AIDS-talk in everyday life: the presence of

HIV/AIDS in men's informal conversation in southern Malawi,' *SSM*, 59 (2004), 292–4.
55 J. Cleland and B. Ferry (eds), *Sexual behaviour and AIDS in the developing world* (London, 1995), pp. 215, 218; M. Mwangi, *The last plague* (Nairobi, 2000), p. 95; J.D. Shelton and B. Johnston, 'Condom gap in Africa,' *BMJ*, 323 (2001), 139.
56 R. Vuarin, '"Le chapeau utile n'est pas dans le vestibule",' in C. Becker, J.-P. Dozon, and others (eds), *Vivre et penser le sida en Afrique* (Paris, 1999), p. 441; I. Bardem and I. Gobatto, *Maux d'amour, vies de femmes: sexualité et prévention du sida en milieu urbain africain (Ouagadougou)* (Paris, 1995), p. 148; UNAIDS, *Report on the global AIDS epidemic 2004*, pp. 70–1; J. Pfeiffer, 'Condom social marketing, pentecostalism, and structural adjustment in Mozambique: a clash of AIDS prevention messages,' *Medical Anthropology Quarterly*, 18 (2004), 88–90; Hearst and Chen, 'Condom promotion,' p. 41.
57 S. Ahmed, T. Lutalo and others, 'HIV incidence and sexually transmitted disease prevalence associated with condom use: a population study in Rakai, Uganda,' *AIDS*, 15 (2001), 2171–9.
58 Malawi, *Knowledge, attitudes and practices in health survey 1996* (Zomba, 1997), pp. 73–4; Zambia, *Demographic and health survey 1996* (Lusaka, 1997), pp. 150–1; Tanzania, *Demographic and health survey 1996* (Dar es Salaam, 1997), pp. 152–3; Zimbabwe, *Demographic and health survey 1994* (Harare, 1995), p. 152; Kenya, *Demographic and health survey 1993* (Nairobi, 1994), p. 132; K. Macintyre, L. Brown, and S. Sosler, '"It's not what you know, but who you knew": examining the relationship between behavior change and AIDS mortality in Africa,' *AIDS Education and Prevention*, 13 (2001), 160–74.
59 G. Kenyon, J. Skordis, and others, 'The ART of rationing – the need for a new approach to rationing health interventions,' *SAMJ*, 93 (2003), 57.
60 UNAIDS, *Report on the global AIDS epidemic 2004*, p. 17.
61 D. Meekers, 'Patterns of condom use in urban males in Zimbabwe,' *AIDS Care*, 15 (2003), 299; E.M. Stringer, M. Sinkala, and others, 'Personal risk perception, HIV knowledge and risk avoidance behavior, and their relationship to actual HIV serostatus in an urban African obstetric population,' *Journal of AIDS*, 35 (2004), 60; N. Kaleeba, *We miss you all* (Harare, 1991), pp. 64–5.
62 A. Buvé, M. Caraël, and others, 'Multicentre study on factors determining differences in rate of spread of HIV in sub-Saharan Africa: methods and prevalence of HIV infection,' *AIDS*, 15 (2001), supplement 4, s12; *Le Quotidien*, 24 November 2004; UNAIDS, 'AIDS epidemic update, December 2004,' p. 4; Walker and others, 'Estimating the global burden,' p. 2183.
63 *AIDS Bulletin*, September 2000, p. 36; Inter Press Service, 24 February 2005, http://allafrica.com/stories (accessed 25 February 2005); UNICEF, 'Children on the brink 2004.' p. 11, http://www.unicef.org/publications/files/cob_layout6_013.pdf (accessed 3 March 2005); South Africa: Department of Health, *HIV/AIDS and STD: strategic plan for South Africa 2000–2005* (Pretoria [2000]), p. 3.
64 Fylkesnes and others, 'Declining HIV prevalence,' p. 911; Alwano-Edyegu and Marum, *Knowledge is power*, p. 19.
65 R. Sabatier, *Blaming others: prejudice, race and worldwide AIDS* (London, 1988), p. 147.
66 Nigeria, 'A report on the UNGASS indicators in Nigeria, January–December, 2002,' p. 4, http://www.unaids.org (accessed 30 November 2003); UNAIDS, *Report on the global AIDS epidemic 2004*, pp. 191–2; Nigeria, 'National policy on HIV/AIDS 2003,' p. 2, http://hivaidsclearinghouse.unesco.org/file_download.php (accessed 21 March 2005).
67 A. Buvé, K. Bishikwabo-Nsarhaza, and G. Mutangadura, 'The spread and effect of HIV-1 infection in sub-Saharan Africa,' *Lancet*, 359 (2002), 2012; UNAIDS, *Report on the global AIDS epidemic 2004*, pp. 191–2; *Le Messager* (Douala), 26 November 2004.
68 UNAIDS, *Report on the global AIDS epidemic 2004*, pp. 191–2.
69 *Ibid.*; UNIRIN, 27 July 2004, http://allafrica.com/stories (accessed 31 July 2004).
70 UNAIDS, *Report on the global AIDS epidemic 2004*, pp. 191–2.
71 UNIRIN, 28 October 2004, http://allafrica.com/stories (accessed 31 October 2004); M. Lejors, 'Soudan: SIDA, la menace cachée,' *Médecine Tropicale*, 64 (2004), 334–6.
72 C. Mulanga, S.E. Bazepeo, and others, 'Political and socioeconomic instability: how does it affect HIV? A case study in the Democratic Republic of Congo,' *AIDS*, 18 (2004), 833; République Démocratique du Congo, 'Plan directeur 2002–2004,' http://www.unaids.org (accessed 29 November 2003); report by Dr François Lepira, November 2003, http://www.msf.org/countries/page (accessed 21 July 2004).
73 UNAIDS, *Report on the global AIDS epidemic 2004*, pp. 34, 191–2; UNIRIN, http://allafrica.com/stories (accessed 11 February 2005).

74 R.M. Anderson, 'The spread of HIV and sexual mixing patterns,' in J.M. Mann and D.J.M. Tarantola (eds), *AIDS in the world II* (New York, 1996), pp. 72, 85.

13 *Containment* (pages 138–57)

1 P. Piot and P. Aggleton, 'The global epidemic,' *AIDS Care*, 10 (1998), supplement 2, s202; UNAIDS, *Progress report, 1996–1997* (Geneva, 1998), p. 18; Great Britain: House of Commons (Session 2000–01): International Development Committee: Third Report, *HIV/AIDS: the impact on social and economic development* (HSC 354: 2 vols, London, 2001), vol. 2, p. 214 (Piot's evidence).

2 UNAIDS, 'AIDS epidemic update, December 2002,' http://www.unaids.org; Mali, 'Plan stratégique national de lutte contre le VIH/SIDA 2001–2005,' http://www.unaids.org (accessed 4 December 2003); Benin, 'Cadre stratégique national de lutte contre le VIH/SIDA/IST au Bénin 2001–2005,' http://www.unaids.org (accessed 30 November 2003); Togo, 'Cadre stratégique national de lutte contre le VIH/SIDA/IST, 2001–2005,' http://www.unaids.org (accessed 30 November 2003).

3 Tanzania, 'National multi-sectoral strategic framework on HIV/AIDS 2003–2007,' http://www.unaids.org (accessed 25 November 2003).

4 République Démocratique du Congo, 'Déclaration d'engagement sur le VIH/SIDA' (2003), http://www.unaids.org (accessed 29 November 2003).

5 Lesotho, 'Monitoring the UNGASS declaration of commitment on HIV/AIDS: country report, January–December 2002,' p. 21, http://www.unaids.org (accessed 21 November 2003); Tanzania, 'National multi-sectoral strategic framework.'

6 World Bank, *Confronting AIDS: public priorities in a global epidemic* (New York, 1997), pp. xv–xvi, 84–5, 142–3.

7 World Bank, *Intensifying action against HIV/AIDS in Africa: responding to a development crisis* (Washington, 1999), pp. vi, 14; A. Whiteside in *AAA*, December 1999.

8 B. Auvert, A. Buvé and others, 'Ecological and individual level analysis of risk factors for HIV infection in four urban populations in sub-Saharan Africa with different levels of HIV infection,' *AIDS*, 15 (2001), supplement 4, s15; E.C. Green, *Rethinking AIDS prevention: learning from successes in developing countries* (Westport, 2003), pp. 33–6.

9 Great Britain, *HIV/AIDS: the impact*, vol. 1, pp. lxxvi–lxxix; vol. 2, p. 64.

10 World Bank, *Confronting AIDS*, p. 10; Great Britain, *HIV/AIDS: the impact*, vol. 1, p. lxi.

11 R. Gallo, *Virus hunting: AIDS, cancer, and the human retrovirus* (New York, 1991), pp. 202, 305.

12 J.M. Mann, D.J.M. Tarantola, and T.W. Netter (eds), *AIDS in the world* (Cambridge, Mass., 1992), p. 813; World Bank, *Confronting AIDS*, p. 179; *AIDS Bulletin*, July l994, p. 17.

13 J.S.A. Stringer, M. Sinkala, and others, 'Comparison of two strategies for administering Nevirapine to prevent perinatal HIV transmission in high-prevalence, resource-poor settings,' *Journal of AIDS*, 32 (2003), 507; B.H. Chi, K. Chansa, and others, 'Perceptions toward HIV, HIV screening, and the use of antiretroviral medications: a survey of maternity-based health care providers in Zambia,' *IJSA*, 15 (2004), 685.

14 M.L. Nolan, A.E. Greenberg, and M.G. Fowler, 'A review of clinical trials to prevent mother-to-child HIV-1 transmission in Africa and inform rational intervention strategies,' *AIDS* 16 (2002), 1991–9; L. Kuhn, 'Beyond informed choice: infant feeding dilemmas for women in low-resource communities of high HIV prevalence,' *Social Dynamics*, 28 (2002), 133–4; J.T. Boerma, A.J. Nunn, and J.A.G. Whitworth, 'Mortality impact of the AIDS epidemic: evidence from community studies in less developed countries,' *AIDS*, 12 (1998), supplement 1, s10.

15 Uganda, *Demographic and health survey 2000–2001* (Entebbe, 2001), pp. 171–2; O. Shisana, L. Simbayi, and others, *Nelson Mandela/HSRC study of HIV/AIDS: South African national HIV prevalence, behavioural risks and mass media: household survey 2002* (Cape Town, 2002), p. 82.

16 G. Walraven, A. Nicoll, and others, 'The impact of HIV-1 infection on child health in sub-Saharan Africa,' *Tropical Medicine and International Health*, 1 (1996), 3–14; *SAMJ*, 90 (2000), 860.

17 G.B. Serengbe, S. Yakoub, and others, 'Aspects épidémiologiques et cliniques du SIDA au complexe pédiatrique de Bangui (Centrafrique),' *Médecine d'Afrique Noire*, 50 (2003), 243–5.

18 V. Sewpaul and T. Mahlalela, 'The power of the small group,' *Agenda*, 39 (1998), 37–8; G.

Seidel, 'Making an informed choice: discourses and practices surrounding breastfeeding and AIDS,' *ibid.*, 69.

19 J. McIntyre and G. Gray, 'What can we do to reduce mother to child transmission of HIV?' *BMJ*, 334 (2002), 219; UNAIDS, *Report on the global HIV/AIDS epidemic, June 1998* (Geneva, 1998), p. 49.

20 D. Wilkinson and J. MoIntyre, 'Preventing transmission of HIV from mother to child – is South Africa ready and willing?' *SAMJ*, 88 (1998), 1304; L.A. Guay, R. Musoke, and others, 'Intrapartum and neonatal single-dose nevirapine compared with zidovudine for prevention of mother-to-child transmission of HIV-1 in Kampala, Uganda,' *Lancet*, 354 (1999), 795–802; *New Vision*, 18 September 1999.

21 F.S. Akiki, 'The focus on women Kampala declaration,' *BMJ*, 324 (2002), 247.

22 M. Magoni, L. Bassani, and others, 'Mode of infant feeding and HIV infection in children in a program for prevention of mother-to-child transmission in Uganda,' *AIDS*, 19 (2005), 433–7.

23 M.-A. Etiebet, D. Fransman, and others, 'Integrating prevention of mother-to-child HIV transmission into antenatal care: learning from the experiences of women in South Africa,' *AIDS Care*, 16 (2004), 37–46; F. Dabis and R. Ekpini, 'HIV-1/AIDS and maternal and child health in Africa,' *Lancet*, 359 (2002), 2097–2104.

24 Botswana, 'Status of the 2002 national response to the UNGASS declaration of commitment on HIV/AIDS' (2003), pp. 11, 42, http://www.unaids.org (accessed 21 November 2003); *Mail and Guardian*, 26 September 2003.

25 Uganda, 'Follow-up to the declaration of commitment on HIV/AIDS (UNGASS): Uganda country report, January–December 2002' (2003), p. 5, http://www.unaids.org (accessed 28 November 2003); UNIRIN, 10 February 2005, http://allafrica.com/stories (accessed 11 February 2005).

26 UNAIDS, *Report on the global AIDS epidemic 2004* (Geneva, 2004), p. 89; Dudu Ginindza, quoted in J. Hall, *Testimonies of hope from people with HIV and AIDS* (Johannesburg, 2002), p. 122.

27 South Africa: Department of Health, 'Essential health care for all South Africans: an investigation into the adequacy of public health financing and the equity of provincial health resource distribution' (September 2003), p. 4, http://www.doh.gov.za/search/index.html; D. McIntyre and L. Gilson, 'Putting equity in health back onto the social policy agenda: experience from South Africa,' *SSM*, 54 (2002), 1647; *Mail and Guardian*, 23 October 1998.

28 A. Grimwood, M. Crewe, and D. Betteridge, 'HIV/AIDS: current issues,' in Health Systems Trust, *South African health review 2000* (Durban, 2000), p. 291; H. Schneider and J. Stein, 'Implementing AIDS policy in post-apartheid South Africa,' *SSM*, 52 (2001), 726; V. van der Vliet, 'AIDS: losing "the new struggle"?' *Daedalus*, 130, 1 (Winter 2001), 163.

29 N. Dodier, *Leçons politiques de l'épidémie de sida* (Paris, 2003), pp. 288–93; H. Marais, *To the edge: AIDS review 2000* (Pretoria, 2000), pp. 38–41.

30 *Times of Zambia*, 6 October 1991; UNAIDS, *AIDS: palliative care* (Geneva, 2000), pp. 14–15.

31 K. Delaunay, 'Des ONG et des associations: concurrences et dépendances sur un "marché du sida" émergent: cas ivoirien et sénégalais,' in J.-P. Deler, Y.A. Fauré, and others (eds), *ONG et développement: société, économie, politique* (Paris, 1998), p. 135.

32 UNAIDS, 'AIDS in Africa: three scenarios to 2025' (2005), p. 44, http://www.unaids.org/unaids_resources/HomePage/images (accessed 7 March 2005).

33 K. Delaunay, J.-P. Dozon, and others, 'Prémices et déroulement de l'Initiative (1996–2000),' in P. Msellati, L. Vidal, and J.-P. Moatti (eds), *L'accès aux traitements du VIH/sida en Côte d'Ivoire* (Paris, 2001), p. 19.

34 V. van der Vliet, *The politics of AIDS* (London, 1996), p. 21; C. Baylies, 'HIV/AIDS and older women in Zambia,' *Third World Quarterly*, 23 (2002), 369–70. See also pp. 100–1.

35 J. Manchester, 'The HIV epidemic in South Africa: personal views of positive people,' MA (Education) thesis, University of London, 2000, pp. 23, 74–7; P. Busse, 'The relationship between the National HIV/AIDS and STD Directorate and the PWA sector/community,' *AIDS Bulletin*, September 1996, p. 13; *ibid.*, May 1997, p. 38.

36 M. Heywood, 'The price of denial' (2004), http://www.tac.org.za (accessed 7 March 2005).

37 P. Das, 'Zackie Achmat – head of the Treatment Action Campaign,' *Lancet Infectious Diseases*, 4 (2004), 467–70; Z. Achmat, 'The Treatment Action Campaign, HIV/AIDS and the Government,' *Transformation*, 54 (2004), 77.

38 UNAIDS, *Stepping back from the edge: the pursuit of antiretroviral therapy in Botswana, South Africa and Uganda* (revised edition, Geneva, 2004), pp. 28–36; Achmat, 'Treatment Action

Campaign,' pp. 76–84; G. Mendel, *A broken landscape: HIV and AIDS in Africa* (Auckland Park, 2001), p. 194.

39 K. Cullinan, 'Khayelitsha women get lucky,' *AIDS Bulletin*, April 2001, pp. 4–5; Dodier, *Leçons*, pp. 293–4.

40 J. Simon-Meyer, 'AZT – the saga continues,' *SAMJ*, 89 (1999), 1244–5; *Mail and Guardian*, 26 November 1999.

41 *AIDS Bulletin*, September 2000, pp. 4–7.

42 *Mail and Guardian*, 1 June 2001.

43 S.C. Kalichman and L. Simbayi, 'Perceived social context of AIDS in a black township in Cape Town,' *African Journal of AIDS Research*, 2 (2003), 33–8.

44 Letter from P.S. Dlamini of Durban in *Mail and Guardian*, 15 September 2000.

45 *Mail and Guardian*, 21 July 2000.

46 M.W. Makgoba, 'HIV/AIDS: the peril of pseudoscience,' *Science*, 288 (2000), 1171.

47 *Cape Times*, 14 September 2000; *Mail and Guardian*, 3 November and 8 December 2000; *AIDS Bulletin*, July 2001, p. 37.

48 Médecins sans Frontières, 'Surmounting challenges: procurement of antiretroviral medicines in low- and middle-income countries' (2003), p. 7, http://www.scanmed_msf.org/documents/procurementreport.pdf (accessed 21 March 2005); P. Bond, 'Globalization, pharmaceutical pricing, and South African health policy,' *International Journal of Health Services*, 29 (1999), 765–92; *Mail and Guardian*, 20 April 2001.

49 *Mail and Guardian*, 26 January, 4 April, and 8 June 2001; V. van der Vliet, 'South Africa divided against AIDS: a crisis of leadership,' in K.D. Kauffman and D.L. Lindauer (eds), *AIDS and South Africa: the social expression of a pandemic* (Basingstoke, 2004), p. 69.

50 *Mail and Guardian*, 26 October 2001.

51 *Mail and Guardian*, 22 October 2004; quotation in M. Martin, 'HIV/AIDS in South Africa: can the visual arts make a difference?' in Kauffman and Lindauer (eds), *AIDS*, p. 127.

52 Judgment in *AAA*, April 2002, p. 12.

53 *Mail and Guardian*, 1 and 22 March 2002; Heywood, 'Price of denial.'

54 'Castro Hlongwane, caravans, cats, geese, foot and mouth and statistics: HIV/AIDS and the struggle for the humanisation of the African' (duplicated [March 2002]), p. 4.

55 *ANC Today*, 19 April 2002; T. Lodge, 'The ANC and the development of party politics in modern South Africa,' *Journal of Modern African Studies*, 42 (2004), 207.

56 South Africa, 'Progress report on declaration of commitment on HIV/AIDS' (2003), p. 6, http://www.unaids.org (accessed 24 November 2003); *Mail and Guardian*, 27 June 2003.

57 *Daily Nation*, 9 July 1996; D.R. Hogan and J.A. Salomon, 'Prevention and treatment of human immunodeficiency virus/acquired immunodeficiency syndrome in resource-limited settings,' *Bulletin of the WHO*, 83 (2005), 140.

58 Health Systems Trust, *South African health review 2002* (Durban, 2003), p. x; L.D. Regensberg and M.S. Hislop, 'Aid for AIDS: a report back on more than four years of HIV/AIDS disease management in southern Africa,' *Southern African Journal of HIV Medicine*, 10 (February 2003), 7–8.

59 *AIDS Bulletin*, July 2001, p. 11; UNAIDS, *The private sector responds to the epidemic: Debswana – a global benchmark* (Geneva, 2002), pp. 12, 34–6; UNAIDS, *Accelerating action against AIDS in Africa* (Geneva 2003), p. 39; *New Vision*, 11 December 2000.

60 N.Z. Nyazema, S. Khoza, and others, 'Antiretroviral (ARV) drug utilisation in Harare,' *Central African Journal of Medicine*, 46 (2000), 89.

61 UNAIDS, *Stepping back*, pp. 41–56; P.J. Weidle, S. Malamba, and others, 'Assessment of a pilot antiretroviral drug therapy programme in Uganda: patients' response, survival, and drug resistance,' *Lancet*, 360 (2002), 34–40; *New Vision*, 26 July 1999, 6 and 9 December 1999; *EastAfrican*, 3 January 2000.

62 Msellati and others, *L'accès, passim*; D. Katzenstein, M. Laga, and J.-P. Moatti, 'The evaluation of the HIV/AIDS drug initiatives in Côte d'Ivoire, Senegal and Uganda,' *AIDS*, 17 (2003), supplement 3, s1–4; C. Laurent, N. Diakhaté, and others, 'The Senegalese government's highly active antiretroviral therapy initiative: an 18-month follow-up study,' *AIDS*, 16 (2002), 1363–70.

63 M. Etchepare, 'La lutte contre le SIDA en Afrique: perspectives et responsabilités,' *Médecine Tropicale*, 64 (2004), 581; UNAIDS, *Accelerating action*, p. 46; Global Fund, 'Progress report – 21 January 2005,' http://www.theglobalfund.org/en/files/factsheets/progressreport.pdf (accessed 17 March 2005); WHO, '"3 by 5" progress report, December 2004,' p. 27, http://www.who/int/3by5/en/ProgressReportfinal/pdf (accessed 17 March 2005).

64   UNAIDS, 'AIDS epidemic update, December 2004,' p. 5; UNAIDS, *Report on the global AIDS epidemic 2004*, p. 132.
65   R. Walgate, 'G8 support for vaccine initiative draws mixed reactions,' *Lancet*, 363 (2004), 2055.
66   R. Gallo, quoted in J. Cohen, *Shots in the dark: the wayward search for an AIDS vaccine* (New York, 2001), p. 8; *Fraternité Matin*, 16 December 1991; P.W. Ewald, *Evolution of infectious disease* (Oxford, 1994), p. 177.
67   D.A. Garber, G. Silvestri, and M.B. Feinberg, 'Prospects for an AIDS vaccine,' *Lancet Infectious Diseases*, 4 (2004), 397.
68   *AAA*, February 1997.
69   J. Esparza and D. Burke, 'Epidemiological considerations in planning HIV preventive vaccine trials,' *AIDS*, 15 (2001), supplement 5, s.50; R.D. Mugerwa, P. Kaleebu, and others, 'First trial of the HIV-1 vaccine in Africa: Uganda experience,' *BMJ*, 324 (2002), 226–9.
70   J. Cohen, 'HIV dodges one-two punch,' *Science*, 305 (2004), 1545–7; *AIDS Bulletin*, March 1999, pp. 4–9, and August 2003, p. 4.
71   *AIDS Bulletin*, October 2004, p. 10; R. Horton, 'AIDS: the elusive vaccine,' *New York Review of Books*, 23 September 2004, pp. 53–7.
72   Uganda: Aids Information Centre, *Annual report 2002* (Kampala, n.d.), pp. v, 1; Great Britain, *HIV/AIDS: the impact*, vol. 2, p. 236.
73   Voluntary HIV-1 Counselling and Testing Efficacy Study Group, 'Efficacy of voluntary HIV-1 counselling and testing in individuals and couples in Kenya, Tanzania, and Trinidad,' *Lancet*, 356 (2000), 103–12; K. Fylkesnes, A. Haworth, and others, 'HIV counselling and testing: overemphasizing high acceptance rates a threat to confidentiality and the right not to know,' *AIDS*, 13 (1999), 2469.
74   *Times of Zambia*, 27 January–4 February 2005; *Standard*, 26 November 2004; *ANC Today*, 5 November 2004.
75   K.C. Goyer and S. Reddy, 'HIV/AIDS and civil rights in Zimbabwe,' *AAA*, June 2002, pp. 5, 16; D. Chiweza, *HIV and AIDS: the last stand* (Harare [1997]).
76   K.M. De Cock, D. Mbori-Ngacha, and E. Marum, 'Shadow on the continent: public health and HIV/AIDS in Africa in the 21st century,' *Lancet*, 360 (2002), 69.
77   WHO, '"3 by 5" progress report,' pp. 18, 29; *Mail and Guardian*, 14 May 2004; *The Post* (Lusaka), 4 June 2004, in http://allafrica.com/stories (accessed 5 June 2004),
78   S.S. Abdool Karim, Q. Abdool Karim, and G. Baxter, 'Antiretroviral therapy: challenges and options in South Africa,' *Lancet*, 362 (2003), 1499.
79   Great Britain: House of Commons (Session 2002–03): International Development Committee: Third Report, *The humanitarian crisis in southern Africa*, vol. 2 (HC116-II: London, 2003), pp. 98–100.
80   UNAIDS, *Stepping back*, p. 10.
81   *Africa Today*, May 2003, p. 24.
82   UNDP, *Botswana human development report 2000* (Gaborone, 2000), p. 9; A.C. d'Adesky, *Moving mountains: the race to treat global AIDS* (London, 2004), p. 202.
83   E. Darkoh, 'Challenges and insights from Botswana's national antiretroviral programme,' *AAA*, December 2003, p. 5; UNAIDS, *Stepping back*, pp. 16–26.
84   WHO, '"3 by 5" progress report,' pp. 52–7; UNAIDS, *Report on the global AIDS epidemic 2004*, p. 109; *Monitor* (Lusaka), 21 November 2003.
85   WHO, '"3 by 5" progress report,' pp. 52–7; Inter Press Service, 23 July 2004, http://allafrica.com/stories (accessed 24 July 2004).
86   Y. Ismail, A. Watt, and others, 'Providing HIV/AIDS care in Mbarara, Uganda,' *Lancet Infectious Diseases*, 3 (2003), 170; WHO, '"3 by 5" progress report,' pp. 52–7; *EastAfrican*, 28 June 2004.
87   C. Wendo, 'Uganda leads way in innovative HIV/AIDS treatment,' *Bulletin of the WHO*, 83 (2005), 244–5; *EastAfrican*, 1 November 2004.
88   *Standard*, 20 July 2004; UNIRIN, 28 April 2005, http://allafrica.com/stories (accessed 29 April 2005); *Addis Tribune*, 28 January 2005; *EastAfrican*, 24 January 2005; WHO, '"3 by 5" progress report,' pp. 52–7.
89   WHO, '"3 by 5" progress report,' pp. 52–7; *Fraternité Matin*, 31 January 2004; *Le Soleil*, 13 January 2005.
90   WHO, '"3 by 5" progress report,' pp. 52–7; UNIRIN, 15 February 2005, http://allafrica.com/stories (accessed 18 February 2005); Médecins sans Frontières, 'Surmounting challenges,' p. 21; *Le Matinal* (Cotonou), 6 March 2004.

91 G. Kombe, D. Galaty, and G. Nwagbara, 'Scaling up antiretroviral treatment in the public sector in Nigeria' (2004), http://www. phrplus.org/Pubs/Tech037_fin.pdf (accessed 15 July 2004); *Newswatch*, 28 February 2005; *Guardian* (Lagos), 1 December 2004.

92 Quoted in C. Bateman, 'Can KwaZulu Natal hospitals cope with the HIV/AIDS human tide?' *SAMJ*, 91 (2001), 367.

93 C. Kapp, 'Antiretrovirals give new hope and new life to South Africans,' *Lancet*, 363 (2004), 1710. See also A. Boulle, D. Coetzee, and M. Darder, 'Reflections and new challenges after four years of HIV services in Khayelitsha,' *South African Journal of HIV Medicine*, 15 (May 2004), 22–4.

94 South Africa, 'Operational plan for comprehensive HIV and AIDS care, management and treatment for South Africa, 19 November 2003,' http://www.gov.za/issues/hiv/careplan19nov03.htm (accessed 7 March 2004).

95 P. Ijumba and others (eds), 'South African health review 2003/04,' pp. 5, 7, http://www.hst.org.za/uploads/files.pdf (accessed 14 December 2004); Treatment Action Campaign and AIDS Law Project, 'Updated first report on the implementation of the operational plan for comprehensive HIV/AIDS care, management and treatment for South Africa' (July 2004), http://www.tac.org.za/Document/ARVRollout.pdf (accessed 11 September 2004); *Business Day*, 4 March 2005.

96 UNIRIN, 23 February 2005, http://allafrica.com/stories (accessed 25 February 2004); WHO, '"3 by 5" progress report,' pp. 52–7; *Mail and Guardian*, 24 March 2005; *Monitor* (Lusaka), 21 January 2003.

97 J. Watson, 'Traditional healers fight for recognition in South Africa's AIDS crisis,' *Nature Medicine*, 11 (2005), 6.

98 *Addis Tribune*, 9 May 2003; *Horn of Africa Bulletin*, September–October 2001, p. 16.

99 Vinh-Kim Nguyen, 'Epidemics, interzones and biosocial change: retroviruses and biologies of globalisation in West Africa,' PhD thesis, McGill University, 2001, p. 249.

100 *Guardian* (Lagos), 10 December 2003 and 10 January 2004; *Namibian*, 27 August 2002; UNIRIN, 5 May 2004, http://allafrica.com/stories (accessed 8 May 2004); *Mail and Guardian*, 21 May 2004.

101 WHO, '"3 by 5" progress report,' pp. 7, 11.

102 UNAIDS, Press release, 18 July 2004.

103 *Standard*, 28 and 29 April 2005; *Namibian*, 7 January 2004; *Lancet*, 363 (2004), 713; *EastAfrican*, 14 March 2005.

104 WHO, '"3 by 5" progress report,' pp. 13, 18, 38; C. Laurent, C. Kouanfach, and others, 'Effectiveness and safety of a generic fixed-dose combination of nevirapine, stavudine, and lamivudine in HIV-1-infected adults in Cameroon,' *Lancet*, 364 (2004), 29–34; C. Laurent, Ndeye Fatou Ngom Gueye, and others, 'Long-term benefits of highly active antiretroviral therapy in Senegalese HIV-1 infected adults,' *Journal of AIDS*, 58 (2005), 14–17.

105 S. Cleary and. A. Boulle, 'Real costs and efficiency of a public sector anti-retroviral project – preliminary findings,' *AAA*, October 2003, pp. 6–7; Hogan and Salomon, 'Prevention,' p. 140.

106 S. Blower, E. Bodine, and others, 'The antiretroviral rollout and drug-resistant HIV in Africa: insights from empirical data and theoretical models,' *AIDS*, 19 (2005), 9–10.

14 *Conclusion* (pages 158–9)

1 UNAIDS, 'AIDS in Africa: three scenarios to 2025' (2005), p. 28, http://www.unaids.org/unaids_resources/HomePage/images (accessed 7 March 2005).

2 *Africa Today*, May 2003, p. 26.

Further Reading

1 General

A good place to start is the latest issue of UNAIDS' biennial 'Report on the global AIDS epidemic' (http://www.unaids.org). An annual 'AIDS epidemic update' is published for World Aids Day (1 December) on the same website. They can be supplemented by documents from the WHO (http://www.who.org), Global Fund (http://www.theglobalfund.org), UNICEF (http://www.unicef.org), and other bodies. African governments, Aids control bodies, and many NGOs have websites.

Important medical research and debate appear in periodicals like *AIDS* and *Journal of AIDS*. *Science*, *Lancet*, and *South African Medical Journal* publish similar articles and more accessible commentaries. Most such periodicals are available online. The online catalogue of the British Library for Development Studies provides links to a wide range of government documents and research reports. Most major African newspapers are available online; a convenient selection of recent articles is available on http://allafrica.com/aids.

M. Essex, S. Mboup, and others (eds), *AIDS in Africa* (2nd edn, New York, 2002) is an up-to-date survey of the entire subject. T. Barnett and A. Whiteside, *AIDS in the twenty-first century: disease and globalization* (Basingstoke, 2002) is a briefer introduction. There are useful collections of papers in P.W. Setel, M. Lewis, and M. Lyons (eds), *Histories of sexually transmitted diseases and HIV/AIDS in sub-Saharan Africa* (Westport, 1999); J. Caldwell. P. Caldwell, and others (eds), *Resistances to behavioural change to reduce HIV/AIDS infection in predominantly heterosexual epidemics in Third World countries* (Canberra, 1999); and E. Kalipeni, S. Craddock, and others (eds), *HIV and AIDS in Africa: beyond epidemiology* (Malden MA, 2004).

S. Sontag, *AIDS and its metaphors* (reprinted, London, 1990) is a wonderfully thought-provoking essay. G. Mendel, *A broken landscape: HIV and AIDS in Africa* (Auckland Park, 2001) contains remarkable photographs. M. Mwangi, *The last plague* (Nairobi, 2000) is a novel set amidst the epidemic. For comparative material on the history of epidemics, see T.O. Ranger and P. Slack (eds), *Epidemics and ideas* (Cambridge, 1992). A more technical account of epidemiology is R.M. Anderson and R.M. May, *Infectious diseases of humans: dynamics and control* (Oxford, 1991).

2 Origins

Accessible scientific accounts of the virus are J.M. Coffin, 'Molecular biology of HIV,' in K.A. Crandall (ed.), *The evolution of HIV* (Baltimore. 1999), ch. 1; J.F. Hutchinson, 'The biology and evolution of HIV,' *Annual Review of Anthropology*, 30 (2001), 85–108; and B.D. Schoub, *AIDS and HIV in perspective* (2nd edn, Cambridge, 1999),

The pioneer account by M.R. Grmek, *History of AIDS* (trans. R.C. Maulitz and J. Duffin, Princeton, 1990) still asks the important questions. The most elaborate (and very long) study of origins is E. Hooper, *The river: a journey back to the source of HIV and AIDS* (reprinted, London, 2000), a remarkable work of research with a contentious hypothesis. For criticism, see J. Cohen, 'Disputed AIDS theory dies its final death,' *Science*, 292 (2001), 615, and the references therein.

Key papers on origins are B. Korber, M. Muldoon, and others, 'Timing the ancestor of the HIV-1 pandemic strains,' *Science*, 288 (2000), 1789–96, and P. Lemey, O.G. Pybus, and others, 'Tracing the origin and history of the HIV-2 epidemic,' *Proc. Natl. Acad. Sci. USA*, 100 (2003), 6588–92.

The evolution and distribution of subtypes are outlined in F.E. McCutchan, 'Understanding the genetic diversity of HIV-1,' *AIDS*, 14 (2000), supplement 3, s31–44, and M. Peeters, C. Toure-Kane, and J.N. Nkengasong, 'Genetic diversity of HIV in Africa,' *AIDS*, 17 (2003), 2547–60.

3 Epidemic in Western Equatorial Africa

Kapita M. Bila, *Sida en Afrique* (Kinshasa, 1988) provides a Congolese perspective on the earliest epidemic. J.B. McCormick and S. Fisher-Hoch, *Level 4: virus hunters of the CDC* (New York, 1999) is a lively expatriate account. The pioneering report was P. Piot, T.C. Quinn, and others, 'Acquired immunodeficiency syndrome in a heterosexual population in Zaire,' *Lancet*, 1984/ii, 65–9.

J. Cohen, 'The rise and fall of Projet SIDA,' *Science*, 278 (1997), 1565–8, outlines its history. Its findings were summarised in T.C. Quinn, J.M. Mann, and others, 'AIDS in Africa: an epidemiological paradigm,' *Science*, 234 (1986), 455–63, and J.M. Mann, H. Francis, and others, 'Surveillance for AIDS in a central African city,' *JAMA*, 255 (1986), 3255–9. The important early papers are collected in D. Koch-Weser and H. Vanderschmidt (eds), *The heterosexual transmission of AIDS in Africa* (Cambridge MA, 1988).

G. Remy, 'Image géographique des infections à VIH en Afrique centrale,' *Annales de la Société Belge de Médecine Tropicale*, 72 (1993), 127–42, is a penetrating survey of the whole equatorial region.

4 The Drive to the East

The original report on Rakai and Masaka was D. Serwadda, N.K. Sewankambo, and others, 'Slim disease: a new disease in Uganda and its association with HTLV-III infection,' *Lancet*, 1985/ii, 849–52. E. Hooper, *Slim: a reporter's own story of AIDS in East Africa* (London, 1990) is a vivid first-hand account. For technical reconstruction of the epidemiology, see R. Stoneburner, M. Carballo, and others, 'Simulation of HIV incidence dynamics in the Rakai population-based cohort, Uganda,' *AIDS*, 12 (1998), 226–8. There is an important unpublished analysis by D. Low-Beer, 'The diffusion of AIDS in East Africa: from emergence to decline?' PhD thesis, University of Cambridge, 1997.

The only overview of Tanzania is Measure Evaluation, *AIDS in Africa during the nineties: Tanzania* (Chapel Hill, 2001). A local study is P.W. Setel, *A plague of paradoxes: AIDS, culture, and demography in northern Tanzania* (Chicago, 1999). The Nairobi epidemic was analysed in F.A. Plummer, N.J.P. Nagelkerke, and others, 'The importance of core groups in the epidemiology and control of HIV-1 infection,' *AIDS*, 5 (1991), supplement 1, s169–76. On Nyanza there is an outstanding thesis by P.W. Geissler, '"Are we still together here?" Negotiations about relatedness and time in the everyday life of a modern Kenyan village,' PhD thesis, University of Cambridge, 2003.

Two good surveys of Ethiopia are Ethiopia: Federal Ministry of Health, 'AIDS in Ethiopia' (5th edition, 2004: http://www.etharc. org/spotlight/AIDSinEth5th.pdf) and L. Garbus, 'HIV/ AIDS in Ethiopia' (2003: http://ari.ucsf.edu/policy/profiles/Ethiopia.pdf). Garbus has an excellent bibliography.

5 The Conquest of the South

The Karonga material is listed in note 1 to chapter 5. For Central Africa there are three excellent overviews with good bibliographies: L. Garbus, 'HIV/AIDS in Malawi' (2003: http://ari.ucsf.edu/ policy/profiles/Malawi/pdf); L. Garbus, 'HIV/AIDS in Zambia,' (2003: http://ari.ucsf.edu/policy/ profiles/Zambia/pdf); and L. Garbus and G. Khumalo-Sakutukwa, 'HIV/AIDS in Zimbabwe' (2003: http://ari. ucsf.edu/policy/profiles/Zimbabwe.pdf). For the extensive research in rural Manicaland, see S. Gregson, R.M. Anderson, and others, 'Recent upturn in mortality in rural Zimbabwe,' *AIDS*, 11 (1997), 1269–80. The epidemic in Botswana is outlined in UNDP, *Botswana human develop-*

ment report 2000 (Gaborone, 2000). For the social context, see D. Meekers and G. Ahmed, 'Contemporary patterns of adolescent sexuality in urban Botswana,' *Journal of Biosocial Science*, 32 (2000), 467–85.

The context and early history of the South African epidemic are analysed in H. Phillips, 'AIDS in the context of South Africa's epidemic history,' *South African Historical Journal*, 45 (November 2001), 11–26, and L. Grundlingh, 'HIV/AIDS in South Africa: a case of failed responses because of stigmatization, discrimination and morality, 1983–1994,' *New Contree*, 46 (November 1999), 55–81. For subsequent growth, see B.G. Williams and E. Gouws, 'The epidemiology of human immunodeficiency virus in South Africa,' *Phil. Trans. R. Soc. Lond. B*, 356 (2001), 1077–86. The most extensive survey is O. Shisana, L. Simbayi, and others, *Nelson Mandela/HSRC study of HIV/AIDS: South African national HIV prevalence, behavioural risks and mass media: household survey 2002* (Cape Town, 2002). Health Systems Trust publishes detailed South African health reviews, available on http:// www.hst.org.za. Among the many studies of sexual behaviour, see especially M. Hunter, 'Masculinities, multiple sexual-partners, and AIDS: the making and unmaking of Isoka in KwaZulu-Natal,' *Transformation*, 54 (2004), 123–53.

6 The Penetration of the West

The HIV-2 epidemic in Guinea-Bissau is analysed in A.-G. Poulsen, P. Aaby, and others, 'Risk factors for HIV-2 seropositivity among older people in Guinea-Bissau: a search for the early history of the HIV-2 infection,' *Scandinavian Journal of Infectious Diseases*, 32 (2000), 169–75.

K.M. de Cock, K. Odehouri, and others, 'Rapid emergence of AIDS in Abidjan, Ivory Coast,' *Lancet*, 1989/ii, 408–11, describes the early HIV-1 epidemic. An original account of society and disease in Abidjan can be found in Vinh-Kim Nguyen, 'Epidemics, interzones and biosocial change: retroviruses and biologies of globalisation in West Africa,' PhD thesis, McGill University, 2001. For expansion from Côte d'Ivoire, see S. Agyei-Mensah, 'Twelve years of HIV/AIDS in Ghana: puzzles of interpretation,' *Canadian Journal of African Studies*, 35 (2001), 441–72; C.M. Lowndes, M. Alary, and others, 'Role of core and bridging groups in the transmission dynamics of HIV and STIs in Cotonou, Benin,' *Sexually Transmitted Infections*, 78 (2000), supplement 1, i69–77; N. Nagot, N. Meda, and others, 'Review of STI and HIV epidemiological data from 1990 to 2001 in urban Burkina Faso,' *Sexually Transmitted Infections*, 80 (2004), 124–9.

The only general study of Nigeria is H.Y. Adamu, *AIDS awareness* (Ibadan, 2001). Senegal's success story is analysed in N. Meda, Ibra Ndoye, and others, 'Low and stable HIV infection rates in Senegal: natural course of the epidemic or evidence for success of prevention?' *AIDS*, 13 (1999), 1397–1405. For social context, see M.L. Renaud, *Women at the crossroads: a prostitute community's response to AIDS in urban Senegal* (Amsterdam, 1997). A.Y. Sawadogo, *Le sida autour de moi* (Paris, 2003) is a view from rural Burkina.

7 Causation: a Synthesis

An explanation stressing gender relations and sexual behaviour is J.C. Caldwell, P. Caldwell, and P. Quiggin, 'The social context of AIDS in sub-Saharan Africa,' *Population and Development Review*, 15 (1989), 185–234. Poverty is stressed in E. Stillwaggon, 'HIV/AIDS in Africa: fertile terrain,' *Journal of Development Studies*, 38, 6 (August 2002), 1–22. A careful study of relationships between disease and socioeconomic status is J.A. Hargreaves, L.M. Morison, and others, 'Socio-economic status and risk of HIV infection in an urban population in Kenya,' *Tropical Medicine and International Health*, 7 (2002), 793–802. Basic data on sexual behaviour are in J. Cleland and B. Ferry (eds), *Sexual behaviour and AIDS in the developing world* (London, 1995).

Accounts of earlier African epidemics include G.W. Hartwig and K.D. Patterson, *Disease in African history* (Durham NC, 1978); M. Vaughan, *Curing their ills: colonial power and African illness* (Cambridge, 1991); R. Headrick, *Colonialism, health and illness in French Equatorial Africa, 1885–1935* (Atlanta, 1994); R. Packard, *White plague, black labour: tuberculosis and the political economy of health and disease in South Africa* (Pietermaritzburg, 1989).

For HIV epidemics in Asia, see B.G. Weniger, Khanchit Limpakarnjanarat, and others, 'The epidemiology of HIV infection and AIDS in Thailand,' *AIDS*, 5 (1991), supplement 2, S71–85; S. Panda, A. Chatterjee, and A.S. Abdul-Quader (eds), *Living with the AIDS virus: the epidemic and the response in India* (New Delhi, 2002); J. Cohen, 'Asia and Africa: on different trajectories?' *Science*, 304 (2004), 1932–8, and connected articles.

For HSV-2, see L. Corey, A. Wald, and others, 'The effects of herpes simplex virus-2 on HIV-1 acquisition and transmission: a review of two overlapping epidemics,' *Journal of AIDS*, 35 (2004), 435–45. The current state of research on male circumcision is summarised in N. Siegfried, M. Muller, and others, 'HIV and male circumcision – a systematic review with assessment of the quality of studies,' *Lancet Infectious Diseases*, 5 (2005), 165–73. Papers reporting the findings of the four cities study are in *AIDS*, 15 (2001), supplement 4.

8   Responses from Above

Jonathan Mann's account of the Global Programme is in J.M. Mann and K. Kay, 'Confronting the pandemic: the World Health Organization's Global Programme on AIDS, 1986–1989,' *AIDS*, 5 (1991), supplement 2, s221–9. His strongest statement of his views is 'The global picture of AIDS,' *Journal of AIDS*, 1 (1988), 209–16. Criticisms include D. Kerouedan and F. Eboko (eds), *Politiques publiques du sida en Afrique* (Bordeaux, 1999); K.I. Hartwig, E. Eng, and others, 'AIDS and "shared sovereignty" in Tanzania from 1987 to 2000: a case study,' *SSM*, 60 (2005), 1613–24. Other national policies are analysed in N. Meda, Ibra Ndoye, and others, 'Low and stable HIV infection rates in Senegal: natural course of the epidemic or evidence for success of prevention?' *AIDS*, 13 (1999), 1397–1405; J.O. Parkhurst, 'The crisis of AIDS and the politics of response: the case of Uganda,' *International Relations*, 15, 6 (December 2001), 69–87; D. Fassin, 'Le domaine privé de la santé publique: pouvoir, politique et sida au Congo,' *Annales ESC*, 49 (1994), 745–75. The basic South African document is NACOSA, *A national AIDS plan for South Africa* (Sunnyside, 1994).

The roles of medical doctors are discussed in L. Vidal, *Le silence et le sens: essai d'anthropologie du sida en Afrique* (Paris, 1996); B. Hours (ed.), *Systèmes et politiques de santé* (Paris. 2001); J. Iliffe, *East African doctors* (Cambridge, 1998), ch. 10; G. Raviola, M. Machoki, and others, 'HIV, disease plague, demoralization and "burnout": resident experience of the medical profession in Nairobi, Kenya,' *Culture, Medicine and Psychiatry*, 26 (2002), 55–86.

9   Views from Below

Evolving popular views are traced in P. Ubomba-Jaswa, *Mass media and AIDS in Botswana: what the newspapers say and their implications* (Gaborone, 1993); A.K. Mutembei, *Poetry and AIDS in Tanzania: changing metaphors and metonymies in Haya oral traditions* (Leiden, 2001); J. Lwanda, 'The [in]visibility of HIV/AIDS in the Malawi public sphere,' *African Journal of AIDS Research*, 2 (2003), 113–26. The *Demographic and health surveys* of each country contain massive information on popular views and understandings. Testimonies from HIV-positive people are contained in J. Hall, *Testimonies of hope from people with HIV and AIDS* (Johannesburg, 2002) on Swaziland; E, Ratsma, E.P. Manjolo, and J. Simon, 'Voices from the epidemic,' *Malawi Medical Journal*, 8 (1992), 60–6; S. Fox, W. Parker, and M. Mundawarara, *Living openly: HIV positive South Africans tell their stories* (Pretoria, 2000).

A sensitive account of stigma, silence, HIV testing, and family conflict is K.J.J. Meursing, *A world of silence: living with HIV in Matabeleland, Zimbabwe* (Amsterdam, 1997). See also Clacherty and Associates, *The role of stigma and discrimination in increasing the vulnerability of children and youth affected by HIV/AIDS: report on participatory workshops* (Arcadia, South Africa, 2001).

S. Heald, 'It's never as easy as ABC: understandings of AIDS in Botswana,' *African Journal of AIDS Research*, 1 (2002), 1–10 is a penetrating analysis of the conflict between moral and medical perspectives. See also A. Wolf, 'AIDS, morality and indigenous concepts of sexually transmitted diseases in southern Africa,' *Afrika Spectrum*, 36 (2001), 97–107; C.B. Yamba, 'Cosmologies in turmoil: witchfinding and AIDS in Chiawa, Zambia,' *Africa*, 67 (1997), 200–23. On indigenous medicine, see R. King, *Collaboration with traditional healers in HIV/AIDS prevention and care in sub-Saharan Africa: a literature review* (Geneva, 2000).

For Christian and Muslim responses, see G. Byamugisha, L.Y. Steinitz, and others, *Journeys of faith: church-based responses to HIV and AIDS in southern African countries* (Pietermaritzburg, 2002); Islamic Medical Association of Uganda, *AIDS education through Imams: a spiritually motivated community effort in Uganda* (Geneva, 1998).

10   *NGOs & the Evolution of Care*

N. Kaleeba, *We miss you all* (Harare, 1991) describes the origins of TASO; this is largely reprinted in E. Kalipeni, S. Craddock, and others (eds), *HIV and AIDS in Africa: beyond epidemiology* (Malden MA, 2004), ch. 19. See also J. Hampton, *Living positively with AIDS: The AIDS Support Organization (TASO), Uganda* (London, 1990). Parallel studies include G. Williams, A.D. Blibolo, and D. Kerouedan, *Filling the gaps: care and support for people with HIV/AIDS in Côte d'Ivoire* (London, 1995); V.C. Mouli, *All against AIDS: the Copperbelt Health Education Project, Zambia* (London, 1992). For women's organisations, see C. Baylies, J. Bujra, and others, *AIDS, sexuality and gender in Africa: collective strategies and struggles in Tanzania and Zambia* (London, 2000); C.F. Ndiaye, 'Women and AIDS in Africa: the experience of the Society for Women and AIDS in Africa,' *South African Journal of International Affairs*, 7, 2 (Winter 2000), 59–66.

Major studies of family care include J.K. Anarfi, 'The condition and care of AIDS victims in Ghana,' *HTR*, 5 (1995), supplement, 253–63; J. Seeley, E. Kajura, and others, 'The extended family and support for people with AIDS in a rural population in south west Uganda: a safety net with holes?' *AIDS Care*, 5 (1993), 117–22; A.F. Chimwaza and S.C. Watkins, 'Giving care to people with symptoms of AIDS in rural sub-Saharan Africa,' *AIDS Care*, 16 (2004), 795–807; M. Steinberg, S. Johnson, and others, *Hitting home: how households cope with the impact of the HIV/AIDS epidemic* (Durban, 2002); O. Alubo, A. Zwandor, and others, 'Acceptance and stigmatization of PLWA in Nigeria,' *AIDS Care*, 14 (2002), 117–26; J. Gruber and M. Caffrey, 'HIV/AIDS and community conflict in Nigeria,' *SSM*, 60 (2005), 1209–18.

For hospital and community based care, see WHO:GPA, *Review of six HIV/AIDS home care programmes in Uganda and Zambia* (Geneva, 1991); K. Hansen, G. Woelk, and others, 'The cost of home-based care for HIV/AIDS patients in Zimbabwe,' *AIDS Care*, 10 (1998), 751–9; G. Woelk, H. Jackson, and others, *Do we care? The cost and quality of community home based care for HIV/AIDS patients and their communities in Zimbabwe* (Harare, 1997); UNAIDS, *Reaching out, scaling up: eight case studies of home and community care for and by people with HIV/AIDS* (Geneva, 2001); C. Stegling, 'Human rights and ethics in the context of home-based care in Botswana,' *Pula*, 15 (2001), 241–8.

The best introduction to palliative terminal care is S. Ramsay, 'Leading the way in African home-based palliative care,' *Lancet*, 362 (2003), 1812–13, on Uganda.

11   *Death & the Household*

The scale of mortality is analysed in R. Dorrington, D. Bourne, and others, *The impact of HIV/AIDS on adult mortality in South Africa* (Tygerberg, 2001). Its impact on beliefs and funeral practices is examined in D. Durham and F. Klaits, 'Funerals and the public space of sentiment in Botswana,' *Journal of Southern African Studies*, 28 (2000), 777–95; C. Nzioka, 'The social meanings of death from HIV/AIDS: an African interpretative view', *Culture, Health and Sexuality*, 2 (2002), 1–14.

A major study of the household impact of death is G.H.R. Rugalema, *Adult mortality as entitlement failure: AIDS and the crisis of rural livelihoods in a Tanzanian village* (PhD thesis, Institute of Social Studies, The Hague, 1999: published in Maastricht). See also his 'Coping or struggling? A journey into the impact of HIV/AIDS in southern Africa,' *Review of African Political Economy*, 86 (2000), 537–45. This should be compared with D. Mather, C. Donovan, and others, 'A cross-country analysis of household responses to adult mortality in rural sub-Saharan Africa' (2004: http://www.aec.msu.edu/agecon/fsz/papers/idwp82forreview.pdf).

E. Guest, *Children of AIDS: Africa's orphan crisis* (2nd edn, London, 2003) is a general account. Major studies include R. Monasch and J.T. Boerma, 'Orphanhood and childcare patterns in sub-Saharan Africa: an analysis of national surveys from 40 countries,' *AIDS*, 18 (2004), supplement 2, S55–65; L. Guarcello, S. Lyon, and others, 'The influence of orphanhood on children's schooling and labour: evidence from sub-Saharan Africa' (2004: http://www.ucw-project.org/pdf/publications/orphans); A. Case, C. Paxson, and J. Ableidinger, 'Orphans in Africa: parental death, poverty, and school enrollment, *Demography*, 41 (2004), 483–508.

The impact of death on agriculture is surveyed in G. Mutangadura, H. Jackson, and D. Mukurazita (eds), *AIDS and African smallholder agriculture* (Harare, 1999). For the Central African famine of 2002–3, see S. Devereux, 'The Malawi famine of 2002,' *IDS Bulletin*, 33, 4 (2002), 70–8, and A. de Waal and A. Whiteside, 'New variant famine: AIDS and food crisis in southern

Africa,' *Lancet*, 362 (2003), 1234–7.

S. Gregson, B. Zaba, and others, 'Projections of the magnitude of the HIV/AIDS epidemic in southern Africa,' in A. Whiteside (ed.), *Implications of AIDS for demography and policy in southern Africa* (Pietermaritzburg, 1998) is a helpful guide to conflicting population projections. The most thoughtful of the doomsday forecasts is A. de Waal, 'How will HIV/AIDS transform African governance?' *African Affairs*, 102 (2003), 1–23.

12 *The Epidemic Matures*

Current estimates of adult HIV prevalences in African countries in 2003 were published in UNAIDS, 'Report on the global AIDS epidemic 2004', pp. 191–2 (http://www.unaids.org).

E.C. Green, *Rethinking AIDS prevention: learning from successes in developing countries* (Westport, 2003), is an excellent introduction to events in Uganda, although with a strong polemical message. See also the review by J.C. Caldwell in *Population and Development Review*, 30 (2004), 159–65. Another explanation in terms of behavioural change is R.L. Stoneburner and D. Low-Beer, 'Population-level HIV decline and behavioral risk avoidance in Uganda,' *Science*, 304 (2004), 714–18.

Initial scepticism was expressed in M.J. Wawer, D. Serwadda, and others, 'Trends in HIV-1 prevalence may not reflect trends in incidence in mature epidemics: data from the Rakai population-based cohort, Uganda,' *AIDS*, 11 (1997), 1023–30. The further scepticism announced in 2005 had not been published at the time of writing.

Evidence of prevalence decline elsewhere is contained in K Fylkesnes, R.M. Musonda, and others, 'Declining HIV prevalence and risk behaviours in Zambia: evidence from surveillance and population-based surveys,' *AIDS*, 15 (2001), 907–16; Ethiopia: Federal Ministry of Health, 'AIDS in Ethiopia' (5th edn, 2004: http://www.etharc.org/spotlight/AIDSinEth5th.pdf); D. Bradshaw, A. Pettifor, and others, 'Trends in youth risk for HIV,' in P. Ijumba and others (eds), 'South African health review 2003/04' (2004), ch. 10 (http://www.hst.org.za/upload/files). This last chapter also surveys evidence of behavioural change. For this see also M. Hunter, 'Masculinities, multiple sexual partners, and AIDS: the making and unmaking of Isoka in KwaZulu-Natal,' *Transformation*, 54 (2004), 123–53. For obstacles to change, see C. Campbell, *'Letting them die': why HIV/AIDS intervention programmes fail* (Oxford, 2003).

Indications of continuing HIV expansion can be found chiefly in UNAIDS reports and the African press. One revealing document is République Démocratique du Congo: Programme National de Lutte contre le SIDA, 'Plan directeur 2002–2004' (http://www.unaids.org).

13 *Containment*

The impact of UNAIDS can be followed in its reports, beginning with *Progress report 1996–1997* (Geneva, 1998). The impasse of the late 1990s is clear in World Bank, *Confronting AIDS: public priorities in a global epidemic* (New York, 1997).

For a general account of perinatal transmission, see G. Walraven, A. Nicoll, and others, 'The impact of HIV-1 infection on child health in sub-Saharan Africa,' *Tropical Medicine and International Health*, 1 (1996), 3–14. The dilemma for African mothers is pictured in G. Seidel, 'Making an informed choice: discourses and practices surrounding breastfeeding and AIDS,' *Agenda*, 39 (1998), 65–81.

Among the many accounts of conflict over antiretrovirals in South Africa, see H. Schneider and J. Stein, 'Implementing AIDS policy in post-apartheid South Africa,' *SSM*, 52 (2001), 723–31; M. Mbali, '"A long illness": towards a history of NGO, government and medical discourse around AIDS policy making in South Africa,' Honours thesis, University of Natal, Durban, 2001 (http://www.nu.ac.za/ccs/files/MbaliThesis.pdf); V. van der Vliet, 'South Africa divided against AIDS: a crisis of leadership,' in K.D. Kauffman and D.L. Lindauer (eds), *AIDS and South Africa: the social expression of a pandemic* (Basingstoke, 2004); N. Nattrass, *The moral economy of AIDS in South Africa* (Cambridge, 2004). For the Treatment Action Campaign, see M. Heywood, 'The price of denial' (2004: http://www.tac.org.za) and Z. Achmat, 'The Treatment Action Campaign, HIV/AIDS and the Government,' *Transformation*, 54 (2004), 76–84. The eventual antiretroviral plan was South Africa, 'Operational plan for comprehensive HIV and AIDS care, management and treatment for South Africa, 19 November 2003' (http://www.gov.za/issues/hiv/careplan 19nov03.htm).

The failure to develop a vaccine is anatomised in J. Cohen, *Shots in the dark: the wayward search for an AIDS vaccine* (New York, 2001). For antiretroviral programmes, see UNAIDS, *Stepping back from the edge: the pursuit of antiretroviral therapy in Botswana, South Africa and Uganda* (revised edition, Geneva, 2004); E. Darkoh, 'Challenges and insights from Botswana's national antiretroviral programme,' *Aids Analysis Africa*, December 2003, p. 5; S, Blower, E. Bodine, and others, 'The antiretroviral rollout and drug-resistant HIV in Africa: insights from empirical data and theoretical models,' *AIDS*, 19 (2005), 1–14. At the time of writing, the most recent continental data on antiretroviral treatment were in WHO, '"3 by 5" progress report, December 2004' (http://www.who/int/3by5/en/ProgressReportfinal/pdf).

Index